AF227640

Raw Foodism: Reclaiming Paradise

© Evan Burns 2026

This book may not be duplicated, republished, shared or distributed without the express permission of the publisher, except for brief quotations in reviews or a similar context. To obtain permissions, review copies, or schedule an author appearance, contact the publisher: editors@emerald-books.com

Hardcover $22.95 US | 32.95 CAD
Hardcover ISBN: 978-1-967628-11-7

Paperback $18.95 US | $26.95 CAD
Paperback ISBN: 978-1-967628-12-4

Library of Congress publication data has been applied for.

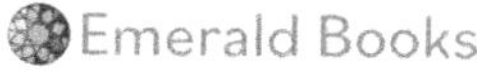 Emerald Books

Raw Foodism:
Reclaiming Paradise

Evan Burns

Contents

SECTION II:

POST-INDUSTRIAL RAW FOODISM

SECTION III:

MODERN AND NEW AGE RAW FOODISM

SECTION IV:

SPIRITUALITY OF NEW AGE RAW FOODISM

Author's Note

This book explores the beliefs and motives of raw foodists throughout the last few thousand years. It is an examination of ideology. This book does *not* seek to evaluate the truthfulness of ideologies nor does it claim to verify the scientific accuracy of the nutritional beliefs of raw foodists throughout time.

"Raw food" refers to any food that has not been cooked or heated above temperatures usually ranging from 115–120°F, by most definitions.

Occasionally, I discuss individuals and groups who may not have been strict raw foodists but who nevertheless demonstrated an intense interest in raw foods.

The word "Earth" is generally capitalized when discussing raw foodists who have granted our planet a godlike status.

I chose to forgo discussion on raw carnivorism and modern raw milk debates and instead focus only on raw veganism, raw vegetarianism, and people who sought to include more raw plant foods in their diet.

Introduction: From Food Flows All Life

Raw food? Food that hasn't been . . . cooked? What could be interesting about that? It may seem like a basic phenomenon that merits no commentary. Wild animals eat raw food. Just about every human has eaten raw foods like fruits, greens, nuts, fermented foods, or breast milk in infancy. Raw foods make up at least a small part of most people's diets. Just about every creature on earth has eaten raw foods. That doesn't seem very notable.

But *conscious* raw foodism—the self-aware purposeful choice to exclude cooked foods from one's diet, or to make uncooked foods the foundation of one's diet, *is* a unique and noteworthy occurrence in history. Not many people have made the choice to shun cooked foods completely nor to substantially minimize them in their diet.

Conscious raw foodism is an ideological choice. Many food choices are ideological anyways.

Cooking is an ancient practice—it's older than civilizations. And the cooking arts are often a central part of our social eating habits and ethnocultural identities. Every culture has signature dishes that are passed down through generations, and they're often cooked foods. In some cultures, cooking a meal is expected to take up nearly an entire day.

Cooking, however, is "risky business," according to modern raw foodist and doctor Gabriel Cousens. And he's not just speaking about the medical or nutritional effects of cooking. There are dangers of cooking, raw food advocates believe, that have far-reaching consequences. Culture, spirituality, politics, ecology, and the aesthetics of our bodies and civilizations are shaped, for better or worse, by whether we eat our food uncooked or cooked, they warn.

If we reject cooked food, both ancient and contemporary raw foodists have believed, we attain a type of power to shape our own destiny and the world around us. That is why peculiar people throughout time have decided to spurn comfort, taste, convenience, or tradition in an effort to gain spiritual and physical empowerment. This book is a collection of their stories, including their motives and beliefs. It gives insight into why so many activists have rejected cooked food, explaining the powers they believed they would gain by doing so.

What raw food are we talking about?

All of the raw foodists mentioned in this book have been either raw vegans or raw vegetarians. Only raw plant foods are consumed by raw vegans; raw vegetarians allow themselves some raw milk or eggs.

In ancient times, we see a few examples of both raw veganism and raw vegetarianism. In the industrial age beginning in the nineteenth century, raw vegetarianism was more common. As we move into the modern and New Age raw foodism of the late twentieth century and early twenty-first, raw veganism takes over.

Raw vegans and raw vegetarians base their diets primarily on vegetables, fruits, nuts, and seeds that have not been heated above a temperature range generally placed at 110–120°F. Among plant foods, occasionally raw sprouted legumes and grains have also been eaten by raw foodists.

Dietary Philosophies

Dietary choices, if a person has any luxury of *choice*, are philosophical choices. Individual and cultural values are evident through the foods we choose to eat. We attach meaning to certain foods, whether we know it consciously or not.

Some discern nutritional value in certain foods and shun other foods for their perceived nutritional uselessness or potential for physical harm. In these situations, bodily health is prioritized. Beliefs about what promotes health or destroys health are revealed.

The supposed spiritual effects of food are another major reason for specific dietary choices. Many religious traditions have rules surrounding food. Think kosher or halal stipulations, or Hindu restrictions on beef. And as we'll see in our story, raw foodists have alleged deep connections between food and the spirit or mind.

For some, non-religious ethical concerns take top priority. Their food discrimination is based on the perceived moral ramifications of consumption—the consumer may have environmental or animal rights concerns, or they may want to fight certain corporate interests.

Sociological, economic, or political explanations can take precedence for these activists.

Even if a person has hardly any conscious ideological motives regarding what they eat, chances are that they still adhere passively to an ideology. If one eats simply for taste, hedonism is the name of the game; pleasure is the philosophy. These people eat to serve their brain's desire for immediate gratification.

Aesthetics comprises another connection between philosophy and food. In Japanese history, for instance, green tea and seaweed were thought to be important for the beauty of an individual's skin or hair.

There is always some purpose behind eating.

RAW FOODISM AND POWER

Philosophy and dietary choices are bound together. This book explores the ideologies and motives behind uncooked movements over time. It is a tour of the beliefs that are built around food as well as how diet is utilized to achieve the life goals of the eater. It examines how many different types of thinking led to conscious raw foodism as well as how raw food has changed people's worldviews.

Through a common thread of raw foodism, we explore the various places and the sometimes surprising individuals and groups who embraced this odd diet. The disparate times, places, and individuals who adhered to the diet are some of the most intriguing aspects of the story. Raw foodism appears in nearly polar opposite ideological and historical contexts. What, to compare two such contexts, does a meek anti-worldly Christian ascetic and a murderous materialist dictator have in common? Why were both monks and Hitler interested in uncooked foods?

The answer is power. Monks sought greater spiritual potential. Hitler believed raw foods would help him create a vigorous Nazi nation. But both, notably, saw raw food as the starting point toward reaching their version of paradise. They argued that diet affects the whole person—both metaphysical and physical parts—and is the gateway to salvation, whether in this world or the next.

There is a materialism that bonds all raw foodists together. Even adherents who have come from extremely different ideological camps have all felt that the body and the food it takes in, affects . . . well, everything.

"Raw plant-foods," in the words of modern raw foodist David Wolfe, "are the most consistent with the physical, mental, spiritual, and idealistic aspirations of the human race."[1] This is a statement, you may be surprised to learn, that both Gandhi and Hitler, two *very* different people who were both interested in raw foodism, would've agreed with.

Raw food was a sacrament of advancement. A sort of magical substance that elevated the eater, embellished her strengths, erased her flaws, and empowered her to accomplish her goals. It was physically cleansing; it healed diseases and cosmetically beautified. It spiritually sanctified; it was jet-fuel for the soul. Some raw foodists have appeared to be electrified with the sense that they experienced a dramatic spiritual rebirth by eschewing cooked foods. Raw food, they held, was a mind-opening awareness tonic and gave the eater a buzz better than a drug high. It helped eradicate toxic emotions and sinful passions.

Raw food, advocates believe, is the source of life. To reject it is death, in many senses, and to imbibe it is to thrive in all things.

The history of raw foodism is a story of how humans have tried to command their destiny through food. It is a story of how people believed utopias could be achieved through the power of eating plants in their most natural state.

---

[1]   Wolfe, David, and Charles Nicholas Good. *Amazing Grace : The Nine Principles of Living in Natural Magic*. San Diego, Calif., Sunfood Pub.; Berkeley, Calif, 2008, 149.

Raw Foodism in the Ancient World

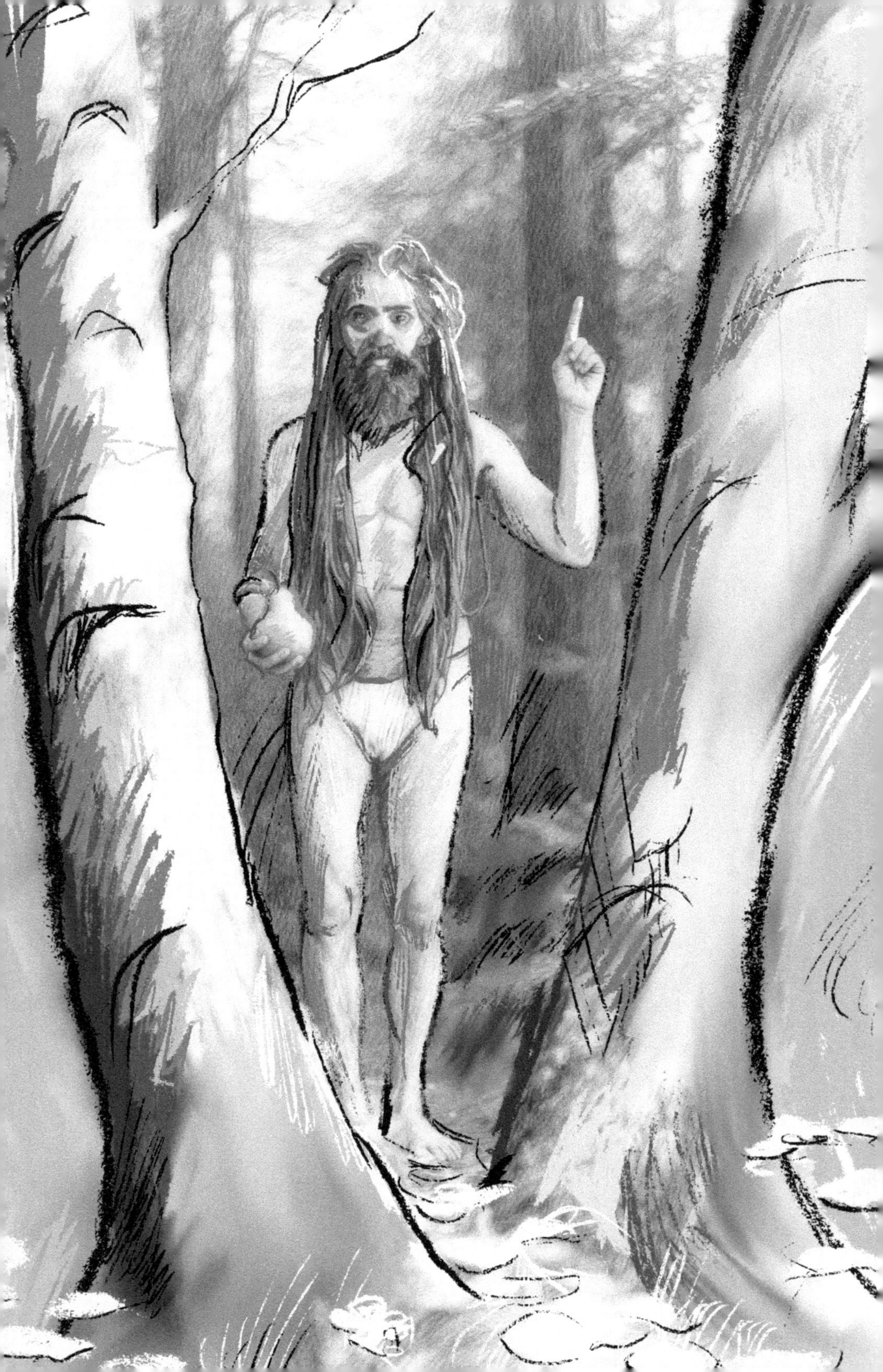

1.
Food of the Rishis

In the ancient forests of India dwelled the first recorded conscious raw foodists. There are no earlier recorded instances of the purposeful rejection of cooked food.

These raw food eaters were holy men and seers, who appear to have believed that raw food was useful in the purification of their spirits.

EATING FOR THE SOUL

Hinduism has long held that food is connected to consciousness and spirituality.

The Chandogya Upanishad, one of the oldest sacred texts of Hinduism, which was composed in the first millennium BCE, holds that "when food is pure, the mind is pure, when the mind is pure, concentration is steady, when concentration is achieved, one can loosen all the knots of the heart that bind us."[2]

It is clear that the authors believed that food quality affected the quality of consciousness, meditation practices, and spirituality. Other food references would be passed down in Hindu texts as well as those texts of Ayurveda (the traditional Indian medical system).

RAW SPIRIT

Raw food, to these ancient Hindu sages, was associated with elite spirituality and devoted ascetics who went the extra mile with their religious questing. Several Hindu texts evidence the usage of raw food.

---

[2]   Cousens, Gabriel. *Spiritual Nutrition: Six Foundations for Spiritual Life and the Awakening of Kundalini.* Berkeley, Calif., North Atlantic Books, 2005, 232.

One of these texts, *Mahabharata* (written sometime between 400 BCE and 400 CE), describes religious seers (*rishis*) living, most likely, on uncooked foods to aid their spiritual practices. "The sages, dwelling in the forest," the text says, "subsisting on fruits and roots, with their senses subdued, and engaged in austere penances, attained to the highest regions of spiritual success."[3] Here we see raw foodism used as a mortification of the body for the empowerment of the soul. We'll see this theme repeated in later Christian contexts as well. Through this physical "penance," the rishis believed they were able to gain powerful spiritual insights. And it was unlikely that the ascetics cooked these "fruits and roots" as they sought complete detachment from worldly comforts.

Another text, the *Ramayana* (circa 500 BCE–100 CE), also refers to forest-dwelling monks "feeding on fruits and roots alone, with leaves for beds," suggesting a minimalist uncooked existence and an intimacy of the seeker with the natural environment.[4]

The later *Bhagavata Purana* (circa 800–1000 CE), also portrays a sage "residing in the forest, tak[ing] wild fruits, roots, and herbs as his food, restraining his senses, and performing penance to purify his soul."[5] Once again, we see the claim that a raw food diet minimizes the "senses" and therefore reduces one's attachments to the world, a is considered a practice of physical "penance" to cleanse as well as empower the soul.

These references to the rishis' diet do indeed seem to specify raw food as the purifying elements. "Ascetics in ancient India," says Patrick Olivelle, a Sri Lanken philologist, "particularly those practicing severe [austerity] in forest retreats, often relied on foraged foods such as wild fruits, edible roots, and fresh leaves. . . . These raw foods," Olivelle says, "were seen as conducive to spiritual discipline, requiring no cooking and aligning with the ideals of detachment from material comforts."[6] Other researchers agree that the rishis were "eschewing cooked food" for their spiritual pursuits.[7] "In Vedic times," says one author, "yogis and sadhus often consumed raw fruits, fresh greens, and sprouted

---

[3]   Ganguli, Kisari Mohan, translator. *The Mahabharata of Krishna-Dwaipayana Vyasa*, vol. 3, *Vanaparva*, sections 25–26. Munshiram Manoharlal Publishers, 2001.

[4]   Griffith, Ralph T.H., translator. *The Rámáyan of Válmíki*, book 3, *Aranyakanda*, cantos 11.23–24. Trübner & Co., 1872.

[5]   Prabhupada, A.C. Bhaktivedanta Swami, translator. *Srimad-Bhagavatam*, book 11, chapter 6, verse 16. Bhaktivedanta Book Trust, 1982.

[6]   Olivelle, Patrick. *The Ascetics of Ancient India*. Oxford University Press, 1998, 126.

[7]   Doniger, Wendy. "Food and Asceticism in Ancient India," *Journal of the American Oriental Society*, vol. 100, no. 3, 1980, 233–240, doi:10.2307/601803.

seeds during meditative retreats, believing these foods enhanced prana and supported mental clarity for spiritual practices." As we'll see, later raw foodists, like Gabriel Cousens, would subscribe to this ancient Hindu belief that raw foods could facilitate spiritual goals.

THE RATIONALE FOR HINDU RAW FOOD ASCETICISM

"O Master, tell me how to find detachment, wisdom, and freedom!"
　—Ashtavakra Gita

In order to escape from the cycle of rebirth, karmic retribution, and suffering, Indian ascetics would "abandon almost all they possessed . . . and withdraw to the forest, separating all links with ordinary society." The Mundaka Upanishad states, "Let the wise, longing for immortality, humbly strive, with mind intent on the self [non-egoic awareness], renouncing all desires for progeny, wealth, and the world."[8] In this context, raw foods can be seen not only as an expression of detachment from the sensory pleasures of cooked food but also from the comfort and community associated with cooking. This was, no doubt, an impressive sacrifice. Imagine eating only roots and fruit in the forest. For most people, these very low-calorie foods, usually lacking fat, protein, and salt would be a form of torturous sensory deprivation if consumed for long periods. These ascetics would have no comfort of the cooking pot, of soft rice, or spiced lentils. It was hard training, depriving the tongue of pleasure and the rest of the flesh of nourishing sustenance. The prize, though, for an emaciated body that spurned pleasures, was spiritual ascendance.

The ascetics' connection of austerity with higher spiritual consciousness could've come from such verses like the following from Maitrayaniya Upanishad: "By the practice of austerity (*tapas*), one destroys impurities, and by the vision of truth, one attains the highest."[9] Similarly, the yoga sutras of Patanjali state, "By austerity (*tapas*), impurities of body and senses are destroyed, and spiritual powers are attained."[10] And what more severe dietary austerity was there than raw foodism?

---

[8]　Gambhirananda, Swami, translator. *Eight Upanishads.* Vol. 2, Advaita Ashrama, 2006.

[9]　Müller, F. Max, translator. *The Upanishads.* Part II, Oxford University Press, 1884.

[10]　Satchidananda, Swami, translator. *The Yoga Sutras of Patanjali.* Integral Yoga Publications, 2012.

The concept of *tapas* was crucial to achieving *moksha* or spiritual liberation and all of the enlightening effects that comprise it like overcoming the illusions of life, realizing one's unity with an ultimate reality or God, and freeing one from the karmic cycle of reincarnation where one has to live out a life of impermanence and suffering. Tapas signified the voluntary mortification of the body and a purifying "penance" in order to "burn away past karma" and liberate oneself.[11]

This self-discipline, like forgoing cooked food and its satiating comfort, was thought to increase one's potential for spiritual liberation. By depriving the body and senses from nourishing sustenance, one's attachment to the "impurities of the body" would be diminished and a rishi would have more bandwidth for spiritual focus. As seen in many traditions, there was a dividing line marked out between the physical and metaphysical realms and in this case, food (especially cooked food) represented the physical realm. "The world where the senses whirl," is where "desire arises" and where ignorance prevents liberation, warns the *Ashtavakra Gita*.[12]

And the ascetics' quest could thrive in more isolated settings, free from the trappings of worldliness and society. Hiding out in the forest and foraging for food was a powerful way to diminish the hold of both society and the physical body on one's consciousness. After all, the "body" and the "world" are "nothing" according to those who have achieved spiritual liberation.[13] To keep withdrawn from society, rishis chose not to accept food from others, especially agricultural products. No grains, no legumes, let alone meat—just wild fruit and roots. Staying away from marketplaces and farms ensured isolation. It was up to the rishis to find enough of these rudimentary foods in the forest to survive.

To minimize food, as we see, was to minimize the importance of material reality in favor of transcendent awareness. As the Ashtavakra Gita says, "For one who knows the self," or pure awareness that is separate and unattached to the material forms of this world, "what need is there for the body, for food, or for anything else?"[14] By minimizing food and eating the lightest, least sustaining edibles like fruit and roots, a rishi could partially sever his connection to the material world

---

[11] Monier Williams (1872). *A Sanskrit-English Dictionary: Etymologically and philologically arranged*. Clarendon Press, Oxford, 363.

[12] Byrom, Thomas. *The Heart of Awareness: A Translation of the Ashtavakra Gita*. Shambhala Publications, 1 Dec. 1990, 12

[13] Ibid., 10.

[14] Richards, John, translator. *Ashtavakra Gita*. John Richards, 1994, www.realization.org/p/ashtavakra-gita/richards.ashtavakra-gita/richards.ashtavakra-gita.html.

as much as possible while still surviving and engaging in spiritual practices. Raw food, in this way, could sustain the ethos of "self-sacrifice" that permeated the culture of Hindu ascetics.[15]

FOOD IN HINDUISM AND AYURVEDA

For thousands of years, the Indian Ayurveda system of medicine has developed theories of how diet and herbs affect the body. Ayurveda, a holistic medicine system that is thought to have begun over 5,000 years ago in India, uses diet, lifestyle, herbs, and spiritual practices to overcome disease. The theories of Ayurveda are deeply intertwined with Hinduism and derive from the Vedas, foundational Hindu texts. Spirituality, the body, and food are all seen to intimately affect each other in Ayurvedic theory. Foods, the system believes, affect consciousness and spirituality.

We find descriptions of the effects of different foods on consciousness. Connected to that, within Hindu texts we find references to which kinds of foods priests (Brahmans) could accept from others.

Different types of foods affect our personalities, it claims, and the energy we give off. Different foods nourish different states of mind, different qualities of being, different *gunas*, as the primal qualities of being are known in Hinduism.

The highest state of being, *sattva*, in which the mind is "clear, peaceful, and harmonious" is nourished by foods that have the most "refined subtle quality."[16] In traditional Ayurveda, these foods, which contain "balanced, harmonious energy" that is transferred to us, include "fruits, vegetables, edible greens, grains, grasses, beans, milk . . . and small quantities of rice or bread."[17] Virtuousness, serenity, and purity are cultivated when these fibrous, antioxidant-filled, and low-glycemic foods are eaten.[18]

Another state of being, *rajas*, signifies a state of passion, energized activity, and self-centeredness. Rajasic foods are stimulating to the nervous system, and "energize us for our worldly activities," and make the mind seek outward and interact with the objects of the world.[19] This could be either good or bad, but often this energizing happens in

---

[15]   Bronkhorst, Johannes. "Historical Context of Early Asceticism." The Oxford History of Hinduism (2020).

[16]   Cousens, 239

[17]   Ibid., 238.

[18]   Gerald James Larson, and Īśvarakṛṣṇa. *Classical Sāṃkhya : An Interpretation of Its History and Meaning*. Delhi, Motilal Banarsidass Publishers, 2014, 10–18, 49, 163.

[19]   Cousens, 238

an unbalanced way and could amplify excessive egocentrism.[20] Foods that stimulate *rajas* include meat, spicy cooked foods, fried foods, butter, cheese, oils, refined flour, sugar, and eggs.[21] These are the delicacies of feisty kings and warriors.

The third *guna*, *tamas*, signifies a state of inertia, ignorance, sluggishness. Tamasic foods generate "a veil of ignorance," "degeneration," or "decadence."[22] These foods are old, stale, overcooked, or leftovers. Modern Ayurveda followers point out that processed or chemicalized foods are also tamasic. Most meat, unless very fresh, falls into this category. Alcohol is also tamasic. It is supposed to be difficult to meditate or to be in harmony with one's mind or environment when consuming these foods.

Comparing these three food groupings and associated states of mind, it's unsurprising that Hindu priests were expected to consume the most spiritual of diets—a sattvic diet, a vegetarian diet composed of harmonious and wisdom-promoting plant foods. And in addition to a sattvic diet plan, eating only raw was going the extra mile: a supercharged spiritual diet that not just ordinary priests but radical ascetics adopted.

According to various Hindu texts, raw food represents a humble sustenance choice—that's why there were some stipulations that priests should accept offerings of raw food for their own consumption.[23] Accepting something raw for personal use (as opposed to being used in offerings, for which food was usually cooked) also ensured that priests wouldn't contact improperly prepared food or items cooked by lower castes.[24,] Uncooked foods could be a welcome part of the priestly diet but such a sattvic diet did not stipulate that plant foods had to be raw. Priests could cook food for themselves after receiving it from others raw.

Accepting donated food in its uncooked state was a sign of humility and piety for a holy person. In the sixteenth century, says one text, "there was a Brahman by name of Ramdas, supremely pious and wise. He used to beg for uncooked food and with it he supported his

---

[20]   Ibid., 238.

[21]   Ibid., 238.

[22]   Ibid., 239.

[23]   Vishvanáth Náráyan Mandlik, et al. *Mānava-Dharma-Śāstra [Vol. 3] with the Commentary of Govindarāja : Being a Supplement to Mānava-Dharma Śāstra with the Commentaries of Medhātihi, Sarvajñanārāyaṇa, Kullūka, Rāghavānanda, Nandana, and Rāmachandra in 2 Volumes.* New Delhi Munshiram Manoharlal Publishers, 1992.

[24]   Mandlik, Olivelle, Patrick, and Richard W Lariviere. *Dharmasūtra Parallels : Containing the Dharmasūtras of Āpastamba, Gautama, Baudhāyana, and Vasiṣṭha.* Delhi, Motilal Banarsidass Publishers, 2005.

family. He was always desireless and contented."[25] The connotations of purity and humility that were assigned to such food, perhaps even if it wasn't consumed raw, laid the groundwork for why ascetics would be attracted to adopting fully raw diets.

RAW HOLY MEN

In Hindu texts, there are occasional mentions of specific exceptional holy men and ascetics who did not eat cooked food. The *Chaitanya Bhagavata*, written in the 1500s CE, mentions that "there was one particular *brahmacārī* who lived in Navadvīpa. He was austere, saintly, and faultless."[26] This young student (*brahmacārī*), dedicated to a celibate and austere existence, "only drank milk and did not eat [cooked] rice."[27] Śrīla Bhaktisiddhānta Sarasvatī Ṭhākura, a prominent Indian guru and theologian, commented centuries later that this young celibate "considered that cooked food destroyed life and [he] took a vow to live only on uncooked foods like milk and mango."[28] The connection drawn between cooked food and destruction could refer to the principle of *ahimsa*, or nonviolence; perhaps an ascetic would not want to kill the life force or prana within the plant or even cook to death the microorganisms on it. It could also refer to spiritual destruction caused by cooked food fueling attachment to the material world.

This specific raw foodist ascetic believed that by adhering to such a limited diet, he would be granted the privilege of witnessing certain holy rites. And although the *Chaitanya Bhagavata* suggests that this sort of raw food austerity is, in itself, not a means to an end, the young ascetic's senior acknowledged that this dedicated *brahmacārī* has "always been a good person" because of the dietary sacrifice that he'd "eaten only fruits" and drank raw milk.[29] "Your body is free from sin," his senior conceded, in a nod to the spiritually purifying effects

---

[25]   www.wisdomlib.org. "Bhaktavijaya: Stories of Indian Saints." *Wisdomlib.org*, 26 May 2024, www.wisdomlib.org/history/book/bhaktavijaya-stories-of-indian-saints. Accessed 9 Feb. 2025.

[26]   www.wisdomlib.org. "Verse 2.23.17 Shri Chaitanya Bhagavata." *Wisdomlib.org*, 28 Mar. 2022, www.wisdomlib.org/hinduism/book/chaitanya-bhagavata/d/doc1107780.html. Accessed 9 Feb. 2025.

[27]   —. "Verse 2.23.18 Shri Chaitanya Bhagavata." *Wisdomlib.org*, 28 Mar. 2022, www.wisdomlib.org/hinduism/book/chaitanya-bhagavata/d/doc1107781.html. Accessed 9 Feb. 2025.

[28]   Ibid.

[29]   —. "Verse 2.23.24 Shri Chaitanya Bhagavata." *Wisdomlib.org*, 28 Mar. 2022, www.wisdomlib.org/hinduism/book/chaitanya-bhagavata/d/doc1107786.html. Accessed 9 Feb. 2025.

of raw food.[30] Raw food had salvific qualities. The indication is clear, in this instance within late Hinduism, that the simplicity of raw food cleansed both the body and spirit of impurities and bad karma.

Ancient Raw Purity

We should keep in mind that within historical Hinduism, the references to specific raw foodists are scattered and there is no broad endorsement of this way of life, besides the rare admirations of ascetics. But it's still valuable for our purposes to see the ancient connections between purity, piety, and raw foodism within the human psyche—traces that become more explicit in the times of early Christian monks. Within Hindu history, we find the first faint clues, obscure sometimes as they are, of the ritual use of raw food and a reverence for the extreme discipline and spiritual dedication that a raw food ascetic accomplishes.

---

[30] —. "Verse 2.23.25 Shri Chaitanya Bhagavata." *Wisdomlib.org*, 28 Mar. 2022, www.wisdomlib.org/hinduism/book/chaitanya-bhagavata/d/doc1107787.html. Accessed 9 Feb. 2025.

2.
The Essenes: Rumors of Living Bread

*"Cook not . . . For I tell you truly, this is
abominable in the eyes of the Lord."*
—Essene Gospel of Peace

Our second group of raw foodists may not be purely historical, but rather mythological. Numerous modern raw foodists have asserted, without much historical evidence, that the Essenes, an ascetic Jewish sect that existed in second century BCE to the first century AD in Judea, were raw foodists.

This assertion largely derives from a highly controversial text called the *Essene Gospel of Peace*, introduced to the world in 1928, by Hungarian philologist Edmond Bordeaux Szekely.

Szekely claimed to have found and translated the manuscripts that he located, written "in Aramaic in the archives of the Vatican, and in old Slavonic in the Royal Archives of the Habsburgs."[31] But there was a problem with his claim: the original copies of the supposed manuscripts were never found. The Vatican also denied that Szekely received access to their archives and most scholars believe his "translation" is fake and that Szekely simply wrote the forged *Gospel.*[32] One scholar, Swedish theologian Per Beskow, called Szekely's gospel "a sheer forgery, written by Szekely himself. It is one of the strangest frauds we know of in the biblical field."[33]

Perhaps Szekely wanted to create a new religion based on dietary rules and lifestyle health practices, using a shadowy ancient sect as a

---

[31] Szekely, Edmond, and Barry Peterson. *The Essene Gospel of Peace: The Complete 4 Books in One Volume.* Audio Enlightenment , 26 May 2018, forward.

[32] Beskow, Per. (1983). *Strange Tales about Jesus: A Survey of Unfamiliar Gospels.* Fortress Press, 84-89. ISBN 978-0800616861, Young, Richard A. (1999). *Is God a Vegetarian?: Christianity, Vegetarianism, and Animal Rights.* Open Court. 5. ISBN 0-8126-9393-0

[33] Beskow, Per. (1983). *Strange Tales about Jesus: A Survey of Unfamiliar Gospels.* Fortress Press, 84-89. ISBN 978-0800616861

template on which to imprint his personal dietary beliefs. After all, Szekely himself was a raw foodist and vegetarian.[34] He argued that 75% of one's food should be consumed uncooked for optimal physical and spiritual health.[35] He also operated a wellness retreat in Mexico, where he taught customers about raw foods and nature therapies like breathing clean air, hydrotherapy, and sunbathing.[36]

Before Szekely publicized the supposed gospels of the Essene sect, there were only a few scattered written sources on the practices and beliefs of the mysterious Jewish sect. The likely facts that we do know about this group come from Jewish philosophers, Neo-Platonists, and early Christian historians in the first through fourth centuries CE. They painted a portrait of the Essenes as an especially virtuous and ascetic community that sought to strictly observe the laws of purity from Leviticus in the Hebrew Bible.[37] They lived in isolated but tightly-knit settlements where they could prevent contact with anyone who did not diligently practice Old Testament laws of purity. To symbolize their purity, they wore white robes.[38] They sought the "power to subdue their passions," banishing all "anger and malice."[39] Their property was shared in common and work duties divided up. Some observed strict chastity and the highest orders among them were unmarried. They intently studied the "mysteries of nature" and the material world as well as theology.[40]

Little is known of their diet or health practices, but the early sources wrote that the Essenes "ate very little animal flesh" and largely limited themselves to "the most simple food" like bread and vegetables.[41] There is also a reference to their study of the body and "medical roots and the property of minerals" and their ability to cure diseases.[42]

Despite indications that the Essenes were frugal eaters and particularly interested in medicine, there is hardly any ancient reference to substantiate Szekely's "translation," which indicated that the Essenes

---

[34]   Albala, Ken. (2015). *The SAGE Encyclopedia of Food Issues, Volume 1*. Sage Publications. 1176. ISBN 978-1-4522-4301-6

[35]   Burton, Tony. "The Visionary Guru Edmond Szekely Lived and Wrote at Lake Chapala in the 1970s – Lake Chapala Artists and Authors." *Lakechapalaartists.com*, 2017, lakechapalaartists.com/?p=8837. Accessed 25 Apr. 2025.

[36]   Young, Richard A. (1999). *Is God a Vegetarian?: Christianity, Vegetarianism, and Animal Rights*. Open Court, 5. ISBN 0-8126-9393-0

[37]   Ginsburg, Christian D. *The Essenes*. Lettel Books, 20 Feb. 2024, 2.

[38]   Ginsburg, 5

[39]   Ibid., 6-7.

[40]   Ibid., 3.

[41]   Ibid., 4.

[42]   Ibid., 25.

were raw foodist vegetarians. Ancient sources, like the Roman-Jewish historian Josephus, mention that "the cook" of their settlements would hand out bread and there according to some sources the Essenes might not have even been strict vegetarians.[43]

However, there's still room for debate over the exact diet of the Essenes, and Szekely may have taken advantage of this lack of clarity. Curiously, the same Josephus as above mentions in another account that "[the Essenes] do not use the same kind of food as the rest of the people . . . They abstain from animal food, and they eat fruits, vegetables, and nuts."[44] If that truly was their diet, perhaps their fare could've been raw in part. And Solinus, a third-century Roman, apparently echoing an earlier historian, claimed that "palm-berries are their food" and that the Essenes "live on fruits and vegetables and the milk of goats."[45] Added to these intriguing descriptions is the more flimsy claim by modern raw foodists that the "bread" that the Essenes ate was made not out of baked flour but of raw, sprouted, sundried wheat.[46]

Against this backdrop of sparse factuality and mystery, Szekely created or "translated" an ancient gospel of raw foodism by reframing the religious traditions of Judaism and Christianity. The new conception of Jesus in Szekely's text was set forth as a dietary apostle who prescribed specific food rules to his followers and nature-therapies to heal their bodies. Szekely would later attempt to institute these un-cooked food and nature therapies at his wellness retreats.

Looking at Szekely's gospel is therefore useful to understand how modern raw foodists view the history of nutrition or read their own dietary beliefs into history. Through the *Essene Gospel of Peace*, a raw food mythos was born and the work gives us insight into the poetics of the diet. With Szekely's publication, raw foodism had seemingly, in the twentieth century, finally had its own dramatic ancient religious text to serve as a foundation for the peculiar way of living.

---

[43]   Ibid., 24.

[44]   Flavius Josephus. *The Antiquities of the Jews*. BoD – Books on Demand, 23 May 2018, Book 18, chapter 1.

[45]   Ginsburg, 30; Gaius Julius Solinus, and Theodor Mommsen. *Collectanea Rerum Memora-bilium*. Berolini, Weidmann, 1958, Chapter 28.

[46]   Zavasta, Tonya. *Your Right to Be Beautiful : How to Halt the Train of Aging & Meet the Most Beautiful You*. Memphis, Tenn., Br Pub, 2003, 37.

A Gospel of the Body

Szekely dismissed canon or traditional New Testament scripture as "hundreds of times rewritten, and hundreds of times transformed." Jesus's words, Szekely wrote in 1937, "as we have them today in the New Testament, have been terribly mutilated and deformed."[47] Nevertheless, he notes, these misunderstood and opaque words of the accepted New Testament had conquered much of the world, as Christianity became the world's primary religion, proving the subliminal spiritual vitality of the true Jesus, despite the fault-filled rendering of his words.

According to Szekely, as a skewed version of Jesus swept the world during "a dark age," the true "gentle Jesus was lost forever in the image of a crucified God." The true meaning and words of Jesus, Szekely claims, "lay neglected beneath the shifting shadows of the desert."[48] Szekely was setting the backstory for his dubious gospel.

Like many raw foodists, Szekely sought a new spiritual perception of the world and wanted to reclaim a more nature-based ethic. "We have proudly separated ourselves," he explained, "from Nature, and the spirit of Pan is dead," he wrote in reference to the Greco-Roman nature god.[49] It was time for man to return to living in harmony with the natural world.

Szekely saw the Essenism that he rendered into print as "the most pure form" of a global spiritual inheritance—a distillation of the most precious wisdom, "the fundamental principles" from a multitude of traditions.[50] He claimed that the Essenes were much more widespread than previously thought and could've existed under other names in other lands outside of the Levant since their ideas resonated with Hinduism, Buddhism, Pythagoreanism, and Stoicism along with other traditions.[51]

With the *Essene Gospel of Peace*, Szekely hoped to "reawaken within the heart of every man an intuitive knowledge that can solve his individual problems and the problems of the world."[52] He wasn't just a disinterested "translator;" he was an advocate for the "eternal vitality" and "profound truths" of his cherished gospel. Szekely's text, according

---

47   Szekely, Edmond, and Barry Peterson. *The Essene Gospel of Peace: The Complete 4 Books in One Volume*. Audio, 26 May 2018, Forward.
48   Ibid.
49   Ibid., 141.
50   Ibid., 145.
51   Ibid.,. 145–46.
52   Ibid., 145.

to him, "speaks for itself"; its importance is self-evident to any con-scious reader.[53]

Diet and the Body in the *Essene Gospel*

"Go, and sin no more, that you may never again see disease."

*"Eating and drinking . . . are the sins of the past. The
wicked creditor is Satan. The debts are diseases."*
—**Book One: The Essene Gospel of Peace**

Szekely described the Essenes as being highly concerned with agri-culture, diet, and health. They were experts, he claimed, in the use of healing plants and herbs. They also held a "vast knowledge of crops [and] soil, which enabled them to grow a remarkable variety of fruits and vegetables in comparatively desert areas and with a minimum of labor."[54] Their supposed expertise in agriculture and plant medicine and their healthy lifestyle "enabled them to live to advanced ages of 120 years or more," Szekely claimed.[55]

Unlike the standard New Testament texts, Szekely's Essenes acute-ly focused on the human body and its health. In his supposed trans-lation of a vow that Essene initiates recited, their focus on the body is straightforward: "I want to and will do my best," he has them saying, "to perfect my body which acts, my body which feels, and my body which thinks."[56] The body, to these Essenes, is not only our sensuous earthly side but is the source of our thinking, spiritual side. Therefore, caring for the body was the central focus of their religious practice.

Those who grow nutritious food and eat pure food—uncooked food, as we'll see—"maketh the Law of the Creator to progress." This Law aims for "all the earth" to be a "garden" where "grass, and fruit soweth the Holy Law." The spiritual and agricultural are practically indistinguishable. Each time healthy food is consumed, the world gets closer to a holy paradise, where there is a radical physiological para-digm shift. When "wholesome green plants and golden grain" and the "medicines" of the earth and the right lifestyle practices are observed, "then shall all the bodily world become free from old age and death,

---

[53]   Ibid., 258.
[54]   Ibid., 147.
[55]   Ibid., 148.
[56]   Ibid., 153.

from corruption and rot."[57] Bodily salvation (good health and freedom from decay) precedes spiritual salvation, when "mercy and truth shall be met together."[58]

The state of one's body is the sign of spiritual progress. In *Book Four* of the *Essene Gospel of Peace*, published two years after Szekely's death in 1979, the opening lines point to the unique bodily excellence of the Essenes. These "Sons of Light" as the text calls them, whether young or old, "all shared in a clearness of eye and a suppleness of body." "For these were signs," that the Essenes faithfully obeyed the dietary and lifestyle "laws" that Szekely's Jesus lays down.[59]

The Essene Jesus claimed that God's precious laws are not in the "pages of books" but "in thy flesh . . . in every part of thy body."[60] Szekely describes the body as a moral experience. The "Law" infuses our bodies and grants us physical and spiritual benefits—"brightness and glory," "communion with the angels," as well as "health and strength of the body" and "long life."[61]

Purity, both physical and spiritual, was what the supposed Essenes sought by obeying the dietary and lifestyle laws laid down by the *Gospel*'s Jesus. After seven years of practicing the right habits, Essenes became like "pure water [that] can mirror forth the light of the sun."[62]

SZEKELY'S NUTRITIONIST JESUS

In Szekely's arrangement, Jesus was an Essene "master"—a healer of body and spirit, the greatest "Healer of Men." In the Essene Jesus's sermons, we find the knowledge, Szekely claims, that humans "needed to cure themselves."[63]

Book one of *The Essene Gospel of Peace* lays out a cosmology: Satan brings disease, while God and his "angels" heal. The greatest healing "angel," the "Mother of the Earth," is a god-like entity that signifies the physically curative power of nature. Satan, or "the prince of all devils," on the other hand, "lies in wait in the body of all the Sons of Men"

---

57   Ibid., 168.
58   Ibid., 169.
59   Ibid., 259.
60   Ibid., 171.
61   Ibid., 177.
62   Ibid., 260.
63   Ibid., 5.

to strike humans with illness if they lose touch with the protective power of the Mother of the Earth.[64]

The Mother of the Earth is a central figure throughout Szekely's gospel and is praised for having the power to "destroy" Satan and his sickness-causing "rule over all your bodies." It is also from this "Earthly Mother" that man receives the wholeness of physical health and "receives his whole body."[65] The Essene Jesus gives this angelic god-like Earth-spirit plenty of respect.

In Szekely's Essene scheme, each person is responsible for initiating his or her own salvation by its personal habits, not the traditional Christian grace of the savior dying for the believer's sins. This salvation, first of the body and eventually the soul, depends on one's relationship with the Earthly Mother angel. People find salvation by following the "laws" of this angel of nature. If they're not followed, you "shall be utterly lost in your grievous sickness, and there shall be," a hell-like "weeping and gnashing of teeth" (a phrase that Jesus also uses in the New Testament.) But if one obeys the Earthly mother's laws, he "shall never see disease."[66] In the cosmic battle over our bodies, the Earthly angel is pitted against satanic disease, which occurs when the Earthly mother is spurned.[67]

Unmistakably, this battle between good and evil is presented as deeply physical throughout *Book One* of the *Essene Gospel of Peace*. "Sins" are regarded largely as dietary and have within them the punishment of having removed "the gifts of the Earthly Mother: breath, blood, bone, flesh, bowels . . . and after all else, life, with which the Earthly Mother crowned [man's] body." Man either "serves death or he serves life," so Essenes should seek to physically preserve themselves and embrace nature's nurturing: "love your Earthly Mother, as she loves your body."[68] Follow the laws of the Earth and her angel that represents its power, and "you shall never see disease," the *Essene Gospel* promises.[69]

Dietary laws help purify the body (the "temple") so that the Earthly Mother's power may infuse the dutiful Essene's physique. Fasting is one critical method of purification to cast out toxins from your body: the "plagues" and "diseases" of Satan.[70] Through water fasting, "unclean

---

[64]   Ibid.

[65]   Ibid., 3.

[66]   Ibid., 179.

[67]   Ibid., 5.

[68]   Ibid., 6.

[69]   Ibid., 16.

[70]   Ibid., 8.

and evil-smelling things of Satan" will be washed out."[71] Physical toxicity is equated with spiritual toxicity. While you fast and pray, the *Gospel* says, while you're starving Satan of the "abominations" which "hitherto defiled" your temple, "the Angels of God protect your body."[72]

The opposites of fasting, "eating and drinking," which are associated with "riotous living," are the "sins" of Satan. By indulging, you are spending life, borrowing credit from Satan and "the debts are diseases."[73] Gluttony is to be vigilantly guarded against and as routine cleansing, Essenes are to fast once every seven days.[74] The Essene Jesus warns that any dietary "evil deed" will be written "in the book of your body . . ." and that "God sees your sins written in the book of your body . . . and is sad in his heart." Every human shows her piety and love of God by the way she treats her body. And God's emotional connection to his creation is dependent on their eating habits. The *Gospel* warns, "feed not Satan, for the wages of sin is death." Sin, food, disease, and death are intimately linked in this "Essene" theology.

When he is not fasting, a good Essene, according to the *Gospel*, should always eat sparingly and "never eat unto fullness."[75] Austerity and not giving into the crude "desires of the body" is a critical bulwark against the body becoming vulnerable to Satan. Even not mixing too many different types of food together and avoiding unpeaceful emotions while eating are important.

THE COOKED HELLFIRE OF SATAN

"Cook not," the Essene Jesus warns, "for I tell you truly, this is abominable in the eyes of the Lord."[76] Szekely's gospel is as clear as it gets when it comes to cooking, which is sacrilegious as well as very harmful to the body. "Eat not anything which fire . . . has destroyed. For burned . . . foods will burn . . . your body also." The evil that comes from without destroys you within. Szekely, or the Essene Jesus, warns readers, "live only by the fire of life, and prepare not your foods with the fire of death, which kills your foods, your bodies, and your souls also."[77] The eater is diminished in spirit and body with every bite. "Kill

---

71   Ibid., 10, 12.
72   Ibid., 26.
73   Ibid., 21.
74   Ibid., 38.
75   Ibid., 36.
76   Ibid., 35.
77   Ibid., 33.

your food," with fire and heat, and "the dead food will kill you also," says the *Gospel.*[78] It can't get any clearer, cooking is a sin against one's own life, a rebellion against the decrees of God, and has deadly consequences. The Essene Jesus was a raw foodist.

If there's any doubt as to the meaning of this "fire" and act of "killing" foods, that is quickly dispelled when the Essenes ask Jesus for clarification as to what the "fire of death" is. "It is the fire which blazes outside your body," Jesus says. "With that fire of death, you cook your foods in your homes and in your fields." In this sense, the gospel is literal, down to earth, and explicitly dietary. But that literal fire also takes on spiritual meaning: it is a "fire of malice" which "destroys" foods, bodies, and "your spirits."[79]

Even the traditional foods of the Middle East, like wheat, were to be eaten uncooked. No baked bread was allowed—for the "fire of death kills the wheat, the bread, and the body."[80] Essenes were directed to sprout their wheat by soaking it in water and then fortify it with the healing forces of nature: "Moisten your wheat that the Angel of Water may enter it."[81] After, dry the wheat, "that the Angel of Air may also embrace it."[82] Raw sprouted foods like this "give strength and youth to your body," and help you live long, similarly to the legendary Methuselah who lived 969 years, according to the book of Genesis, the gospel claims.

Besides raw wheat grain, *Book Four* of the gospel endorses eating grass, including wheat grass, the leaves of the wheat plant. It's advice that would, conveniently, earn the endorsement of twentieth-century raw foodists and wheatgrass advocates like Ann Wigmore (and Szekely himself).

The "most precious gift of your Earthly Mother," the gospel declares, "is the grass beneath your feet" and in the "brightness of the green color of the blades of wheat."[83] The "grass which you tread upon without thought" is full of the "power" of the Earthly Mother.[84] Wheatgrass is a superfood. By consuming grass raw, the power of the Earth enters one's body.[85] Potent nutrition and the life force of nature is contained in green plants, but especially grass, even though it is

---

[78]   Ibid.

[79]   Ibid.

[80]   Ibid., 34.

[81]   Ibid.

[82]   Ibid.

[83]   Ibid., 269.

[84]   Ibid.

[85]   Ibid., 271.

usually ignored as a food source. Grasses are secret stores of goodness and the source of life itself. "Here is the secret, Sons of Light; here in the humble grass . . . here is the Stream of Life which gave birth to all creation," the Essene Jesus proclaims.[86]

Consuming grass raw is an important path to entering "into the deathless way," i.e. becoming practically immortal in this earthly realm. This state of bodily immortality is connected with holiness. In a similar way to how modern raw foodists extract the juice from grass with machines, Essenes were instructed to juice the grass, in a sense, with their own teeth: "chew well the blades, for the Son of Man has teeth unlike those of the beasts," Szekely's Jesus tells followers.[87] It's hard to digest, but if you can distill its liquid essence, you will receive its power.

Fasting and avoiding meat and cooked foods purifies the body and paves the way to *spiritual* cleanliness. "No one can reach the Heavenly Father unless through the Earthly Mother."[88] Szekely alters the Biblical Jesus' saying that no one comes to the father except through him. In this new Essene rendering, nature holds the power to connect humans with God. Contact with God is intensified as "your body become[s] as perfect as the body of your Earthly Mother," nature, "is perfect."[89] Following the laws of nature will make one perfect in spirit and form, the Gospel declares to dutifully hygienic Essenes.[90] Because of their corporeal purity, Essenes will "be able to bear the light of our Heavenly Father," to be vessels of God.[91]

HEALED BY NATURE

Along with its raw foodist dietary injunctions, the *Gospel* demands adjunctive nature therapy for Essenes. These nature therapies demonstrate the *Gospel*'s unerring faith in the healing power of the natural world. It's no wonder why the Essene Jesus would warn followers to not dare cook their food, which could corrupt the perfection of nature—plants in their raw state.

Along with consuming raw foods (as the angel of nature intended), Szekely's Essenes were to get fresh air, bathe in sunlight, and drink clean water from streams. The "Angel of Water," as it "flows through all

---

86 Ibid., 272.
87 Ibid., 274.
88 Ibid., 12.
89 Ibid., 40.
90 Ibid.,
91 Ibid., 15.

your bowels" will "forgive all your past [dietary] sins" and as it "runs out from your body," it will carry away "unclean and evil-smelling things," washing out toxicity that has built up.[92] The detoxifying power of sunbathing is evident by how the Angel of Sunlight empties "your body of all evil-smelling and unclean things which defiled it."[93] Additionally, by bathing one's feet in "clayey mud" next to rivers, Essenes "embrace the Angel of Earth" so that it "may draw out from your bones all uncleanness."[94] Nature, in its many forms, will cleanse away any bodily problem.

A RAW FOOD MYTHOS AND THE CONQUEST OF DEATH

Some modern raw foodists have accepted the Essene Gospel as being historically true and its mythos remains powerful to this day. Raw food eaters have been inspired by the sayings of the gospel and the possibility that some ancient sect did actually know the spiritual and physical powers that could be unlocked by uncooked plant food. Nevertheless, Szekely himself, the practitioner of the gospel's tenants and most likely the creative author of them, was no shining example of thriving longevity.

Despite writing a wellness guidebook called *The Conquest of Death*, which preached radical lifespan extension, Szekely died at the unremarkable age of seventy-four. His death was portrayed as a peaceful exit during sleep in 1979 in Costa Rica. But hardly any details about his death are available, which makes one wonder whether he had suffered a long-term illness or died suddenly from a heart attack. Some have speculated that he was poisoned but fringe claims like that sound like raw foodists attempting to cope with an early death of someone who had promised a life without disease and flirted with the idea of earthly immortality.

But still the attraction of this raw food scripture lives on. Raw food advocates are tempted to believe that there was a wisdom tradition of their own dating back millennia. The Essene mythos would also influence people to believe that there were also hidden references to raw food in the Bible. Activists would claim that the "bread" referred to

---

92   Ibid., 10.
93   Ibid., 11.
94   Ibid., 24.

and revered in Biblical scriptures actually refers to the loaves prepared with uncooked sprouted grains.

Myths like these, signifying that we have lost touch with God's instructions for natural and uncooked living, were to play a powerful role in the minds of future raw foodists.

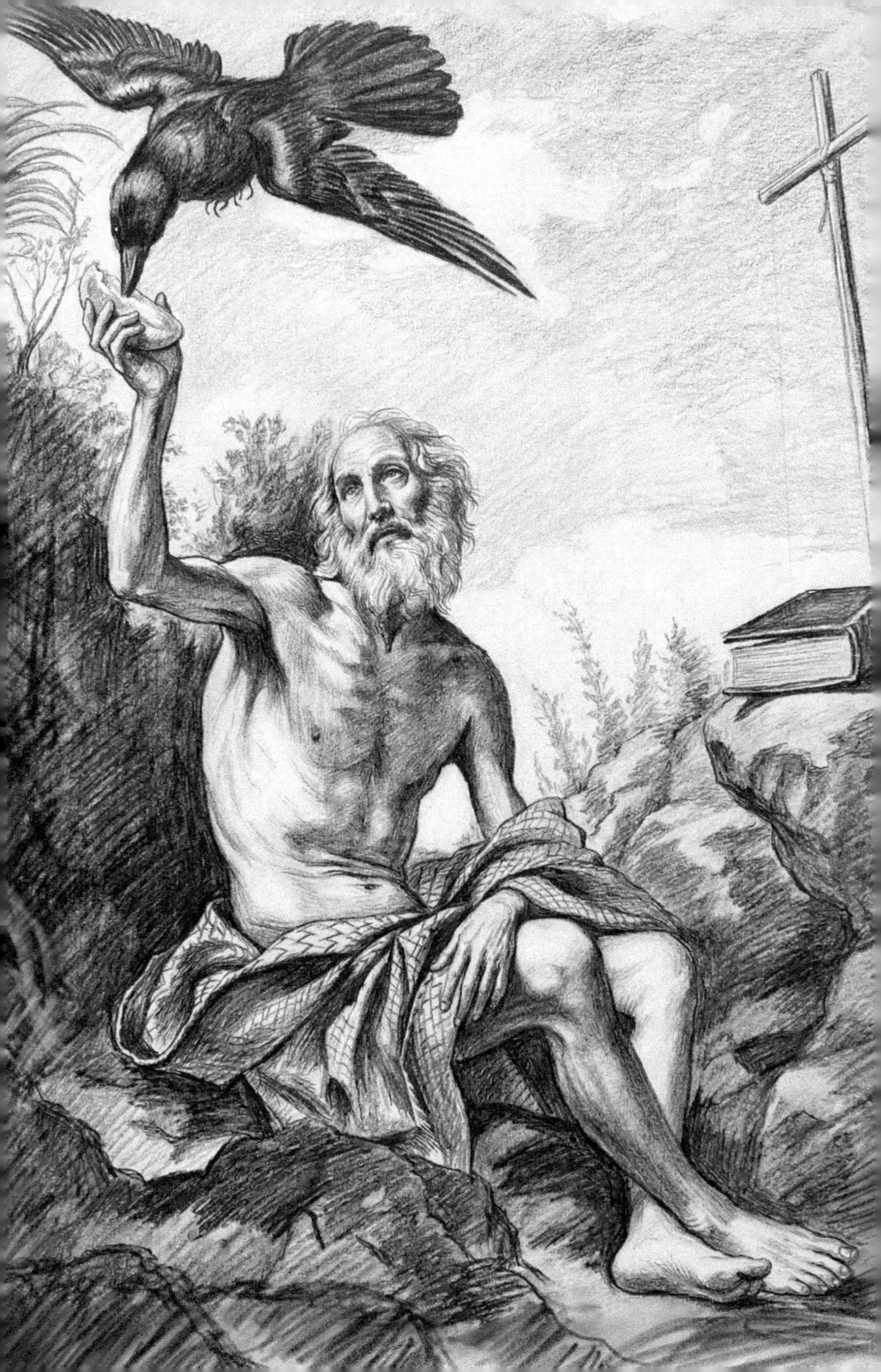

3.
The Desert Fathers: Overcoming the World and Pleasing God

From the third to fifth centuries CE, Christian monks of the Egyptian deserts might've taken austerity even more seriously than the Hindu raw foodists. Brutal extended fasts as well as the long-term diets of unflavored raw vegan food were marks of their self-chastising lifestyles.

Among the stories of these monks, we find explicit references to completely uncooked diets and the rationales for adopting such a way of eating.

The Desert Fathers, as they're known, were some of the first Christian monks. They lived simple lives of brutal penance and complete devotion to God (instead of the world—for the two things were seen in opposition). These monks lived in little cells in the desert, far from civilization's temptations. And to accentuate their anti-worldliness, some of them committed to eating no cooked food for years on end.

THE WORLD OF THE DESERT FATHERS

In the late antiquity of the Near Eastern world, a new spiritual reality was unfolding. Christianity was ascending in influence, shaping people's worldviews, and impacting their daily habits. The teachings of Jesus, his apostles, and the early church leaders were pervading social structures and inspiring people to become martyrs and sacrifice their lives in defiance of the "pagan" Roman political authorities who were ordering their Christian deaths.

As Christianity became widely known, devotees turned to a different form of sacrifice, one that didn't require their immediate deaths. As time went on, there was less of a threat (or opportunity) of being martyred, so some Christians decided on the next best option of proving their dedication: asceticism. Abandoning their communities and the infrastructure of civilization, extremely devoted Christians exiled themselves to the remote deserts of Egypt (and occasionally Syria or Palestine). They began severe regimens of prayer and material abstinence free from the distractions or temptations of cities. These people became known as the Desert Fathers.

A fundamental dichotomy existed in their minds: the world was in opposition to God. The more one spurned the world and its material cares, the greater his dedication was to God. Food, sex, and money were obstacles to be spiritually overcome. What's more, these earthly indulgences, even food, often represented sin and death itself (which are intertwined in Christian theology).

Being absorbed in the concerns of the world not only threatened one's tranquility in this life, but more importantly, separated one's mind from God and threatened to condemn one to painful judgment in the afterlife. Thus, they thought, an ascetic lifestyle could strengthen their spiritual existence, increase their peace of mind, and help them attain salvation in the afterlife.

Food choices were a critical part of that asceticism. Raw foodism, the most severe dietary restriction, would be practiced by a minority of the most dedicated monks.

In considering the lives of these desert raw foodists, we'll examine specific ways that the diet was acted out and the ideological contexts that led to these practices.

A Tale of Two Influences: The Bible and Greco-Roman Philosophy

Both the Bible and certain aspects of pre-Christian philosophy greatly influenced the minds of the desert monks and can give insight into why some adopted raw foodism.

Influence of the Bible

Two themes of Biblical literature are especially helpful in examining the ascetics' motivations for austere raw food diets (which we'll explore in more detail, momentarily): the notion that the desires of the flesh are in opposition to the Holy Spirit and the poetic imagery of the gluttonous "belly" as emblematic of sin.

The Gluttonous Belly

"And put a knife to your throat if you are given to gluttony."
—Prov. 23:2

Sometime around 50 CE, the apostle Paul, the primary figure, behind Jesus, of the New Testament, wrote to the Christian church in
Philippi, Greece. One of the lines from his letter is filled with grief. He
laments those who have succumbed to the sensual earthly world at the
expense of their spiritual dedication to Christ:

> "For many, of whom I . . . tell you even with tears,
> walk as enemies of the cross of Christ. Their end is
> destruction, their god is their belly, and they glory in
> their shame, with minds set on earthly things." [95]

What is remarkable about this is Paul's connection of the "belly"
and appetite with sin as well as its connection with damnation, the
worship of false gods, and rebellion against the true God. Again, in
his epistle to the Romans, Paul reiterates a clear dichotomy between
serving God and serving the belly: "For they that are such serve not
our Lord Jesus Christ, but their own belly."[96] Certainly, desert ascetics
had in mind this Pauline binary choice: either serve God or serve the
"belly" of earthly desires.

In the Old Testament, there are traces of the belly theme as well.
In the book of Job, we see expressions of the belly/sin connection in
descriptions of the wicked: "They conceive mischief, and bring forth
vanity, and their belly prepareth deceit."[97] The wicked slaves to the
belly, the Book of Job continues, are held captive by their own sin,
punished by their own desires. The state of the "belly"—whether it is
at peace or tormented with desire—acts as an indication of spiritual
health. The belly expresses wicked insatiability—the wicked man "shall
not feel quietness in his belly," and when a wicked man is "about to fill
his belly, God shall cast the fury of his wrath upon him."[98] There is no
peace for the sinful belly.

Throughout the Bible, the belly poetically reflects the state of a
person's soul. Proverbs states, "The righteous eateth to the satisfying of

---

[95]   Phili. 3:18-19
[96]   Rom. 16:18
[97]   Job 15:35
[98]   Job 20:20; Job 20:23

his soul: but the belly of the wicked shall want."[99] Once again, those submerged in sinful habits are cursed with insatiable desire. But in the New Testament, those cleansed of sin, like those who believe in Christ, "out of his belly shall flow rivers of living water," as Jesus says.[100] The belly, later taken literally sometimes, was seen as the crux of the battle between good and evil and the desert monks, thoroughly immersed in Scripture, knew that if they were to be victorious, they could not lose on this battleground. They felt they had to prove their mastery over earthly temptations to prove their dedication to the unseen Creator of the world. Therefore, they waged war on not only gluttony and the pleasure of the taste buds, but, even more fanatically, they refused themselves the honor of even being adequately nourished. Put starkly, salvation was pitted against food.

Rebuking the Gluttonous Belly and Embracing the Raw

The Lausiac History (written in 420 CE) is a collection of stories about the Desert Fathers. In it, we read about one monk named Macarius the Alexandrine who, nearing age 100, was heard in his living cell verbally fighting with the devil—and his own belly. Macarius chastised himself for desiring oil and wine. Then, he was heard denouncing himself (and/or, ambiguously, the devil) as "old eater."[101] Even at the end of his life, Macarius was still fighting against the great Tempter, who was most clearly symbolized by the desire for food. In this vignette, where food and drink were emblematic of evil and sin, it is implied that any indulgence could throw the enjoyer into the devil's grasp.

Prior to his end-of-life fight with the belly/devil, Macarius was dedicated to a raw food diet. At one point, he "resolved not to eat anything treated with fire for seven years. . . Apart from raw cabbage (if there was any) and steeped [sprouted] lentils, he ate nothing." [102] Macarius's raw food diet became even more intense during Lent season, as it's claimed that he didn't allow himself water and consumed only uncooked cabbage leaves on Sundays, and that only "to give the impression that he was eating," so as to not become too proud of his

---

[99]   Prov. 13:25

[100]   John 7:38

[101]   Palladius, Bishop Of Aspuna, and John Wortley. *Palladius of Aspuna : The Lausiac History*. Athens, Ohio, Cistercian Publications ; Collegeville, Minnesota, 2015, 46.

[102]   Ibid., 38.

asceticism.[103] Macarius's dedication to Christ went further than that of the more typical ascetics around him and was proven by his avoidance of cooked food. The breaking of fasts would've offered him little material comfort as he chewed on practically tasteless uncooked cabbage leaves. A simple piece of cooked bread that other monks munched on might indulge the body too much and give the devil a foothold, he must've felt.

For some monks like Macarius, the desires of the belly were a distraction from Scripture recitation and prayer, and even worse, could be a sign that the belly and Satan, instead of God, were ruling over them. For the most dedicated ascetics, even the little attention required to prepare cooked food indicated too much servility toward the belly.

In rebellion to their fleshly needs, these monks would become like the "birds of the air" whom God provides for, that Jesus alluded to. They would consume only what arose naturally from the ground, without any human effort in altering it. Like those birds, they would graze on God's earth—in some cases, eating only what herbs grow in the wild.

The "illustrious deacon" Evagrius, for example, took his raw food diet to the extent of unendurable malnourishment. Palladius relates, "In the sixteenth year of this way of life without cooked food, on account of a malady of the stomach, his flesh needed to partake of something cooked."[104] After a long self-denying war on his belly, using the weapon of low-calorie and bland raw foods, Evagrius relented to the hardy and sustaining cooked foods out of necessity for his health.

THE DESIRES OF THE FLESH

> *"But put on the Lord Jesus Christ, and make no*
> *provision for the flesh, to gratify its desires."*
> —**Rom. 13:14**

Added to the poetics of the belly as a generator of sin was the New Testament's clearly expressed dichotomy between the desires of the flesh and godliness, a conception that the Desert Fathers took very seriously.

The New Testament offers stark warnings against succumbing to evil desires, which originate from "earthly nature." In addition to Ro-

---

[103]   Ibid., 39.

[104]   Ibid., 98

mans 13:14 warning to make "no provision" for this nature, Colossians 3:5 more dramatically tells readers to "put to death what is earthly in you: passion, evil desire." Similarly, 1 Peter 2:11 reminds Christians to "abstain from the passions of the flesh, which wage war against your soul."

1 John 2:16 summarizes the theological view that, "all that is in the world—the desires of the flesh and the desires of the eyes and pride of life—is not from the Father but is from the world."

The themes of the world versus God, and of the flesh versus spirit, had a tremendous effect on early Christians. Take one moving articulation in the epistles of the early Christian martyr Saint Ignatius, who in the battle to detach himself from the material world before his imminent death by wild beasts in the Roman Colosseum, declared that he could be proven to be a true follower of Christ "when I am no more visible to the world. [For,] nothing visible is good." As he rebuked the world and its trappings, similar to the desert monks, Ignatius declared, "My lust has been crucified, and there is no fire of material longing in me." This attitude would seem heroic to many Christians.

Dying to the Flesh

The material "world" symbolized the sinful desires that posed a threat to the soul. Refrains like "hate the world and all that is in it"; "Flee from the glory and repose of this world"; and "flee from men and you shall be saved" filled the writings of the monks. All these sayings followed the tone of the apostle Paul, who in Galatians 1:4, referred to "this present wicked world."

Aside from seclusion and "fleeing from men," food practices were of course critical to containing this world's hold over the monks and the wicked flesh that enveloped their spirits. Prolonged fasting and limiting one's diet to raw food were expressions of a monk's "hating his own life," as referred to in the Gospel of Luke, and rejecting the sinful world.

Abstemiousness in General

*"By no means is the soul humbled unless you reduce its
food or restrict it to feeding only when necessary."*
—**Saying of the Desert Fathers**[105]

"Fasting is the mother of all virtues, because it gives birth to them."
—**Saying of the Desert Fathers**[106]

Food was clearly a problem in the minds of the Desert Fathers. Any enjoyment of it was an obstacle to spiritual growth. The quote above about humility and fasting suggests that a monk wouldn't even have a chance at reaching Christian humility if he ate liberally. One's relationship to food was spiritually crucial to the rest of one's struggle against temptation. Fleshly desires would run wild and sexual lust would seethe if the flesh were invigorated and emboldened from plentiful nourishment.

It's not surprising, therefore, that fasting was a "most bitter medicine" to starve the flesh of its desires. A Desert Father, Abba John Colobos, said that "the enemy [Satan] submits to [the monk], reduced by famine. So it is with the passions of the flesh too: if a person exists with fasting and hunger, the Enemy wastes away from his soul."[107] For Colobos, the enemy—sinful flesh (and Satan)—was starved into submission similar to the way an army starves "a city of the enemy" to make it surrender. Sin had less hope of flourishing if it wasn't physically fed.

When a monk wasn't fasting for days at a time, his food intake was to be strictly controlled, lest the flesh rear its dangerous head. Because the elders in the desert monk colonies were acutely aware of the connection between sinful passions and food intake, they undertook years of experimentation and self-reflection and refined their rules surrounding sustenance into a science: "The elders tested all these things and concluded that it was good to eat each day, but in small quantities."[108] They had tested various timetables for fasting—three days, four days, a week and settled on the notion that fleshly desires would best be quelled by consuming one sparse meal a day.

---

105   Wortley, John. *An Introduction to the Desert Fathers*. Cambridge, United Kingdom: Cambridge University Press, 2019, 87.

106   Ibid., 89.

107   Ibid.

108   Ibid., 90.

A monk wasn't required to eat raw but his fare was expected to at least be strictly vegan, plain tasting, not pleasurable, and often consist only of long-stored dried bread, although occasionally vegetables or lentils were also consumed.[109]

This disciplined dietary regimen felt sufficient to many monks in its ability to restrain the flesh. But for an elite few, raw foodism offered an even more aggressive path to starving out evil.

Disempowering the Flesh through Raw Foodism

The writer of the Lausiac History, Palladius, praises the desert ascetic Ammonios for his ability to ward off his earthly passions, even to the extent of genitally torturing himself when erotic impulses arose. Another central indication of Ammonios's pious zeal was that almost all of his "fare at table was raw" from when "he was a young man until his death."[110]

The most extreme monks, it seems, were dedicated to raw food, as we see in similar examples. The sometimes-raw foodist Evagrius, for instance, would stand naked in the freezing cold of his cell as a self-punishing attempt to ward off "the demon of fornication." In the life of the priest Philoromus, we see a similar connection between the defeat of the flesh and the practice of raw foodism. In his early adulthood, he fought against "fornication and gluttony . . . He drove out these passions by shutting himself up and wearing irons, and by abstinence from corn-bread and all things cooked by fire. After persevering in this course for eighteen years, and accomplishing victory over lust, he sang the hymn of triumph to Christ."[111] Raw foodism was clearly an aid, even a purifying medicine, used in the torturous struggle to starve out sexual impulse and sin in general.

Raw foodism played a central role in Philoromus's "rejection of the world," as Palladius describes it. Philoromus demonstrated uncommon scorn for many of the cares and desires that affected most people and would show his courage in speaking with "boldness" to earthly authorities like the Byzantine emperor Julian (for which he suffered gruesome torture). But in regard to the most challenging temptation, sexual lust, Philoromus only achieved victory by refusing cooked food for eighteen years to starve this "passion" out of his body and mind.

---

[109]   Ibid.

[110]   Palladius, Bishop Of Aspuna, and John Wortley. *Palladius of Aspuna : The Lausiac History.* Athens, Ohio, Cistercian Publications ; Collegeville, Minnesota, 2015, 26.

[111]   Ibid., 107.

Occasionally, whole communities would embrace the spiritually cleansing effects of going raw. In one Egyptian ascetic settlement, many monks would eat "nothing cooked" for all of Lent.[112] In this case, we have evidence of a widespread temporary adoption of raw food to chastise the flesh to commemorate the forty days that Jesus spent fasting in the desert and fighting temptation. All cooked food, even the plainest fare, was occasionally considered too tasty, too luxuriant, too strengthening for the abstinence-themed season of Lent. So it was appropriate, in this case, for monks to temporarily give it up in an act of deference for Jesus's suffering.

One of the most important reasons for abstaining from cooked food was to display exceptional discipline and show one's willingness to sacrifice physical needs and to hope that the "old self was crucified."[113] That is, the carnal self dies to its desires and figuratively assumes the cross that Jesus literally suffered.

As Palladius makes clear, the "disturbances [of the world]" imperiled the goal of the monks' "desire for immortality."[114] Every fleshly desire, including every comforting piece of cooked food that was given up, reassured the monks of their salvation and proved their love for the Creator.

THOSE WHO FELL: GIVING IN TO THE FLESH

> *"We asked therefore what was the reason why the men*
> *who lived there in the desert, were some of them deceived*
> *in their mind and others shattered by lust."*
> **—The Lausiac History**

If abstemiousness and raw foodism chastised the flesh into meekness, then gluttony (especially of cooked food) led to the flesh conquering the spirit. Monks who failed to dietarily discipline their bodies were warned that by "overeating and knocking back wine like this," they would "fall into the mire" of sexual profligacy.[115] If the flesh was emboldened with food, sexual sin followed, and the monk would lose, at least temporarily, the battle against evil. As one monk who lived in the fifth century CE, John Cassian, wrote, "But now we have to deal with

---

[112]   Ibid. 38.

[113]   Romans 6:6

[114]   Palladius, Bishop Of Aspuna, and John Wortley. *Palladius of Aspuna: The Lausiac History*. Athens, Ohio, Cistercian Publications ; Collegeville, Minnesota, 2015, 53.

[115]   Ibid., 69.

Gluttony, that is the desire of the palate, against which our first battle is. He then will never be able to check the motions of a burning lust, who cannot restrain the desires of the appetite."[116]

Food was at the core of spiritual health. The sexual sin that nourishing food could foment was taken as a serious threat and one monk went so far as to describe it as "physical death."[117] This most insidious of temptations could sever one from God. There are stories of the monks being harassed by the "demon" of lust, seething in their stone cells, battling this great enemy sometimes for decades on end.

To give into food could fell a monk to these desires of the body.

"This disaster," as the *Lausiac History* calls the wayward path of satisfying the appetite of the belly, fell on a monk named Ptolemy, who "diverged so greatly from the straight way" and "constant communion of the mysteries," having "given himself over to gluttony and drunkenness." Ptolemy surrendered to the base desires of flesh, instead of the elevated spiritual path of constantly keeping the appetite for food in check. The result was wantonness, being "puffed up with pride." Lost souls such as these, the *History* warns, are met with destruction—they "fall like leaves, away from the godly path"[118]

MORAL MOTIFS FROM THE CLASSICAL WORLD AND RAW FOODISM

Christianity's integration into the mainstream culture of the Roman Empire in the third, fourth, and fifth centuries CE did not completely erase the influence that classical (pre-Christian) Greco-Roman values had on people, including monks. Holdover morals and symbolic paradigms from ancient Greek culture and non-Christian philosophy still influenced the psyche of even the most devout Christian ascetics.

And at least a few of these paradigms played into the aversion to food and dedication of some ascetics to a raw food diet.

---

[116]   Cassian, John. 2019. "St. John Cassian. St. John Cassian's Institutes: Gluttony." OrthoChristian.com. 2019. https://orthochristian.com/119858.html.

[117]   Wortley, John. *An Introduction to the Desert Fathers*. Cambridge, United Kingdom: Cambridge University Press, 2019, 44.

[118]   Palladius, Bishop Of Aspuna, and John Wortley. *Palladius of Aspuna : The Lausiac History*. Athens, Ohio, Cistercian Publications ; Collegeville, Minnesota, 2015, 70.

Dietarily Starving the Passions and Attaining Apatheia

"Death is a cessation from . . . the tyranny of the passions,
the errors of the mind, and the servitude of the body."
—Marcus Aurelius, Emperor of Rome and Stoic philosopher

The opening pages of the *Lausiac History* demonstrate how Greco-Roman ideas—especially Stoic philosophy—seeped into the Desert Fathers' worldview. The book on the monks' lives states that its purpose was to be a "perpetual medicine against . . . irrational desire—anger, agitation, grief, and irrational fear."[119] Palladius, the author, sought to ignite readers with courage to "still" their minds which are usually "tossed hither and thither."[120]

The language that the *Lausiac History* uses about "irrational desires" and agitated movements of the mind is similar to that of the Stoics, if not appropriated directly from them. Discussions about "passions" and "agitations" could be plucked right from the writings of such Roman Stoics as Aurelius and Epictetus. Aurelius wrote that "the mind which is free from passions [negative emotions] is a citadel," a sure and safe refuge, and wrote that he revered people who were "free" from passions.[121] Fellow Stoic Epictetus talked of "passions that torment" and defined them as impulses "that cause a person to act irrationally or without due consideration. The early Greek Stoics, before Epictetus and Aurelius, described passions as perversions of the intellect.[122]

Palladius refers to passions frequently in his *Lausiac* narrative and explains that one of the goals of a Christian monk's life was to attain the Stoic ideal of "apatheia," a serene state of mind devoid of agitating passions.[123] He was on the same page as so-called pagan philosophers as to what day-to-day spiritual goals should be.

Their goal of mental peace, articulated in Stoic terms, fit nicely with the desert monks' conception of sin and salvation. The passions led people to sin; they were the emotional, intellectual, and even bodily sources of sin. And sin separated people from God and imperiled their salvation. Both Aurelius and Paul, Stoic and Christian, respectively urged people to "yield not to any lusts and motions of the flesh," and

---

[119]   Ibid., 2

[120]   Ibid., 3

[121]   *Meditations*, 6.16, *Meditations*, 4.1, *Meditations*, 4.48

[122]   Diogenes Laertius and Charles Duke Yonge. *The Lives and Opinions of Eminent Philosophers*. United States, Andesite Press, 2015, 47

[123]   Palladius, Bishop Of Aspuna, and John Wortley. *Palladius of Aspuna : The Lausiac History*. Athens, Ohio, Cistercian Publications ; Collegeville, Minnesota, 2015, 3.

"walk by the [Holy] Spirit, and you will not gratify the desires of the flesh."[124] "For the desires of the flesh," Paul wrote, "are against the Spirit, and the desires of the Spirit are against the flesh."[125]

The dual psychic pressure, from the Bible and from "pagan" writings, weighed on the monks and influenced their daily habits, including eating. This intersection of ideologies is evident by the *Lausiac History*'s praise of the most devout monks as also "the most devoid of passion."[126] If the desires of the flesh imperiled the monks' mental peace and eternal salvation, they had better act. And what better way than to stop feeding the problem? That's why fasting and severely limiting food intake, Palladius details, were the go-to dietary weapons against the passions of the mind and body—weapons used to "break down the insolence" of lustful desires.

Monks who emaciated their bodies with severe fasting and subsisting on raw food were lauded for being "advanced so far in apatheia" because they controlled their fleshly passions. One monk was, heroically, so thin that "the sun shone through his bones."[127] Conversely, gluttonous people were referred to as "the impassioned."[128] Food intake was directly correlated to one's spiritual state.

Palladius praises monks who fought passions with "spiritual discipline" like working, reciting prayers, and bodily torture, but he singled out practices "concerning food," to starve out passion and sin.[129] One Ethiopian monk, a Desert Father named Moses, strictly limited his food intake in an effort to prevent him from "burning up" with sexual desires.[130] Moses had a metaphor for passions and sin that could easily be applied to food intake: Dogs (or sin) will hang around a butcher's shop if they receive meat, but "if the shop is closed and no one gives him anything, he no longer comes near it."[131]

Food was dangerous fuel for the passions and there was shame surrounding it because of this. One monk named John of Lycoplis triumphantly claimed that he had lived forty-eight years in an isolated cell without seeing the temptations of women or gold, and equally

---

124   *Meditations*, Book 6, 30.

125   Galatians 5:16-17.

126   Palladius, Bishop Of Aspuna, and John Wortley. *Palladius of Aspuna : The Lausiac History*. Athens, Ohio, Cistercian Publications ; Collegeville, Minnesota, 2015, 94.

127   Ibid., 117.

128   Ibid., 113.

129   "Palladius, the Lausiac History (1918), 35-180. English Translation." 2025. Tertullian.org. 2025. https://www.tertullian.org/fathers/palladius_lausiac_02_text.htm.

130   Ibid., 50.

131   "Palladius, the Lausiac History (1918), 35-180. English Translation." 2025. Tertullian.org. 2025. https://www.tertullian.org/fathers/palladius_lausiac_02_text.htm. Chapter XIX

important, he says, "I did not see anybody chewing, and nobody saw me eating or drinking."[132]

It was virtuous, after all, to feel shame around food, and thus to practice severe austerity. This made raw foodism a welcome option for those seeking to minimize food's hold on their life. One monk, Poseidon, who took up raw foodism and succeeded in his battle against the passions, was described as "meek" and "extremely spiritually disciplined."[133] He was said to have existed for a time on "small dates and wild herbs." Once, he found a "basket of fresh grapes and figs," a treasure trove of nourishment by his standards, that sustained him for two months.[134]

The fact that Palladius singled out instances of raw foodism shows that this way of eating was a badge of honor within the community of monks. Palladius found such dedicated discipline as worthly of being recorded for posterity. It was a feat that earned as much acclaim as athletic accomplishments, which is another motif of dually pagan and Biblical morality that influenced the Desert Fathers—that of the spiritual athlete.

DISCIPLINED DIETARY ATHLETES

"Every athlete exercises self-control in all things. They do it to receive a perishable wreath, but we an imperishable."
—1 Corin. 9:25

"No man, in my opinion, has a more profitable difficulty on his hands than you have, provided you will but use it, as an athletic champion uses his antagonist."
—Epictetus, Stoic Philosopher

The theme of the victorious athlete that loomed large in the minds of monks originated in the classical Greek world but bled into the later Christian New Testament. This archetype was prominent throughout the ancient Mediterranean and larger Greek world, including the Near East into the time of the New Testament. That's why the Desert Fathers often viewed their ascetic struggles figuratively as those of an athlete engaged in a long struggle to win a prize. And as we know, food

---

[132] Palladius, Bishop Of Aspuna, and John Wortley. *Palladius of Aspuna : The Lausiac History*. Athens, Ohio, Cistercian Publications; Collegeville, Minnesota, 2015, 85.
[133] Ibid., 86.
[134] Ibid., 86.

practices were one of the most important daily paths to attaining their spiritual prize.

Classical "pagan" culture and early Christian culture shared the perception of the athlete as a symbol of intense discipline and glorious victory. Epictetus, a Greek Stoic philosopher described a person who achieves a state of serene passionlessness, *apatheia,* as able to "achieve mastery over yourself, just as an athlete competes for glory in the Olympics." [135] To "make progress in the virtues," he also says, you have to live "a life of discipline. Think of the athlete, who does not indulge in luxuries, does not drink wine, nor give in to sleep or laziness, but instead trains in a way that makes him strong and tough."[136] Similarly, the New Testament of the Bible often alludes to spiritual athletes who suffered "painful" "discipline."[137] The apostle Paul addresses Christians, saying, "Do you not know that in a race all the runners run, but only one receives the prize? So run that you may obtain it."[138] "Everyone who competes in the games goes into strict training," Paul reminded. Continuing with a reference to athletic feats combined with quelling the body's desires, he declared, "I strike a blow to my body and make it my slave so that after I have preached to others, I myself will not be disqualified for the prize."[139]

So it's no surprise that monks sought to prove themselves as heroic athletes, seeing that both the Greco-Roman and Christian influences are so obvious. Considering this, we might ask who among the Desert Fathers were the most meek, austere, and deprived? Who was "running" the hardest race? Arguably, who else but those who were relentless in their fasting and those who consumed only raw foods for years.

The monks who lived on steeped lentils, wild herbs, occasional fruit, and raw vegetables—those who suffered what most people would consider a horrifyingly tasteless and an arduous calorie-restricted diet—these were the monks who often earned mention in Palladius's narrative. He described his conception of ascetic monks, calling them "invincible athletes" who were "our holy and immortal spiritual fathers" and trained strenuously to "please God with much mortification of the body."[140]

---

[135]   Discourses 2.2

[136]   Discourses 1.2

[137]   Heb. 12:11

[138]   1 Cor, 9:24

[139]   1 Cor. 9:24-27

[140]   "Palladius, the Lausiac History (1918), 35-180. English Translation." *Tertullian.org,* 2025, www.tertullian.org/fathers/palladius_lausiac_02_text.htm. Accessed 14 Feb. 2025.

Palladius called the ascetic feats of monks, "contests of the arena" and noted that he recorded only the "main contests and achievements of the noble athletes and great men."[141] This signifies that Palladius felt that long-term raw foodism was an "achievement" worth mentioning, as evidenced by his numerous descriptions of these types of dietary "contests" in his *History*. Those who rejected the comfort of even simple cooked food would be ranked among the athletes of the "highest life," athletes of Christ.[142] These were the ascetics who, Palladius says, "I have been privileged to see with my own eyes in the he arena of piety.[143]

Eternal glory, and even earthly glory (though they might not have admitted it), awaited dedicated monks like those who sought out raw food "contests." Those who "engaged in contests with demons a thousand times and more" (and who did that more than the malnourished raw foodists?) earned a "famous name" in the records of "the athletes of Christ."[144] The daily renunciation of the world, their bodies, pleasing food, and each hunger pang that came with it, was a "contest" to test the dedication of the aspiring athlete. Would the ascetic give in to hearty food or cooked food, or maintain his anti-worldly endurance? The desert monks would've been well aware of the book of Hebrews which warned to lay aside any "sin which clings so closely, and let us run with endurance the race that is set before us." After all, like an athlete in the arena, the Book of Hebrews says, "we are surrounded by so great a cloud of witnesses."[145] The contest was on. The spirit of the Greek and Roman athletic games prefigured the new ascetic contests of the Christian era. God and men watched. Those eyes were staring, with either dreadful judgment or reverent praise, to see how and what monks ate. And eating raw was one of the most effective ways for the monkish "athlete" to perform successfully in this cosmic arena.

---

[141] Ibid.,
[142] Ibid.
[143] Ibid.
[144] Ibid.
[145] Hebrews 12:1 (ESV)

4.
Raw Food Inverted: Ancient Chinese Medicine

From the Desert Fathers, we move back in time, to account for a different type of ancient view on uncooked food. In this chapter, we study an instance of the disapproval of raw foods within the context of ancient Chinese medicine. We'll also look at the attempt of a modern raw foodist and believer in ancient Chinese medicine principles to assert the value of raw foods within this hostile context.

ANCIENT ANTI-RAW FOODISM

As long ago as 5,000 years, Chinese hermit-herbalists in the misty mountains of northern China, meditated on the nature of the universe. They generated theories of how the cosmos functioned—what kept it in a state of balance. They also mused on what they saw as a microcosm of the cosmos: the human body. Through experimentation and evaluation, they sought to discover what kept the body healthy and identified herbs and dietary practices that supposedly nourished vigor and longevity. Eventually, systems of thought surrounding food and herbs developed into what's generally known as traditional Chinese medicine (TCM).

"They listened to plant wisdom," wrote modern raw foodist Rehmannia Dean Thomas, who is a follower of TCM.[146] There's a problem within TCM, though, as it relates to raw food. For anyone familiar with the traditional tenets of this system, it would be shocking to see raw foodism and TCM being practiced simultaneously. Often, these

---

¹⁴⁶ Rehmannia Dean Thomas, and Janabai Owens Amsden. *Raw Chi : Balancing the Raw Food Diet with Chinese Herbs*. Berkeley, California, Evolver Editions, 2014, 2

two philosophies are seen as incompatible, because for a few thousand years, the proponents of TCM have rejected raw foods.

YIN, YANG, AND RAW FOOD

> *"Some other scholars believe that 'other foods' refer to foods that tend to damage the spleen and produce dampness."*
> **—Yellow Emperor's Inner Cannon**

In China, raw food has been seen, since ancient times, as throwing the energy systems of the body out of balance. Traditionally, TCM has held that eating raw foods was too risky because it might cause what's known as the spleen meridian to become too "dampened," stifling the ability of the digestive "heat" that is needed to produce energy from and "cook down" food we eat to produce chi.[147] As you can see, cooking is innately seen as a good thing in TCM, as the linguistics of it are built into its essential physiological theories.

CHINESE MEDICINE'S BROADER PHILOSOPHY AND VIEW ON RAW FOOD

TCM, during its development, drew some inspiration from the ancient Chinese philosophy of Daoism, which places emphasis on harmony and balancing the cosmic energetic forces of yin (passive, receptive, darkness) and yang (active, positive, light). When yin and yang are in balance within a body, the flow of chi is vibrant.

Chi is often defined as the "vital life force" energy that permeates all living things and sustains life. Rehmannia Dean Thomas, the raw foodist previously mentioned, says that chi "gives rise to epochs and ecosystems" and is "a crucial requirement for the maintenance of health and vibrancy throughout all stages of our lives."[148] Life tends to thrive when chi is flowing freely through us.[149] Sickness and disease often occur when chi is constricted. And that theory is at the foundation of TCM.

Within Chinese medicine, there are five energy meridians or systems: liver, kidney, lung, heart, and spleen. But the spleen governs all

---

[147]   Thomas, Amsden, 23

[148]   Rehmannia Dean Thomas, and Janabai Owens Amsden. *Raw Chi : Balancing the Raw Food Diet with Chinese Herbs*. Berkeley, California, Evolver Editions, 2014, 2.

[149]   Thomas, Amsden, 2

the other meridians. Represented visually, the other meridians surround the spleen system at the center of it all, "the center of our cosmology," Rehmannia says.[150] The spleen system is not represented by a specific season like the other meridians, as it is active all year round, "governing" the metabolism and producing chi.[151] The blood receives chi from this spleen system.

When we consume raw food, many Chinese medicine advocates believe, we are handicapping the energetic flow of chi through our "spleen" and the rest of the body. "Raw, uncooked foods are classified as yin," Rehmannia explains. They are "watery and cooling" to the body and can dampen the flow of chi and obstruct metabolic function.[152]

The foundational texts of TCM concur. The *Huangdi Neijing* ("Inner Canon of the Yellow Emperor"), a text written by multiple ancient physicians and scholars around the third century BCE, argues that cooked food, as opposed to raw, is generally considered to be more easily absorbable by the body because it requires less digestive energy to break down the raw elements. If food is already cooked, the process of assimilation is already half done for the eater, which makes it less taxing for the digestive system.

In the *Inner Canon,* cold and raw foods are thought to be disruptive to the flow of chi through the digestive system or the digestive "fire" or "yang" of the spleen and stomach energy meridians. To preserve the efficient flow of chi, food should be cooked and warm. Cold and raw foods dissipate warmth and weaken the stomach and spleen by concentrating "cold" energy there, leading to discomfort and digestive troubles. Warm, cooked foods support the digestive energy flow; raw foods block it, leading to trouble. The eater of raw or cold foods is at greater risk, the *Inner Cannon* claims, of digestive disorders and may become weak. The skin will lose its glow and the person will be prone to sickness.[153]

Other foundational TCM texts testify to the supposed danger of raw foods. More than 1,500 years after the *Inner Cannon* was written, the *Zhen Jiu Da Cheng (The Great Compendium of Acupuncture and Moxibustion),* published in 1601, states that raw, cold foods harm the stomach chi because indigestion can form if "dampness" is accumulated.[154] Only warm, cooked foods support the stomach's digestive func-

---

[150]   Ibid., 18.

[151]   Ibid., 18.

[152]   Ibid., 31.

[153]   Hicks, Angela. *The Huangdi Neijing: The Yellow Emperor's Classic of Medicine.* Singing Dragon, 2013.

[154]   Li, Gao, and Bob Flaws. *Li Dong-Yuan's Treatise on the Spleen & Stomach : A Translation of the Pi Wei Lun.* Boulder, Co, Blue Poppy Press, 2004.

tion.[155] Centuries before that, the *Pi Wei Lun (Treatise on the Spleen and Stomach)* warned that cold and raw foods consume the spleen's warmth and when that happens, the spleen can't transform food into chi.

RECONCILING OPPOSITES: CHINESE MEDICINE AND RAW FOODISM

Despite TCM's generally negative view of raw foods, modern raw foodists who have an appreciation for Chinese medicine have attempted to reconcile a "living foods" diet with TCM theory. Rehmannia, one of those raw foodists, has written about the conflict between TCM and raw food. As a Daoist herbalist, he believes that people can still thrive on a raw food diet if they make use of Chinese herbs that fight the "dampness" that can occur as a result of consuming uncooked foods. By using certain herbs, he believes, people can maintain the heat of their digestive system, or in other words, the ability to generate life energy from the food they eat.

After all, besides his love for Chinese medicine, Rehmannia believes strongly in the virtues of raw foods. "Raw food is the gift of Gaia, our Mother Earth, to humankind and all animals, great and small, through all time," Rehmannia proclaims.[156] He's not about to give up the high esteem he has for raw food. "The incredible healing power that raw food has on the human body is clear," he continues.[157]

Because Rehmannia personally healed by adhering to a raw food diet and because he's also deeply dedicated to TCM and completed an eight-year traditional master-pupil apprenticeship under a Daoist master herbalist, he is acutely aware of the perceived conflict between TCM and raw food and wishes to bridge the gap.

In Rehmannia's mission to reconcile TCM and raw foodism, he seeks to "see through the collective dogma of the past and [in]to the deeper teachings of TCM in order to serve the needs of the present."[158] TCM practitioners have been shortsighted. Centuries of "dogma," in his mind, have obscured the true meaning of TCM teachings and unnecessarily caused a sweeping condemnation of uncooked foods. He

---

[155]　Yang, Jizhou, and Sabine Wilms. *The Great Compendium of Acupuncture and Moxibustion : Zhēn Jiŭ Dà Chéng. Volume 1*. Portland, Oregon, Chinese Medicine Database, 2010.

[156]　Thomas, Amsden, xi.

[157]　Ibid.

[158]　Ibid., xii.

seeks to make a "powerful case" for the inclusion of raw foods into Chinese medicine.[159]

"Many of us interested in the raw food diet," Rehmannia regrets, "have had the experience of visiting our acupuncturist and seeing a finger waving in our faces, 'No raw food. Damp spleen!'"[160] His goal is to soften this categorical dismissal of raw foods. Even his mentor, a master herbalist of Chinese medicine, dismissed the idea of a raw food diet. "Not a good idea," he said. "Too cold. Vegetables and fruits are cooling . . . they will . . . dampen the spleen."[161]

Despite these experiences, Rehmannia's intuition told him that there was something exceptionally valuable in the raw food diet. He had to find a way to reconcile these beloved but supposedly conflicting ways of life.

CHINESE HERBS AND RAW FOOD

> *"The raw food movement is vital and important, but there are some potential detriments to a raw food diet. Modification is the message nowadays."*
> **—Rehmannia Dean Thomas**

Rehmannia was curious to test the wrist pulses (a TCM technique of measuring the energy patterns in the body) of raw foodists and examine their physical characteristics to see how healthy the diet was. After feeling the pulse of a strict raw vegan, he found a confounding result—her pulse "was *very* strong" and "thriving," stronger than many "conscientious omnivores."[162] Her spleen/pancreas were strong, working well as governors of the digestion and yet there were signs of "dampness," of some chi "stagnation."

The idea struck Rehmannia to encourage raw foodists to use TCM herbs as a preventative measure against the potential dampness and excessive moisture retention they could be at risk for. "Drying" herbs, taken in a hot tea, could be the perfect balancing complement to a very vibrant but damp raw food diet. If this regimen were followed, raw eaters could experience the vitality of a raw food diet without the potential drawbacks. And in the process, Rehmannia could spawn a renaissance, a "paradigm shift" within Chinese medicine, initiating it

---

[159]   Ibid., xiii.
[160]   Ibid., 10.
[161]   Ibid., 11.
[162]   Ibid., 12.

to become more accommodating to uncooked food and redefine its accepted doctrine.[163]

There was no way, he thought, that raw food was completely incompatible with TCM. Daoist philosophers, after all, had some beliefs that were similar to modern-day raw foodists. They believed that in order to honor the gods that bring harmony inside the human body, they were to avoid "grains, meat, and wine"—foods not looked highly upon by raw vegans.[164] Thoughts like these served as a starting point for questioning commonly accepted interpretations of TCM theory.

Rehmannia attempted to reconcile popular raw food theories with the TCM theoretical framework. The living enzymes in raw foods are chi, he posited. They're an important form of "nutritive chi"—a concept in Chinese medicine referring to the gathering of chi energy from food that's consumed.[165] "When our chi is sufficiently supplemented" by the food we eat, especially raw foods, "our inner wellspring of vitality bubbles over" and we are filled with energy. The accumulation of chi makes for excellent health and enriches our life experience with "self-empowerment" and "satisfying adventures in the creative and procreative realms."[166]

By consuming raw food enzymes, "packets of chi" are released into our bodies. These vibrant "catalysts" for metabolic activity are "wiped out by heavy cooking and processing."[167] Many people, Rehmannia claims, who eat cooked foods have weak spleen chi because their food is "devitalized" and without enzymes. Much cooked food also lacks micronutrients and is toxified with synthetic agricultural chemicals.[168] Bodies run sluggishly and eventually have to dip into their "deeper reserves of *jing*"—adrenal energy and storage of chi, causing a loss of vitality and "rapid aging."[169]

Rehmannia also holds that organic raw food is great for enhancing energy, because of the lightness of the food and for cleansing the body, as there's so little toxicity from additives, synthetic agricultural chemicals, or harmful compounds generated by cooking.[170]

Another way, he believes, in which raw foods can strengthen chi is by generously supplying beneficial bacteria to the gut that have not

---

[163] Ibid., xiii.
[164] Ibid.,xiii.
[165] Ibid., 6.
[166] Ibid., 6-7.
[167] Ibid., 9.
[168] Ibid., 28.
[169] Ibid., 29.
[170] Ibid., 30-33.

been destroyed by cooking. Conversely, many "overcooked" foods can proliferate harmful bacteria. Good bacteria are deeply involved in the assimilation and production of nutrients that build chi and thus "could be considered part of the spleen meridian."[171]

Raw food is very vitalizing, Rehmannia holds, and conducive to good health, as long as enough warmth is maintained in the spleen meridian. That's why it's important for raw foodists to preventatively use herbs that "have been shown to cultivate and protect chi" and "tonify the spleen."[172] These drying herbs "turn up the fire under the stomach," and "the Chinese have a near religious reverence" for them. They are, Rehmannia claims, the perfect complements to the wet cooling energy of raw foods.

Even in the absence of drying herbs, Rehmannia notes, some men may benefit from raw foods because they are high-yin foods which "can help cool and moisten" the masculine yang energy if it becomes too hot.

BALANCING RAW YIN WITH YANG HERBS

Rehmannia tested his drying herbs regimen on a raw foodist community in Santa Monica, California. Uncooked enthusiasts would consume his "spleen chi tea" to complement their diet, break the cycle of dampness, and "light the internal fires" to boost chi.[173] The Californian raw food eaters loved the ginseng, poria, citrus peel, cinnamon, jujube date, codonopsis, atractylodes, and others that would supposedly invigorate their spleen chi, and Rehmannia remained convinced that these herbs helped balance the potential downsides of raw foods.

Still, it's a tough task to spread any "paradigm shift" in such a massive sphere like Chinese medicine, which influences at least over a billion people worldwide. It'd take a big ideological transition for such an ancient system to be reevaluated by its adherents and uncooked foods to not be seen as harmful to the body's energetics. Nevertheless, Rehmannia's quest to reconcile two different dietary theories evidences the depth of raw foodists' beliefs in the healing efficacy of uncooked food.

---

[171]   Ibid.,.33.

[172]   Ibid., 39.

[173]   Ibid., xii.

The Struggles of Raw Foodism

Rehmannia saw his efforts as successful, on a small scale, at sowing some seeds of doubt about whether raw food should be considered untouchable within TCM. He defended this maligned food group within ancient Chinese medicine while remaining faithful to the system's general notions. Still, the debate rages within TCM and the wider world regarding the value or harm of raw foods and the TCM perception of raw foods highlights the uphill battle that raw foodism often faces in its struggle against the civilizational habit of cooking.

Because cooking is so entrenched in a society's traditions, the advocate of uncooked foods often finds himself in rebellion against established norms, whether in a larger cultural context or a more niche context like that of TCM. And as the story of raw food's place within traditional Chinese medicine shows, there are systems that are hostile to leaving things raw. Uncooked food advocacy is most often assigned to the extremities of history, as an abnormal interest.

The story of TCM and Rehmannia shows that unlike other ancient belief systems, like those of some Christian and Hindu monks, there existed a thought system in which raw food was vilified. And the majority of humans follow that line of thought today; at the least they would be unwilling to dispense with cooking entirely.

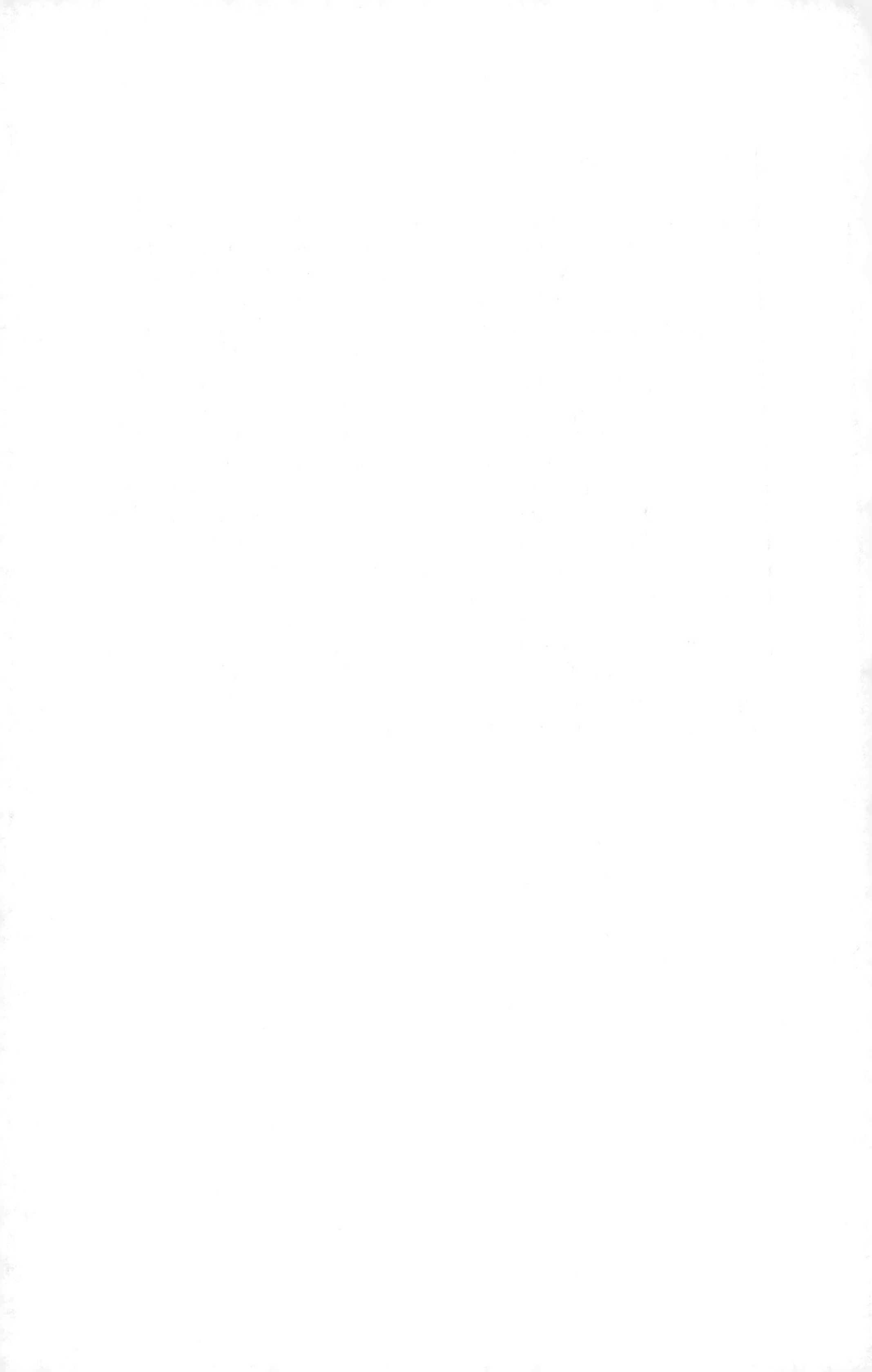

Post-Industrial Raw Foodism

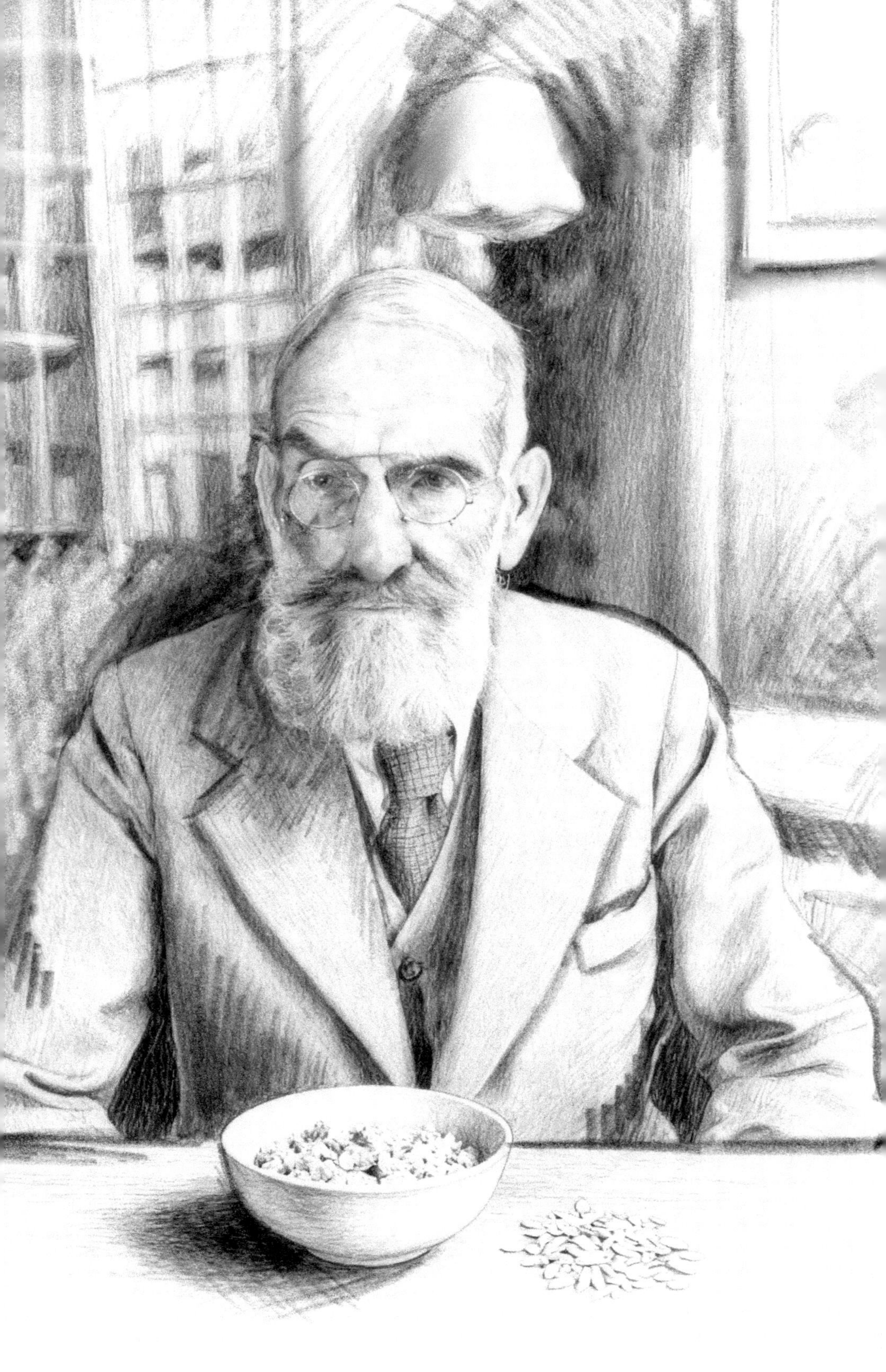

5.
Max Bircher-Benner: The "New Physician"

There is a long gap in the history of raw foodism, between the Desert Fathers of the early Common Era and the 1800s, when certain unconventional physicians began considering the healing potential of uncooked plant foods.

After the Industrial Revolution separated humans more and more from nature, Western writers, artists, and physicians yearned to get back in touch with nature and return humanity to a more wholesome existence. In nineteenth-century Europe and America, there were movements to embrace natural living and to revere non-industrialized peoples around the globe for their purity and cultural advantages over degenerate "civilized" industrial societies.

Max Bircher-Benner, a Swiss physician born in 1879, was part of this nature-forward movement. After experiencing a civilizational hellscape of rampant drug addiction and ill health as a young physician, he sought out solutions in unorthodox corners of medical thought.

EXPERIENCING DEGENERATE CIVILIZATION

In 1890s Zurich, Switzerland, a young, demoralized Bircher-Benner stumbled upon a horrific scene that seemed to encapsulate his feelings of hopelessness. He had been called to an apartment, where he discovered a murder-suicide. A dead mother was hanging from a door, having just suffocated her two children. The woman had been anguished by her unsupportive morphine- and alcohol-addicted husband. Worrying about her financial future, the wife saw no other way out of her distress.[174]

---

[174]   Bircher-Benner, Max. *The Physician of the Future*. Germany, Bircher-Benner, 2015. 37.

Poor health and drug addiction (including alcoholism) were endemic in the industrial quarter where Bircher-Benner worked. In these relatively poor and polluted areas of Zurich, where people worked long hours in poor conditions, many suffered from "diseases of the gastro-intestinal and cardiovascular organs . . . rheumatism, nervous diseases, neuroses," among other maladies. Bircher-Benner felt insufficient to heal his patients in this disease- and drug-plagued time. "The illness of these people weighed heavily on me," he reflected, "all the more since . . . my therapeutic measures were insufficient."[175]

But his experience with one patient changed the trajectory of his thought and career. The woman in this case languished in bed, emaciated by malnutrition and a distended and malfunctioning stomach. The case was "hopeless" in Bircher-Benner's mind. But a chance encounter with a "German natural healer and vegetarian" changed that. The man recommended that Max treat his patient with a diet of mostly raw vegetables.[176]

Within weeks of starting the peculiar diet, the patient healed her digestion, gained strength, and rose from her bed. Paradoxically, Max was "shattered" since he had to shed his "prejudice" against vegetarianism and recognize his ignorance.[177] Ideologically he felt defeated. "The vegetarian had won." But the initial egoic disappointment gave way to a new and exhilarating mission and outlook. As the months passed and Bircher-Benner tested this new raw food diet on recalcitrant patients and his own family members, it became clear that the vegetarian healer had handed him a shockingly effective regimen—one that seemed to heal a variety of disorders.

He had known nothing about the "nutritional science" of raw food previously, but now, he saw that there was something unique about its effects. He had, though, somewhat of a background in the practice of abstinence, which he would later connect to raw food therapy. Abstaining from food was responsible for his own triumph over a childhood illness. At age eleven, he had been debilitated by an inflammatory intestinal condition but had fasted for ten days, subsisting only on water, and had healed completely.

But it was in adulthood that the power of abstinence truly sank in and became integrated in the raw-food treatment of his patients. His heartfelt mission to heal the world intensified and after seeing the miraculous effects of uncooked diets, he felt like he had the tools to complete his work. He had found nature's secret, the ultimate medicine.

---

175   Ibid.

176   Ibid., 41.

177   Ibid., 38.

Bircher-Benner sought to make sense of what happened. Why did uncooked foods seem to heal people from deadly illnesses? How did raw foods work their magic? In his quest of understanding, as well as advocating for raw foodism, he utilized his wide-ranging reading in medicine and philosophy.

THE PHILOSOPHY OF BIRCHER-BENNER

Bircher-Benner felt strongly about his mission to heal the suffering around him, and articulated his fight against disease and enfeeblement in grandiose language filled with religious and mythological references. The Desert Fathers no doubt would have approved of his fervor; although his passion, unlike theirs, was dedicated to rehabilitating the human body and not solely to spiritual and ascetic ends. But similar to the monks, Bircher-Benner used Christian imagery to justify his prescription.

Bircher-Benner also extracted insights from other philosophies in his effort to understand his mission as a raw foods healer. Many centuries had passed and many new philosophies articulated since the desert "contests" of the early Christian monks. Bircher-Benner read widely of the literature of the intervening years and we can see it influencing his thought.

Purification through "Abstinence"

In Bircher-Benner's writing, we see a Christian-like crusade against death as well as an ascetic strain in avoiding physically harmful things.

Religious imagery saturates the mission statement of this self-described "new physician," who is in a fight against death and the devil. The ideal healer, he says, "increases in knowledge and skill, his insight and experience, in an unceasing fight against disease, death, and the devil."[178] Bircher-Benner employed the *topos* of the devil to represent threats to the health of the body. The devil and his effects—disease and death—needed to be defeated by the "new physician" similar to the Biblical theme of defeating these same foes. Isaiah 25:8, for instance, states, "[God] will swallow up death forever; and the Lord God will wipe away tears from all faces."

---

[178] Ibid. Ch. 1

In the figure of Bircher-Benner's "new physician" is a poetic echo of Christ. During his life, Jesus was said to have physically healed many people. He also defeated death and the devil by giving believers eternal life. Hebrews 2:14 states that "through death [Christ] might destroy him that had the power of death—that is, the devil." The new Christ-like physician was charged with the "rescue of mankind" in the words of Bircher-Benner. But, this new savior, unlike Jesus, "does not need to let himself be crucified," wrote Bircher-Benner, borrowing a quote from Nietzsche.[179]

It's unlikely that Bircher-Benner thought he could completely defeat "death" in the here and now, but his language makes clear that the ideal physician was engaged in an epic task to at least alleviate suffering and minimize disease. In an age in which momentous medical discoveries were being made, especially against bacterial and viral diseases, Bircher-Benner felt proud to be a part of the "never-ending efforts of the human spirit to understand life, health, the causes and meaning of disease and suffering," he wrote. A "guide to health, protector of life; this is what the new physician should be."[180] Like Christ, the new physician would heal and bring life where there was disease, death, and (dietary) sin.

Cleansing the patients' old habits was a main feature of Bircher-Benner's crusade against disease. The state of the body depended on austerity and discipline. Without purifying the patient of toxic foods and habits, there was little opportunity for one's health to flourish. Abstinence was the foundation of the raw foodism that Bircher-Benner preached. The body had to be purified of disease-fomenting toxins and cooked food before the earth's and God's highest quality nutrition—raw food—could nourish and invigorate the body.

"I lack words to describe the great benefits of abstinence," Bircher-Benner mused. Abstinence was the "first great step of medicine towards causative therapy" and disease prevention.[181] By first avoiding things that harm the body, we strike at the core causes of illness.

Bircher-Benner was first exposed to abstinence as a way of life when he came into contact with natural healers who abstained from alcohol. He would later write that this fight against alcohol was the first great step towards disease prevention. To have a chance of successfully fighting disease, alcohol abstinence taught him, one would have to stop ingesting toxic substances.

---

[179]   Ibid., Ch. 7
[180]   Ibid.
[181]   Ibid., Ch. 2

The apostles of purity, the "important physicians and priests" calling others to abstinence, were trailblazing this quasi-religious path toward bodily purification. Bircher-Benner and his dietary revolution would follow. Water would replace alcohol and raw food would replace the corrupted cooked foods of the dystopian so-called "civilized" era—an era disconnected from God and nature, in Bircher-Benner's mind, and one that the new physician messiah would have to remedy.

Abstinence from "Civilized" Lifestyles

Understanding Bircher-Benner's coming to raw foodism requires an understanding of his worldview, a worldview particularly associated with the nineteenth-century Western world—that industrialized societies had pathologically severed themselves from nature, causing devastating spiritual and physical consequences.

The early to mid-nineteenth century witnessed a renaissance in the literary world. There was a tidal wave of authors questioning the way that "civilized" society was constructed and the habits and institutions of industrializing Europe and America. In America, writers Ralph Waldo Emerson and Henry David Thoreau urged readers to get back in touch with the liberating effects of the natural world and break the civilizational chains that imprisoned them. Emerson's 1836 essay "Nature" established his literary career and outlined his mystical belief that nature was full of transcendental wisdom and that God pervaded the natural world. Bircher-Benner mentions Emerson as an ideological influence and tellingly, Bircher-Benner's hero Friedrich Nietzsche hailed Emerson as "the most gifted of the Americans."

Alongside commentators like Emerson, artists as well as writers like Herman Melville, in his Polynesian adventure stories, extolled the virtues of primitive societies and meditated on the pernicious aspects of Western civilization. Melville made readers question whether the West was really better off than societies that were considered "savage." Questions of health and quality of life entered the musing. Would you rather be a pristinely healthy, vibrant, athletic Polynesian with a glowing complexion, nearly naked and always outdoors, in a world without the technological advantages of nineteenth-century America—or a sickly white person entrapped in factory toil, heavy clothes, oppressive cultural mores, and suffocating coal smoke, albeit with access to the advantages of trains, steam engines, and other machines?

More Westerners were reconsidering their reflexive high regard for their own civilizations as well as how they were living, and their relationship (or lack thereof) to the natural world. Writers had triggered civilizational self-examination and self-criticism.

Bircher-Benner was born into the generation succeeding these thinkers and was influenced greatly by their worldview. He was convinced that modern Western man had been severed from a harmonious relationship with nature, resulting in widespread pathology, both physical and mental. Both lifestyle and diet had contributed to the ill health and "disordered life of civilized man." "Civilized mankind," he mocked gravely, is "a continuous increase in sickliness . . . discontent . . . and failed existences." Western Europe was a sickly industrial dystopia. The West had severed "the relationships of the human organism with the inanimate environment." Too much clothing and internal dwelling had caused "the theft of light that is committed against the human body." The first step to regaining health was to return to "air bathing and sun bathing" and to "return to natural order." After all, "sunlight is the medication" and the "artificial light" that man attempted to replace it with is a violation of the "laws of order" set down by nature.[182] Bircher-Benner's claims sound similar to Emerson, who wrote previously, "To the body and mind which have been cramped by noxious work or company, nature is medicinal and restores their tone."

"Add bad air to bad food," says Bircher-Benner, and you make way for "the downfall of the Western world." Bircher-Benner looked all around him and witnessed the physiological "disaster that civilization has caused" and the plunge in personal quality of life.[183] Westerners, in the late 1800s and early 1900s, had little chance of enjoying their unique technological advantages if they were ill and drug addicted.

Alongside the national misery that such unnatural lifestyles entailed, even international geopolitics suffered as a result of industrial living. Bad habits and bad food were connected with Western countries' irrational aggression toward their national neighbors and insatiable colonial exploitations overseas. Studies had shown, Bircher-Benner claimed, that rats who were deficient in calcium from bad diets became overly aggressive. "Bad air," bad lifestyles, and "bad food" had caused a "distance from God and therefore fear of life and an urge to destroy." The behavioral repercussions of man's severance from nature caused ripples throughout the entire world. A miserable worker in an industrial district of Zurich and a rapacious European soldier or merchant domineering foreigners in the Far East were both acting out the consequences of unnatural "civilized" living and degenerate food.

---

[182]   Bircher-Benner, Max. *The Physician of the Future.* Germany, Bircher-Benner, 2015, Ch. 4.
[183]   Ibid.

Severance from nature begat suffering for such people and that suffering spread outward to others whom they came into contact with. As Emerson wrote in the preceding generation, "As we degenerate, the contrast between us and our house [nature] is more evident. We are as much strangers in nature, as we are aliens from God."

"Cooked" Civilization

"Therefore, raw food is the healing food par excellence, and therefore it is used for every disease, no matter its name, as a first-class healing measure."
—**Bircher-Benner**

The sickliness of society proved that it was out of sync with the "laws of order" of nature as Bircher-Benner called them. The medical community didn't help much. It made no connection between food and the widespread ill health and drug addiction. But Bircher-Benner and a few others felt they were becoming aware of the *causes* of the maladies of civilization.

In "1895–1900, medicine knew very little about the relationships between food and disease," Bircher-Benner later wrote. But his years of medical observation and experimentation had taught him to make connections between health and nutrition. In his writings, he described the corrosive effects of the unnatural foods that the "civilized" world excelled at—cooked and processed foods.

Cooking, he wrote, was considered "progress" but it has "weakened and degenerated" "civilized man." The "devalued food" of civilization was a major cause of "physical and mental problems." In his denunciation of this food, Bircher-Benner referred to the physical changes that it undergoes when it's cooked and lamented the "excessive masses of [toxic] heat-changed proteins" that people consumed. This was most likely a reference to advanced glycation end products (AGEs), toxic sugar-altered proteins that can be generated by cooking, which were discovered in the early 1900s, before Max wrote his *Physician of the Future* book. Perhaps Bircher-Benner was aware of these toxic compounds. The new physician deduced that "the total of diseases [and] suffering is most predominant by far in civilized mankind" where people's diets consisted largely of "animal meat, white bread" and "lots of sugar." He also considered early animal studies which, he claimed, showed that primates developed chronic colitis after eating "heat-treated food."

Hundreds of positive experiences of enforcing raw food diets on patients had solidified Bircher-Benner's suspicions about cooked foods, meat, and processed foods. He found it ironic that cooking had long been considered a simple advancement yet was hindering human health and eroding life quality.

He was realizing that cooking had actually been a step backward, a corruption of the delicate characteristics and biological perfections of the ideal food of nature. At the least, cooking was clearly unnatural in the purest sense, as animals don't cook. Beyond that, he began to consider the sentiment that the natural world had near-divine wisdom and whether food should be left alone and consumed in its original unheated state. Did raw food contain properties that were not yet understood? Did it have a magic to it? Over the years, Bircher-Benner developed theories as to why raw food caused the healing transformations he was witnessing in his patients.

SEARCHING FOR CAUSATION IN THE FOOTSTEPS OF EMERSON AND NIETZSCHE

> *"This feeble human being has penetrated the vast masses*
> *of nature with an informing soul and recognized itself*
> *in their harmony, that is, seized their law."*
> **—Ralph Waldo Emerson**

When Bircher-Benner started his career, shortly after 1890, "there was no insight-relationship between diagnosis and therapy," in his words.[184] The Western science model, in his mind, offered hardly any pragmatic knowledge about the causes of degenerative disease. Progress had been made on certain viral and bacterial diseases but all the supposed scientific prowess of Western civilization could not yield any usable insight into the connection between diet, lifestyle, disease, and long term health.

The primary medical paradigm in Switzerland, in Bircher-Benner's mind, had an antiquated reductionist "anatomical" view of the body. Taught to be a physician in the context of this clueless school of thought, Bircher-Benner felt "insufficient" in his care for patients and the results of his conventional therapies were "getting more and more depressing. The "limited horizon of exact natural sciences" had, according to another physician that Max revered, "clouded our view of clinical reality.[185] The scientific community was only throwing medications at diseases, without addressing the root causes of those diseases.

---

[184]   Ibid., Ch. 3
[185]   Ibid.

Bircher-Benner was frustrated with medicine's refusal to "look these causes in the eye." "Tangible causes" must be found and physicians ought to base their therapies on these causes.[186]

The tired and impotent old system that left him feeling powerless as a doctor had to be left behind. Like his philosophical hero, Nietzsche, whom he called, "the great overcomer and far-seer," Bircher-Benner would overcome mainstream thought and create a new value system. Where nutrition had been utterly ignored before, "Insight into the field of nutrition" would be the source of power in healing patients.[187]

Bircher-Benner's philosophical influences, Emerson and Nietzsche, were on the same page with him regarding the limits of nineteenth-century science.

Emerson thought Western science was impotent to a certain extent: "Empirical science is apt to cloud the sight . . . to bereave the student of the manly contemplation of the whole."[188] The science of that day was losing sight of the forest through the trees. The reductionist "half sight of science," Emerson critiqued, caused people to lose valuable holistic insights by getting lost in less significant details. The "hundred concerted experiments" of short-sighted scientists were relatively inept, even compared to intuitive "untaught sallies" into the mysteries of nature. This was an ethic that Bircher-Benner absorbed. The "new physician's" mind would make these "sallies" into the schoolroom of nature and "finally perceive these connections" between health and the human's relationship with nature.[189]

Nature became Bircher-Benner's ultimate guide for achieving good health. He had seen patients, for instance, whose severe religion had led them to suppress their natural sex instinct, develop physical disorders. Those who did not "obey the laws of life" could face emaciation, stomach problems, insomnia, among other issues. By following the "order" of nature, these problems could be corrected. Raw foodism would fulfill nature for Bircher-Benner, not squash its instincts, as in the case of the Desert Fathers.

"The permanence of natural laws" are to be "sacredly respected," wrote Emerson. Respect them and find them, Bircher-Benner would. That way, the "life disorder" that he witnessed could be made a "well-ordered life."[190]

---

[186]   Ibid.

[187]   Ibid.

[188]   Emerson, Ralph Waldo. *Nature: Original*. Independently Published, 2023.

[189]   Bircher-Benner, Max. *The Physician of the Future*. Germany, Bircher-Benner, 2015, Ch. 4.

[190]   Ibid., Ch. 5.

Both Bircher-Benner and Emerson felt that reconnecting with the benevolent genius of nature was the way to heal mankind physically and psychically. Emerson urged people to be "embosomed for a season in nature, whose floods of life stream around and through us," and feed off "the powers they supply." Nature, in this scheme, is the source of highest knowledge. It was more capable of granting insights than anything else.

"In the woods, I feel that nothing can befall me in life—no disgrace, no calamity which nature cannot repair," Emerson proclaimed. Nature, he felt, was made for humans and could heal just about any of our woes. "All the parts" of nature "incessantly work" for the profit of man. If people would only get back in touch with nature, Emerson felt, they would see that "the endless circulations of the divine charity nourish man."

Bircher-Benner, of course, sought to access the "nourishing" power in nature that Emerson poeticized. It soon became clear that the most powerful way to absorb the Emersonian "profit" and "divine charity" from nature was to eat it.

Lifestyle changes provided part of nature's healing power—the sensory therapy of being in nature, looking at, smelling, or hearing "natural objects," getting exposure to sunlight, and exercising in the aromatic air. But consuming the perfection of natural law through raw foods was the most intimate way of imbibing its power. If there was "an occult relation between man and the vegetable," in Emerson's words, what better way to receive the occult rites than to ingest them in their original unadulterated state? Raw plant food was the most direct way to living out the "perfectness and harmony" of nature. "Nature stretcheth out her arms to embrace man," Emerson claimed, so receive that love and care, added Bircher-Benner, through the mouth.

RAW FOODS: CURING CIVILIZATION AND REUNITING THE MAN WITH NATURE

Bircher-Benner's experiences with raw food healing patients cemented his idea that only raw food could "regenerate" man from the disorders caused by civilization: "Why does raw food heal? What is the difference between raw and cooked food?" he asked himself. Raw plant foods seemed to have the ideal "quality." "Nutritional science had previously only evaluated the energy value of food *quantitatively*, i.e. by the amount of calories," Bircher-Benner explained.[191] Now thought

---

[191]   Bircher-Benner, Max. *The Physician of the Future*. Germany, Bircher-Benner, 2015, Ch. 4.

pioneers like him were becoming aware of what was more important than just the amount of calories in food—they started to consider how those calories were organized.

Bircher's theory of food quality involved the Creator of the universe. God oversaw the process of food quality control: "Our engineer . . . processes his material with a secure selection in quantity and quality." Raw plant foods, the foods designed by him, were the highest quality. God infused these foods with "wonderful forms" and "high-energy designs." They contained energetic patterns that nourished. They were full of perfectly "charged" compounds—God knew "every element and every compound" in them. Raw foods were even suffused with a moral meaning, intelligently designed, and "ordered . . . according to purpose and a plan."[192]

Sunlight was central to Bircher-Benner's theory of raw food since it was the source of plants' perfect energetic organization. He was confident that these edible energy patterns of raw food were "identical to that of sunlight" and that "we eat solar energy in the plants." The sun transferred its life energy—the "highest-organized energy present in the universe"—to us through raw food. Through sunlight energy, God made raw plant food "with comprehensive knowledge and skill," as it contains perfect "quantity and quality" of nutrients. The ideal combinations of macro and micronutrients were "planned" for human consumption. But most "civilized" people in the West sadly rejected this medicine of our Creator and ate pathologically altered foods that either have their fiber removed (like white bread) or contain toxic heat-induced "altered proteins."[193]

To reclaim bodily vitality, humans had to consume food that was energetically designed for their flourishing. What better medicine could there be than ingesting what God had designed with purpose and exact and ideal proportions of energetic "organization." By consuming the sun's life force, structured into plants, people could ingest nearly magical healing potentials. This food, because of the sunlight's electrical organization, could heal our cells and "strengthen the reduced electrical potential of the cells," often depleted from consumption of lifeless cooked food. "Light is the fuel of life," said Bircher-Benner, and was also transformed into the known micronutrients that our bodies use: "mineral compounds, vitamins, hormones, enzymes."[194]

---

[192]   Ibid.

[193]   Bircher-Benner, Max. *The Physician of the Future*. Germany, Bircher-Benner, 2015, Ch. 4.

[194]   Ibid.

The end result of this energetic and micronutrient transfer from plant to humans would be the body's army of fierce cells ready to perform with stamina and have the "highest power to fight" off illnesses.[195]

Within the energetic power of raw food, Bircher-Benner believed, was also its higher "redox potential" or ability to donate electrons. He could've been referring to the antioxidant capacities of plant food, an impressive awareness for his time.

Purity was another attribute of raw plant food. Bircher-Benner argued that it didn't contain the toxic substances found in cooked food. Uncooked food, it was argued, had the "lowest internal resistance" and caused the least strain on the body (an idea still adhered to by modern-day raw foodists). Raw food didn't zap the body of energy, stress it, or damage it. It was "protective and healing food."[196]

Bircher-Benner made clear that the medicinal effect of raw plant food, which "borders on the miraculous" was "entirely different" from even some cooked vegetarian foods. Just because a food wasn't an animal product, didn't mean it was healthy. Processed food had no place in Max's dietary program. Grains stripped of their fiber like table sugar, "white bread," and "pastry" were "disorganized, partially demineralized, and depleted in vitamins" and certainly not healthy.[197]

As for meat, the human body was not designed for it. Max claimed that by evidence of the body's dental characteristics and "construction of [its] digestive organs," it was designed for a more plant-based "fruit eating" diet. "All serious and unbiased researchers" agreed with this, he claimed.[198]

"Food energy" had "its highest value in plants." Meat was pathetically low-energy food because it "captures only negligible amounts of sunlight." Even carnivorous animals often reject the muscle meat that humans seemed to be so fond of eating. These animals first devour the blood, "then the intestines, then fat and bones." Swiss and Western eating habits, including the particulars of eating meat, were "downright unnatural" in every way.[199]

All these explanations of the efficacy of raw plant food helped Bircher-Benner justify why he'd seen such dramatic healings in his patients. At a later stage in his career, after forty years of success in professionally utilizing this diet, his confidence in the medical efficacy of raw food had been cemented, "with astonishing success on thou-

---

[195]   Ibid.
[196]   Ibid.
[197]   Ibid.
[198]   Ibid.
[199]   Ibid.

sands of patients."[200] Raw food, in his experience, was proven to be the most effective medicine on the planet.

Spiritually Reordering "Civilized" Minds

"Everything starts in the physiological."
—Bircher-Benner

Raw food could also heal the spiritual maladies of civilization, in addition to the physical. Eating God-designed food could cure this unhealthily "civilized" creature of his "distance from God" and "fear of life" mentioned previously.[201] Pathological spiritual states and behavioral failings could be remedied by an actual ethical value transfer—from plants into humans.

Bircher-Benner believed that whatever we eat, we are absorbing the food's personality and its spiritual quality— "every food introduces a piece of soul of the plant or animal . . . we receive not only chemical substances . . . but also mental values and lack of values," he said.[202]

In his mind, arguably, if you're eating processed grains, you're receiving the deranged values of "unnatural" foods created through greedy expediency. Whole grain is morphed into a white flour, so as to be more shelf-stable and give the consumer a quick hit of fiber-less sugar. By eating this abuse of nature we could adopt more harmful, expedient, and abusive traits. If you're eating meat, perhaps you could absorb the fear of the slaughtered animal. On the other hand, if you're eating lettuce, fruit, raw oats, or wild plants in their natural state, you're assimilating the Creator's benevolence and harmonious vitality. Materiality underlies spirituality—hence, Bircher-Benner's claim that "everything starts in the physiological."[203] We have the choice of eating "devalued" cooked food, meat, or refined starches or the value-filled raw items that nourish and elevate our souls.

In Bircher-Benner's claim about the transfer of the "soul" and "mental values" of the plants or animals we eat, we see an echo of Emerson's belief that every "object" in nature is imbued with moral meaning. "All things"—all natural objects—"with which we deal, preach to us," wrote Emerson. "All things are moral."

---

[200] Ibid.

[201] Ibid.

[202] Ibid., Ch. 6

[203] Ibid.

And most poetically relevant to Bircher-Benner's arguments, Emerson wrote, "moral sentiment . . . grows in the grain." "Every natural fact is a symbol of some spiritual fact," Emerson said, and "shall hint or thunder to man the laws of right and wrong." Through nature, Emerson and Bircher-Benner believed that God's spiritual qualities were administered to us. ". . . Throughout nature, spirit is present," Emerson said. The "Supreme Being puts it forth through us," and through the food we eat, would add Bircher-Benner.

Bircher-Benner also quoted his much beloved Nietzsche in describing the effect of diet upon mental life: "I believe," the philosopher said, "that the vegetarians with their requirement of eating less and more simply have done more good than all of our moral systems together."[204] The material and dietary basis of spirituality was not to be disputed.

The moral uplifting that a raw food eater experienced would also help in healing their body, Bircher-Benner felt. The "unconditional rest of the mind," fostered by raw foods, was an important part of physical healing. Along with consciously ridding the mind of toxic and frantic thoughts, people should fill their bellies on the harmonious vibrations of edible morality. Physical as well as mental healing would follow.

INDIVIDUALISM AND WILLPOWER

"[He was] a person of iron diligence, complete devotion, immense willpower, and a strange nose for the truth . . . obeying his own conscience unconditionally."
—Dr. Ralph Bircher on his father Max Bircher-Benner

To get to the point of actually having the courage to prescribe raw food to his patients, Bircher-Benner had to develop a sense of individualism and willpower in overcoming the pressures of society and the medical profession to submit to norms.

Bircher-Benner saw his vocation as a war-like struggle. His enemies were the obstacles of cultural tradition and medical orthodoxy. Swiss culture took great comfort in cooked food and alcohol. The raw doctor would be fighting quite the uphill battle in convincing a Swiss person to give up bread, noodles, veal and the like. "By long custom" and erroneous presumptions in his home country, "everything raw was

---

204   Bircher-Benner, Max. The Physician of the Future. Germany, Bircher-Benner, 2015, Ch. 8.

strictly forbidden because it was considered difficult to digest." How wrong were the Swiss and German cultures, thought Bircher-Benner.

Without a doubt, he faced aggressive criticism within the medical community because his dietary and lifestyle "causative therapy" differed starkly from the usual protocol of medicating symptoms with pharmaceutical drugs. He noted that his "efforts met terrible resistance": "Hell was unleashed against me," Bircher-Benner lamented, "even my colleagues turned on me."[205]

The opposition pained him but generated a heroic struggle. He envisioned apparitions from Greek mythology: "Legendary creatures of antiquity appeared before my eyes." Ancient Greek statues of the Trojan priest Laocoon writhing as he's attacked by serpents filled his head. "Mankind in its sequence of generations, surrounded by powers destroying life!"[206] Bircher-Benner was up against the powers of disease and disapproving doctors.

Against such challenges, he developed his spiritual powers. "Only divine powers are able to strengthen the man within the physician" so that he did not cower before the "serpents" he faced.[207]

Luckily he had developed an individualism that could've been considered one of those "divine powers." Early in adulthood, the experience of being mocked for rejecting alcohol, he said, "made me independent and strong in my character, in thought and in action." By steadily adhering to this frowned-upon abstinence, he learned that he had the power to overcome pressure. From this experience of sneers and laughter from those who thought he was no fun, he "learned to resist, to go against the masses." Only a man with a "strength of consciousness" could have the fortitude to be a raw food pioneer. The heroic healer, the new physician, "must have fought through a thicket of prejudice and bias," and Bircher-Benner proved that he was brave enough to do so.[208]

To see clearly, the new physician had to overcome the shortsightedness of civilization and the surrounding culture that "limits our independence" so that we no longer have independent thought. If too influenced by the norms around us, we become like everyone else, we become "mass men," Bircher-Benner bemoaned. It was imperative that a good physician "overcome" the "training" of civilization and the fear,

---

205   Ibid., Ch. 1.

206   Ibid.

207   Ibid.

208   Ibid.

Bircher-Benner noted, of "being different from all of my friends and acquaintances."[209]

Despite the pressure of the mob, the new physician "grows slowly with the understanding" and the confidence that he will change patient's lives dramatically. "The [new] physician needs much more comprehensive knowledge and skill" than previous medical authorities because he will fight against the tide of orthodoxy. He will not be able to "rely on any authority or professor" to defend him.[210]

When Swiss doctors declared, "Mr. Bircher has left the borders of science!," and mockingly labeled him the "raw food apostle," he had enough fortitude to continue on his lone path.[211] Bircher-Benner was also willing to suffer pay cuts in addition to a lack of respect. He detailed how a tax commissioner and merchant were shocked at how little he earned in attending to less well-off patients.

"Existing dietetics" and "self-important" critics had to be overcome if humanity was to make any physiological progress. Bircher-Bircher likened his novelty of thought and professional isolation to those of other trailblazing explorers of the past. "All of these healing attempts with a raw-vegetable diet were Columbus voyages on new paths."[212] Emerson would have been proud of Bircher-Benner's individualistic gumption and it's no wonder, once again, that the two were of a similar mind. Emerson's *Self Reliance* essay echoes Bircher-Benner's individualistic proclamations and reads like a guiding map for the new physician's career and struggles. "Trust thyself . . . great men have always done so," Emerson proclaimed. "Whoso would be a man," Emerson urged, and a "new physician" (one might add), "must be a nonconformist."[213]

Emerson's words truly sound like a roadmap for Bircher-Benner's overcoming of the professional critics that surrounded him. "A man is to carry himself," he said, "in the presence of all opposition." It was natural for unorthodox paradigm-changers to be spat upon by the conformist physicians of reflexive tradition—"For non-conformity, the world whips you with its displeasure," Emerson warned.[214]

If the new physician would stay steady on his path and not waver under pressure, he would inaugurate a new era of meaningful medical

---

209   Ibid.
210   Ibid.
211   Ibid.
212   Ibid., Ch. 3
213   Emerson, Ralph Waldo. "Self-Reliance." *Essays: First Series*, Project Gutenberg, 8 Feb. 2006, www.gutenberg.org/files/16643/16643-h/16643-h.htm#SELF-RELIANCE. Accessed 27 Apr. 2025.
214   Ibid.

progress. There could be, as Emerson describes in his ode to *Nature* a fresh "philosophy of insight and not of tradition."[215] Raw food, Bircher-Benner felt, was insight and what Nietzsche's Zarathustra called the "stream of life" and in proving so, he had overcome stale tradition and what Nietzsche's sister called "the whole horror of that loneliness to which, perhaps, all greatness is condemned."[216]

Passing

The courageous Bircher-Benner, in his "Columbus voyage," of raw food experimentation, allegedly helped heal hundreds of sick patients.

In 1939, on the eve of the Second World War, Bircher-Benner died in Zurich, aged seventy-one. It's said that he had a congenital heart defect, probably caused by his premature birth after his mother was affrighted by a fire in her neighborhood.[217]

After his death, Bircher-Benner's "muesli" concept of a cereal consisting of raw oats, dried apple, and nuts has become a symbol for healthy eating and has been adopted by naturistic movements and innumerable health food stores as a dietary staple.

Bircher-Benner started his career with a sense of powerlessness. He was a physician who felt helpless in healing his patients. But a fortuitous meeting with a natural healer had led him to witness the transformative power of raw food on hundreds of sick. Raw food had given him power as a physician and a confident sense of purpose.

---

[215] Ralph Waldo Emerson. *Nature*. 1841. Woodland Hills, Cailf., Regatta Press, 2010.

[216] Nietzsche, Friedrich . *Thus Spoke Zarathustra*. Evergreen Books, 2017.

[217] Meyer-Renschhausen, Elisabeth, and Albert Wirz. "Dietetics, Health Reform and Social Order: Vegetarianism as a Moral Physiology. The Example of Maximilian Bircher-Benner (1867–1939)." *Medical History*, vol. 43, no. 3, July 1999, 323–41, doi:10.1017/S0025727300065388.

6.
Arnold Ehret

Arnold Ehret was another explorative Germanic nutritionist. He was born just one year before Bircher-Benner, in 1866. These two men helped set the ideological stage for modern raw foodism. And although Ehret died in 1922, his theories about detoxification influenced a multitude of twentieth- and twenty-first-century raw foodists ever since.

Ehret had an insatiably curious mind and believed the maxim that "ignorance is the only tragedy of existence."[218] This attitude was reflected in his radical nutritional experiments on his body to prove the dietary assumptions of society wrong. He set world records for lengthy water fasts. His conclusions led him to preach the importance of not only fasting but raw food and fruitarianism.

Alternative ways of eating first caught Ehret's attention around the time that he turned thirty, when he "collapsed under the burden" of work and "chronic kidney inflammation."[219] To solve his ills, he tried out "naturopathy and vegetarianism."

After adopting a raw fruitarian diet, Ehret's "sense of health increased to unimaginable levels," he claimed.[220] He put his stamina to the test by performing weeks-long walking treks and bicycle rides. He noticed that whenever he ate cooked food, "so-called 'good food,'" he felt slovenly and a disturbing discomfort. After these experiences, he was hooked on a mostly raw regimen.

---

[218]   Ehret, Arnold. *Arnold Ehret Works (3 Books in 1): Mucusless Diet Healing System & Rational Fasting & 49 Day Fasting Experiment* . Independently Published, Oct. 2023.

[219]   Ibid., 11.

[220]   Ibid., 13.

Ugly Bodies and Decrepit Civilization

People in the highly industrialized Germany of the late 1800s were neither healthy nor beautiful according to Arnold Ehret.[221] All over, he observed the "white color of corpses and sunless culture men." Their pallid color signified malnutrition and the "white corpse color of dead-cooked, false food material" that they fed on. White bread, meat, and other colorless food were staples for these people of "culture," and made them appear like pale vampires, drained of any vitality and pigment in their appearance. This was the price they paid for not eating enough fruits and veggies.

The human figure had become "deformed" by unnatural lifestyles and even the sense of beauty of the average German had been "dulled." Fat, wrinkled, and pale bodies suffered from lack of sunlight, colorful food, and "poor circulation."[222] Bald and gray heads, "robbed of the glorious . . . hair ornament" were like "living skulls," signifying the "alarming deformation of man."[223]

Health and beauty had been destroyed by the "adverse effects of culture," especially cooked food.[224] "Indians" of the Americas and "negros" had much less gray hair and wrinkles, even in advanced age than his fellow countrymen, he noted.[225] The "ideal beauty and health of man, living completely under natural conditions" had been lost to civilization.[226] The fallen, decrepit modern man could "hardly imagine with what beauty and with what abilities the paradisiacal 'godlike' man" of the distant past was endowed.[227]

Little did these Germans know that, if they were raised from childhood forward with "living sun food," i.e. raw fruit, they would be able to reclaim their health.[228] Fruit could retrieve the "red colored" vibrancy of the flesh that healthy humans were supposed to have—the "sensual emblem of life" – and counteract the "slow decline of the universe" that occurred ever since humans forsook their ideal plant-based Edenic diet.[229]

---

221   Ibid., 58.
222   Ibid., 59.
223   Ehret, 60.
224   Ibid., 65.
225   Ibid., 65.
226   Ibid., 61.
227   Ibid., 69.
228   Ibid., 71.
229   Ibid., 72.

As we saw with Bircher-Benner, the medicine of the time didn't have answers to this perceived aesthetic and health crisis. But Ehret believed he did. "With the influence of my dietetics," he proclaimed, "I can guarantee that the most severe hair loss will be stopped."[230] His claims were extremely ambitious. "If someone would live from youth without mucus"—his word for toxicity that occurred from low-quality cooked foods—"even only from fruit, it would be just as sure that he could neither age nor become ill."[231]

Utopian Health and Unimaginable Pleasures

"When man deviated from the only correct food with the Fall, the whole misery of his existence began; this is written exactly in the Bible."
—Arnold Ehret

Ehret's rendering of human history is a key to understanding his dietary beliefs. Like numerous raw foodists throughout our story, he believed in the Biblical storyline of human history. All was well and without suffering until people left behind the blueprint of the garden of Eden.

And, of course, dietary habits were central to Adam and Eve's utopian existence. Life was perfect in the "fruit orchard," as Ehret described it. This belief, along with his personal experiment, cemented his belief that the "natural" "paradise" diet of humans was only fruit and leafy greens – "the divine clean food of the Genesis," as he said.[232] Utilizing his hopeful outlook, Ehret believed that his contemporaries could reclaim the Edenic paradise if they adopted the diet that was adhered to in such a garden.

Ehret believed that unnatural eating was responsible not only for "deformed" bodies but also acted as the "root cause of all evil in the world."[233] Ehret referred to this diet-focused thesis as "the whole epitome of all knowledge," which was "the solution of all questions" as well as to how humans could be physically and spiritually "raised to paradisiacal perfection" again. He had cracked the code of the universe, he believed, and could solve humanity's problems with only fruit and vegetables.

---

[230] Ibid., 68.
[231] Ibid., 69.
[232] Ibid., 9.
[233] Ibid.

"All sickness," Ehret proclaims, all "pain sorrow and suffering, all passions, alcoholism . . . all 'evil,' the whole social struggle . . . slavery, aging, and perhaps even death itself, all . . . moral heresies, but especially pessimism, in short, all degeneracy, comes, except in a few circumstances, from wrong, unnatural food and from overeating."[234] No wonder Ehret felt strongly about nutrition—the fate of the world hinged on it

All of modern humans' bad nutritional habits, including cooking, refining, and overeating, seemed to stem from the mindset of a deep "distrust" toward nature and "life" and from the attitude that a "cook" can create foods "more perfect than an apple or banana."[235] To regain physical and spiritual health, Ehret made clear, humans must obtain "confidence in nature and in life."[236]

Ehret's History of World Degeneracy

Everything degenerated when fruit began to be shunned in favor of fire-cooked food. Ehret's conception of the fall of humanity echoes the Biblical narrative but is explicitly nutritional. Clothing had to be invented to cover up the shame of marred bodily beauty, damaged by the invention of cooked food.[237] The "regular meals" of "dead-cooked material" also sunk the "cultured man" into spiritual misery.[238] "Everything cooked," warned Ehret, is "almost worthless" and ironically people can, in a sense, "starve to death by eating all day long" because of this bankrupt nutrition.[239]

Every modern human invention was tainted by the cooked smut of civilization. Even the thoughts of society were toxic. Philosophy and science created by sick bodies and minds could be regarded as "pathological" and ignorant. Their answers to the most critical questions of life were "answered with as many yeses as nos."[240] The supposed rationality of civilized humanity is corrupted to its core. The beliefs of cooked-food civilization should be questioned since they arise out of toxified brains. If "decomposed cellular or food material or [other poisons] circulate in the blood and in the brain" of even the

---

234   Ibid., 10.
235   Ibid.
236   Ibid., 11.
237   Ibid., 22.
238   Ibid., 17.
239   Ibid., 19.
240   Ibid., 21.

most talented Western scientists and philosophers, can the integrity of their thoughts really be trusted?[241] Without pristine physiology, enlightened thought is not possible. "Thinking is pathological in itself as long as (man is not completely healthy!)," he warned.

Ehret agreed with famed philosopher Jean-Jacques Rousseau that humans needed to return to an uncorrupted natural state. "Give me a group of mentally and physically degenerated people. I want to make them healthy in the forest, to speak with Rousseau, by fasting and fruit diet."[242] Ehret, though, notes that spiritual ills and the end of "equality and fraternity" came not because of the invention of private property like Rousseau claimed, but from "inequality of nutrition."[243]

"The pure natural diet," which Ehret sometimes refers to as a "strict fruit diet," consisting only of uncooked fruits, could be the saving grace of humanity, as a heavily cooked diet is the culprit of nearly every societal problem.[244] That's why mere vegetarianism, which Ehret initially tested on himself, was not sufficient to heal the body. Common cooked-food vegetarians had the "exact resemblance of the Munich beer bellies" of meat eaters, and even meat caused less "mucus" production than "strong-flour-containing" cooked vegetarian foods.[245] Rawness was the solution. If only humanity would embrace the foods of the Garden of Eden, could the world reclaim "health, beauty and unimagined power, without pain and suffering, exactly as it was written in the Bible."[246] This was Ehret's "paradisiacal" vision.

But modern humans appeared to be the only creatures stupid enough to reject the "plentiful sun kitchen" of foods that were designed for us.[247] Apparently, humans felt that the foods of God's garden were not good enough for them. Did we really need to refine and cook things and eat animal flesh when plants, raw and unprocessed, could bountifully supply all our needs? "The vegetables, the salads themselves, the marvelous fruits and berries . . . are worth covering a god's table," Ehret wrote.[248] But humans were no gods and exchanged the "living energy cells" of fruit for the "killed food" of fallen civilization.

---

[241]   Ibid.

[242]   Ibid., 22.

[243]   Ibid., 23.

[244]   Ibid., 31.

[245]   Ibid., 41,44.

[246]   Ibid., 40.

[247]   Ibid., 53.

[248]   Ibid., 52.

Even just bananas and coconuts, he claimed, were scientifically proven to contain all the sustenance that a human needs.[249]

But as long as people remained in this self-imposed cooked hell, they stay spiritually degenerate. Since behavior is shaped by what we eat and the "nature" of the blood that nourishes our brain is critical for proper cognition, pathological cravings develop out of the deranged consumption of cooked malnutrition.[250] "Spiritual evils" arise.[251] "Meat produces" a general and ominous "demon thirst" for vices of all sorts; it gives birth to prostitution and alcoholism.[252] A vague "hunger for love" permeates the soul.[253] A vicious cycle is born. More and more must be cooked, fried, and baked to fill the love-shaped hole and give the eater a quick pleasure hit. That is how cooked food addiction reinforces the cycle of human fallenness.[254]

But the choice to exit this vicious cycle is ours. If one sticks to Ehret's "paradisiacal diet"—"fruits and greenleaf vegetables and their perfectness as human food," he or she will be brought "higher and higher, into physical and mental conditions never before experienced."[255] Only a "modern representative of asceticism," as Ehret described himself, could lead humans to a complete healing. The spirit of his spiritual raw foodist ancestors, the Hindu rishis and the desert monks, was alive in him. "Were not the greatest of mankind, the prophets, ascetics?"[256] Ehret believed that he, the prophet of the age, had arrived.

CLEANSING THE BAD

"I dare say there may not be another man in history who has studied, investigated, tested and experimented on fasting as much as I did."
—Arnold Ehret

Some of Ehret's fasts lasted over forty days. By them, he attempted to show the new nutritional ideal. The seer, emptied of the burden of civilized food, envisioned paradise on earth in which everyone would

---

[249] Ibid., 53.

[250] Ibid., 10.

[251] Ibid., 20.

[252] Ibid., 42.

[253] Ibid., 24.

[254] Ibid.

[255] Ibid., 198.

[256] Ibid., 43.

be physically beautiful and have a "perpetual" lifespan.[257] "If we do not break the machine with much food, we could live much more healthy lives and build heavenly civilizations."[258]

Ascetic fasting was key to Ehret's protocol. Cleansing the sins of civilization was an important foundation for successfully adhering to an Edenic raw diet. When Ehret first experimented with a fruit diet in northern Africa, he noticed that his healing progress was slowed because he ate too much and didn't fast.

He practiced what he preached. Ehret set a world record with a harrowing forty-nine-day water fast.[259] He did it in public view and under the supervision of government officials—being watched by passersby all day and night.[260] "I have degraded myself," he wrote of his sacrificial experiment, "by letting myself be locked up in a glass cell . . . and let the public gawk at me."[261] Citizens of Cologne watched him when he was reading, sleeping, and resting. "I was not able to sleep quietly for half an hour during the entire forty-nine days" because of constant interruptions from the public.[262] But Ehret was set on proving that he could survive and even thrive without food for long periods.

In one year, he boasted that he fasted for a total of 105 days out of the 365. And his experiment of food abstinence, he believed, not only didn't harm his health, it actually improved it.[263] Alongside a raw diet, fasting had far-reaching benefits for society, Ehret believed. "If combined with the pure natural diet," fasting will be "the only infallible way in which all evils could be eliminated from the world!"[264]

He saw himself as leading the charge. Comparing himself to revered religious figures, Ehret claimed that many Catholic saints had existed for years on nothing but water and that there is "tremendous proof that vitality does not depend primarily on food, but rather from an unobstructed circulation."[265] As evidence, Ehret walked for fifty-six hours continually after a ten-day fast.[266] People certainly did not need bread, meat, nor other cooked food to be strong, he felt he had shown.

---

[257]   Ibid., 47.

[258]   Ibid.

[259]   Ibid., 7.

[260]   Ibid., 5.

[261]   Ibid., 5.

[262]   Ibid., 8.

[263]   Ibid., 9.

[264]   Ibid., 10.

[265]   Ibid., 179.

[266]   Ibid.

The "Mucusless Diet Healing System"

"Only nature heals, cleanses, decongests."
—Arnold Ehret

Ehret is still controversial for his opposition to the "germ theory" of disease. This fruitarian argued that pathogens like bacteria or viruses were not responsible for some illnesses.[267]

In place of pathogens, Ehret believed that "mucus" was the "common and main cause of all diseases."[268] Although Ehret did hedge his claim by saying that "mucus" was not "always" the cause of all diseases but it is always present in every case. All disease, he felt, was ultimately characterized by the "clogging of the smallest blood vessels" with mucus.[269]

Although he claimed to see mucus in the urine and feces of unhealthy people, Ehret often used the term in a vague way to denote toxicity—especially the toxicity that he believed resulted from eating cooked food. Such food often became, in the intestines, a "gelatinous mucilage" substance that gradually made the digestive system sticky and "slimy" with the "glue" of cooked refined grains and meat. This then set the stage for pathogens to thrive.[270] Mucus is the vague, almost metaphorical residue or "waste" of "wrong food of civilization" that clogs capillaries and bowels. "Every disease," claimed Ehret, is "constitutional constipation," caused by the "sticky" things left behind from cooked starches and protein.[271]

One's level of vitality depended upon the lack of "obstruction" in the body (some later raw foodists would also use this term). This "obstruction" was responsible for nearly all physical problems, in addition to the spiritual.

Cooked, mucus-producing food triggered the "overgrowth of white blood cells" that signify bodily inflammation and this overgrowth often causes death, Ehret believed. "Mucus coming from the cultured food" caused "the symptoms of old age: hair loss, wrinkles."[272]

Fructose, on the other hand, the main sugar in fruit, is the "highest form of fuel" and left only traces of plant fiber behind which would be

---

267 Ibid.,.33.
268 Ibid., 34.
269 Ibid., 37.
270 Ibid., 35.
271 Ibid., 99.
272 Ibid., 46.

"immediately excreted."[273] This fruit sugar leaves no stickiness behind, Ehret claimed.[274] Once he started eating fruit and gave up bread, milk, and cheese, he no longer needed a handkerchief to blow or wipe his nose.[275]

Cooked food produced such toxic buildup in the body, he thought, that his fruitarian cure must be done with great caution if danger was to be avoided. A new raw foodist could detoxify too rapidly and face a "cellular collapse."[276]

The mucusless diet that Ehret promoted, consisted of the "ideal food": "raw fruits and, if desired, raw green-leaf vegetables." But since switching to such a perfect diet quickly could be risky, he allowed some cooked, steamed, or baked fruits, vegetables, and grains on a transitional diet that eased people off the food of "culture."[277] Such was the supposed difference between a cooked and raw diet. If one had a very toxic body, intense sickness or even death could result from fasting or an immediate switch to a raw food diet.[278] Partial allowance of cooked food was for the "slowing down of the elimination" of the "too aggressive" detoxification symptoms.[279] Fasters can die "suffocated in and with their own waste," he warned.[280]

By allowing cooked food during the transition period, Ehret tried to separate himself from the shortsighted "propaganda of the Raw Food Movement." In seeking to differentiate himself from dogma, he claimed that his mucusless diet was "clinical," not some ideology based purely on faith.

Nevertheless, Ehret was fervently dedicated to his utopian portrait of the raw diet and made extremely optimistic claims concerning societal change and longevity that hardly anyone in his time or after would've considered soberly "clinical."

An Untimely Death

Ehret certainly did not fulfill the "perpetual" lifespan that he believed possible on a paradise diet. In the 1910s, just before the outbreak of

---

273   Ibid., 35.
274   Ibid., 35.
275   Ibid., 38.
276   Ibid., 44.
277   Ibid., 159.
278   Ibid., 109.
279   Ibid., 166.
280   Ibid., 181.

World War I, he had moved to California—which would later become a major hub of raw foodism in the late 1900s and early 2000s.

Sunny California, with its abundant fruit, was much more amenable to Ehret's lifestyle than grey Germany. In this American state, he was likely to find more cutting-edge thinking and higher quality foods. It was the "new world" after all and a gathering place for alternative health practitioners. Ehret became a popular consultant, public speaker, and writer in his new home.

But on October 10, 1922, in Los Angeles, two days after one of Ehret's most successful and highly attended public speeches, he was found unconscious on the pavement at the age of fifty-six.

The most commonly accepted explanation for his death is that it was an accident—he slipped on the wet and oily pavement, fell back, and hit his head. Some said he wasn't used to his new shoes, some guessed that perhaps his routine fasting had left him lightheaded and dizzy (from lack of macronutrients, vitamins, or electrolytes), and others put forth darker theories, intuiting that representatives from the meat, dairy, and medical industries that his raw food program threatened played a role in his sudden death.[281]

What's certain is that Ehret's detoxification theories have inspired alternative health thinking for subsequent generations. And future raw foodists were to keep alive his optimism, in thinking that they could heal the world.

Next chapter, we continue our theme of turn-of-the century German-speaking raw food advocates, but with a darker turn—the notorious genocidal Führer of Nazi Germany.

---

[281] "Arnold Ehret. *Bionity.com*, 2025, www.bionity.com/en/encyclopedia/Arnold_Ehret.html. Accessed 19 Mar. 2025.

7.
Hitler: Rebuilding the German Race with Raw Food

"It's probable that, in the old days, human beings lived longer than they do now. The turning-point came when man replaced the raw elements in his diet with foods that he sterilizes when he eats them."
—Adolf Hitler

In the 1920s, Germans were recovering from the hellish experiences of World War I. They were also dealing with hyperinflation and widespread drug use. Culturally conservative Germans were alarmed at Berlin becoming a chemically "experimental capital" where morphine, heroin, and cocaine were widely used and were relatively socially accepted. Berliners were heavily medicating the pain that reverberated from the tumultuous events of the preceding years. The war was lost, as was nearly everything of national importance and so any type of self-medication seemed permitted.[282]

During this era of cultural lassitude and intoxication, Nazi Party members lamented the drug abuse and "moral decay" of Germany. They wanted to clean up the nation's act, remove any "un-German" chemical poison from the streets, and purify the population to fit their imagined view of the Aryan race.[283] And when the Nazis cemented their national power in the early 1930s, forming a coalition with traditionalist conservatives, they would institute an aggressive war on drugs. Their program would also expand to a national health project. The new ruling party wanted Germans to become the master race. They wanted Germans to prove they were an abnormally vigorous,

---

[282]   Ohler, Norman, and Shaun Whiteside, *Blitzed : Drugs in the Third Reich*. Boston, Houghton Mifflin Harcourt, 2017, 18.
[283]   Ibid.

intelligent, healthy, and beautiful ethnic group, while pushing away—annihilating—those they believed to be inferior.

RECLAIMING THE GERMAN BODY

The new Nazi regime was on a mission to reclaim the physiological excellence of the German race, which had embarrassingly lapsed, in their view, after the First World War. In order to justify its racial propaganda and physically rehabilitate the nation, the party demanded that Germany be cleansed of poisonous foreign influences, both chemical and cultural. After that, Germans had to be replenished and rebuilt with quality nutrition. Only then could German minds and bodies regain their innately superior strength.

CLEANSING OUT THE "POISON"

In this physiological war, drugs were connected to culturally and biologically dangerous "subhuman" racial elements in German society. As authorities made the claims that Jews, Romanis, Slavs, and the disabled were no longer welcome in the society they were building, they also disallowed the toxic drugs that the Nazis accused Jews of promoting.

Historians Norman Ohler and Shaun Whiteside point to an "intersection between anti-Semitic propaganda and anti-drug policy."[284] Many in the Nazi apparatus, from experts in medical journals to authors of children's books attacked the presence of the Jewish "infection" and "poison" that they alleged plagued the country.[285] In addition to being hated, Jews were blamed for rampant drug proliferation. This was another excuse to try to oust Jewish Germans from the country. The Nazi Central Office for Combating Drug Transgressions charged Jews with playing "a supreme part" in the drug trade, while the Office of Racial Policy claimed that Jews were innately prone to drug-addiction and often sought cocaine or morphine to calm their "excited nerves."

Nazi propaganda also accused Jews of poisoning the German mind and habits with a sociological theory that the body and its rights

---

[284]   Ibid.

[285]   Ibid.

belonged to an individual instead of the German people.[286] The Jews, the Nazis claimed, taught Germans that they could do what they liked, follow pernicious desires, and ingest whatever drugs they felt because an individual's body belonged to him or her alone. Conversely, a German book argued that this individualism was "Irreconcilable with the Teutonic German idea that we are the bearers of the eternal legacy of our ancestors, and that accordingly our body belongs to the clan."[287] Put simply, "You are nothing, your people are everything," the Nazi propaganda reiterated.[288] "There will be no license, no free space, in which the individual belongs to himself," Hitler is supposed to have said.[289] With the Nazi rise to power, bodily autonomy was over, and Germans were to put their bodies in service of the regime's national ideal.

Under the Nazis' hygienic regimen, there would be no more aimless pleasure-seeking nihilism. "National Socialism is the determination to create a new man," Hitler decreed. He argued that the repair of the post-World War I mentality as well as social and economic problems would occur simultaneously with the physical cleanup of each citizen. All Germans would be required to dedicate themselves to the common effort. "The time of happiness as a private matter is over," and the "concept of personal liberties of the individual . . . had to disappear," the Nazis declared. Every German was "organically connected" to the exclusive national community."[290]

By 1933, there were aggressive anti-drug laws in place. Drug consumption that *wasn't* authorized by the state (as forms of meth *would* be, for instance), was severely penalized, and Germans were ordered to turn in family members and acquaintances who consumed forbidden drugs.[291] The state usurped all authority in deciding who could use what. Nazi officials would be free to experiment on or torture with any substance they wished but the private citizen had no such choices. The Reich Health Office inserted itself into the health choices of the citizenry and warned of the "damage that could be inflicted by alcohol and tobacco," and Hitler was no less physiologically focused. He

---

[286]   Ibid., 19

[287]   Ibid.

[288]   Johann Chapoutot. "The Nazis and Nature: Protectors or Predators?" *Vingtième Siècle. Revue D'histoire*, vol. 113, no. 1, 2024, 29–39, shs.cairn.info/journal-vingtieme-siecle-revue-d-histoire-2012-1-page-29?lang=en.

[289]   Hicks, S. R. C. (2006). Nietzsche and the Nazis. Rockford, IL: Ockham's Razor Publishing, 111.

[290]   Ibid.,107

[291]   Ohler, Norman, and Shaun Whiteside, *Blitzed : Drugs in the Third Reich*. Boston, Houghton Mifflin Harcourt, 2017, 15-16.

mused that the "premature hardening of veins and arteries" could be among the dangers of smoking.[292]

A new era of intense bodily-focused hygiene had begun. The Führer often mused about what habits Germans should be practicing. "Certain hygienic practices are good for a man—fasting, for example," he declared in one mealtime conversation with other officials.[293] Certain types of food were also ideal, the government proclaimed.

NUTRITIONALLY REBUILDING GERMANS

The government project for national "racial hygiene" and bodily health moved onto nutrition.[294] Public health campaigns were unleashed. Healthy eating and anti-drug educational programs, occupational health regulations, bans on carcinogens in water and food, and restrictions on asbestos and smoking were aimed at protecting German bodies and rebuilding them anew.[295] The Nazi administration started fixating on anti-cancer research, initiating a quest to defeat the disease. The Ministry of Agriculture and Nutrition urged Germans to adopt more plant-based and whole-food diets and reduce alcohol and tobacco consumption.[296]

Institutional concern with nutrition had military bureaucrats pondering whether troops would perform better when given brown or white bread. Cutting-edge systematic drug experiments were tested on those troops.[297] Institutes like the Research Institute of Defense *Physiology* were created, where Hitler was willing to be administered experimental intestinal flora transplants, receive chamomile enemas, and get daily injections of vitamins, herbs, and hormones.[298]

A publication from the German Ministry of Agriculture and Nutrition attributed bad nutrition habits for rising rates of cancer, rheumatism, and other diseases.[299] The plant-centered diet that the Nazis urged the public to adopt was seen as crucial to the productivity and well-being of the populace (at least, those who weren't target-

---

[292]   Ibid., 17; Linge, Heinz. *With Hitler to the End.* Simon and Schuster, 1 Sept. 2009.

[293]   Hitler, Adolf, et al. *Hitler's Table Talk, 1941-1944 : His Private Conversations.* New York, Enigma Books, 2008. 85.

[294]   Aboul-Enein, B. H. (2013). Preventive Nutrition in Nazi Germany: A Public Health Commentary. *Journal of Health Ethics, 9*(1). http://dx.doi.org/10.18785/ojhe.0901.10

[295]   Ibid.

[296]   Ibid.

[297]   Ohler, Norman, and Shaun Whiteside, *Blitzed : Drugs in the Third Reich.* Boston, Houghton Mifflin Harcourt, 2017, 47.

[298]   Ibid., 115.

[299]   Aboul-Enein, B. H. (2013).

ed for murder). So-called Aryans would return to eating "as in old-en times"—mostly veggies, fruits, legumes, and whole grains.[300] And cutting-edge research and regulation regarding environmental health and disease-lifestyle links would also aid Germans to achieve the new health ideal.[301]

The Exemplar of the Reclaimed German Body

Against this backdrop of the war on "seductive poisonings," the quest to halt hedonistic cultural decay, and the attempted nutritional reha-bilitation of the German people, the Nazis sought to promote an ex-emplar for every German to follow. Authorities wanted to broadcast the image of an ideal, pure, disciplined, and healthy person. And they created this image in the person of the Führer himself.

By the early 1930s, Hitler was portrayed by political allies as aus-tere, unsullied, untempted by worldly pleasures, and a "model for an entirely healthy existence." Legend claimed that after WWI, in a righ-teous act of self-care, the Führer threw his last pack of cigarettes into the Danube. It was said that "he mortifies [his] body in a way that would shock people like us! He doesn't drink, he practically only eats vegetables."[302] These narratives of purity and self-control were spread in German mass media to rally the populace to imitate its leader.

The authoritarian Führer was portrayed as competent and as un-sullied as possible. He was immune to Jewish and "foreign" health-de-stroying temptations while staying totally dedicated to the success of his country and cleaning up Germany's social and economic problems. He was tirelessly productive and biologically pure.

As far as his personal habits were concerned, there was some truth to these projected images of Hitler. He was mostly a vegetarian, al-though his doctor gave him medicine made with animal parts.[303] He ranted against smoking, "poison," and the importance of health during his private mealtime conversations. He helped personally fund studies on the effects of smoking.[304] He had an intense interest in his personal health and performance. His daily vitamin injections were so import-

---

300 Ibid.

301 Ibid.

302 Ohler, Norman, and Shaun Whiteside, *Blitzed : Drugs in the Third Reich*. Boston, Hough-ton Mifflin Harcourt, 2017, 14.

303 Ibid.

304 Smith, George Davey. "Lifestyle, Health, and Health Promotion in Nazi Germany." *BMJ*, vol. 329, no. 7480, 16 Dec. 2004, 1424–1425, https://doi.org/10.1136/mj.329.7480.1424. Accessed 4 Apr. 2020.

ant to him and his personal physician that wobbly government train rides had to be halted so that he could receive the needles on stable footing.[305] He was not too keen on drinking, and only gave into the habit, having an after-dinner drink, later in WWII, when his stresses seemed unbearable.

As we'll see, his austere reputation proved no longer relevant as his drug addictions mounted during the war. Nevertheless, the image of the Nazi dictator as a venerated ascetic was used to inspire people to follow the government's physiological plans. And despite the Führer's later drug addictions, he always maintained his interest in the therapeutic effects of diet—even raw food.

RAW FOOD AND THE LAWS OF NATURE

> *"We shall learn to become familiar with the laws by which life is governed, and acquaintance with the laws of nature will guide us on the path of progress."*
> —**Adolf Hitler** [306]

> *"As in everything, nature is the best instructor."*
> —**Adolf Hitler**[307]

Hitler's insistence on raw food was unmistakably tied to his practically religious devotion to what he considered to be the "laws of nature." His casual conversations, recorded by secretaries during meals, are filled with instances of his reverence for this supposed law, which he believed should've been a guidepost for Germany in seizing power.

To seize power, Hitler claimed, one must accept "the principle that nature herself gives all the necessary indications, and that therefore one must follow the rules that she has laid down."

It was a high compliment for Hitler to describe someone as "deeply immersed in the realities of nature."[308] It signified a person's wisdom, acute awareness, and adherence to the necessary facts of life. "Salvation," in his mind, "consists in the effort that each person makes to understand Providence and accept the laws of nature." He perceived

---

[305]   Ohler, Norman, and Shaun Whiteside, *Blitzed : Drugs in the Third Reich.* Boston, Houghton Mifflin Harcourt, 2017, 115.

[306]   Hitler, Adolf, et al. *Hitler's Table Talk, 1941-1944 : His Private Conversations.* New York, Enigma Books, 2008, 5.

[307]   Hitler, Adolf, 396.

[308]   Ibid., 295.

nature, similarly to some raw foodists throughout time, to be like a god, deserving of homage.

The "natural order" or similar phrases were invoked to praise people who succeeded in the Führer's eyes. Nazi discourse was filled with appeals to the authority of nature and the dire consequences of not conforming to its dictates. "What we need are men gifted with a sixth sense, who live in nature and with nature," Hitler said of the functionaries he wanted to lead his empire.[309] "University studies" within the Reich, "should turn out men who are fitted for life and capable of ensuring for the State the preservation of natural law."[310] By understanding and adhering to "natural law," Germans would win the power struggle of existence, because nature was "constantly deciding the supremacy of one creature over another by means of a constant struggle," Hitler explained.[311]

Hitler attempted to use nature to justify everything from genocide to dietary prescriptions.

Because of his view of natural law, Hitler viewed raw food and dietary practices as part of the constant power struggle that nature had ordained for the planet. Nature constantly tested people's physical resilience, which dietary habits largely contributed to. Whether a person consumed raw food or not was, in Hitler's mind, part of that biological litmus test. A person eating an unnatural diet will lose out in the struggle of the survival of the fittest, whereas someone eating a natural diet that's in tune with the "intimate harmony of things," as Hitler described natural law, will thrive. In order to have vigor and survive, a person must follow, as he said, what "Nature thus teaches us—that a rational diet should be based on eating things in their raw state."[312] People who ate too much cooked food were liable for physical weakness and would be naturally punished for their irrational choices.

Cooked food weakened an organism and made it susceptible to disease. Hitler declared, "Nature, in creating a being, gives it all it needs to live. If it cannot live, that's either because it's attacked from without or because its inner resistance has weakened."[313] By eating unnatural "sterilized" and "debased" cooked food, an individual weakens his or her "inner resistance."[314] This person becomes one of the "incorrectly nourished organisms" with a weak immune system. Hitler further il-

---

[309]   Ibid., 62.
[310]   Ibid., 375.
[311]   Ibid., 396.
[312]   Ibid., 443.
[313]   Ibid., 115.
[314]   Ibid.

lustrates the connection between diet and "inner resistance": "We all breathe in the microbes that give rise to colds or tuberculosis," but not everyone develops the diseases. Only a strong body nourished by good food can overcome viral and bacterial threats.[315] Therefore, anyone who impiously spurns the laws of nature does so at their own peril and doesn't deserve compassion: one must never have pity on those who have lost their vital force."[316] Nature has no pity on those who turn their back on it, nor should we.

Each person must either live in "harmony" with the laws of nature and include raw foods in their diet or be weakened, drained of vitality, and die early like those German peasants who only eat food that has been "cooked and re-cooked, and thus deprived of all its virtues," as Hitler warned.[317]

Eating raw food, for Hitler, unlike the Desert Fathers, was certainly not a means of honoring the Christian God. Christianity was a "rebellion against natural law," according to Hitler.[318] Natural law, not traditional religious belief nor any devotion to a personal Creator, was the sacred source of truth. If he were to give a definition of "God," Hitler would likely apply his description of the "dominion of natural laws throughout the universe."[319] Of natural law, he said, "Let's seek inspiration in these principles, and in the long run we'll triumph over religion . . . The man who lives in communion with nature necessarily finds himself in opposition to the Churches."[320]

Through raw food, the Desert Fathers rejected the world and the desires and needs of the body. Through raw food, Hitler paid homage to the flesh and sought to strengthen it in its battle for survival. Caring for the body was, in a sense, embracing the world, of paying tribute to its laws, whereas the desert monks sought to overcome the world.

HEALTHY GERMANS AND SOCIETAL PRODUCTIVITY

"Bear witness to our will, our industry,
our ability . . . German Workers, to the work!"
—Adolf Hitler[321]

---

315   Ibid.

316   Ibid., 396.

317   Ibid., 236.

318   Ibid., 15.

319   Ibid., 6.

320   Ibid., 61.

321   Linge, Heinz. With Hitler to the End. New York: Simon and Schuster, 2009, 183.

Along with Germany's adherence to natural law, economic productivity was at stake when it came to raw food consumption.

Raw food, Hitler felt, could be important in maximizing the productive potential of Germans in war and in work. Increasing economic output and being efficient in military campaigns were crucial to the Führer. Germans needed to prove, he felt, that they were of the master race by winning the struggle for supremacy over other peoples.

And the medical community and government were acutely aware of the connection between productivity and bodily health.

The "strengthening" of the country took on an intense and destructive energy with the ascendancy of the Nazis. People who were accused of possessing hereditary illnesses were registered, sterilized, or murdered. Citizens were supposed to be healthy and productive. And if a German was beyond utility for the regime, the German economy, and the war effort, there could be deadly consequences for him or her.

RAW FOOD AS INTEGRAL TO GERMAN THRIVING AND PRODUCTIVITY

"During the Ice Age, circumstances compelled [man]...to have his food cooked, a habit which, as one knows to-day, has harmful consequences."
—Adolf Hitler[322]

In the Führer's casual hours, food was often on his mind. Over meals, Goebbels and Hitler worried about food transport and how to efficiently get fresh vegetables to poorer workers. Goebbels "expressed the fear," Nazi secretaries recorded, that poorer Germans would be left nutritionally lacking as "the wealthy would send their servants . . . into the country and buy up all the fruit and vegetables, while the Berlin workman would then have nothing to buy in the fruit and vegetable stalls of the local market."[323] The logistics of ensuring equal access to fruits and veggies and the implications for the productivity of the working class were worthy of being discussed.

In other mealtime conversations, Hitler clearly denoted cooked food and meat as destroyers of human health and performance. Articulating a simple insight from the natural world, in one conversation, Hitler declared that "the dog, which is carnivorous, cannot compare in

---

[322] Hitler, Adolf, et al. *Hitler's Table Talk, 1941-1944 : His Private Conversations*. New York, Enigma Books, 2008, 231.
[323] Ibid., 531.

performance with the horse, which is vegetarian."[324] He also discussed how the often-victorious armies of the Roman Empire preferred a grain-based vegetarian diet and "had recourse to meat only in times of scarcity."[325] Meat was not needed for optimal martial performance and it even weighed armies down in his opinion. "Japanese wrestlers," he claimed, "who are amongst the strongest men in the world, feed exclusively on vegetables."[326] A "vegetarian diet," has "obvious advantages," he summarized.[327]

Critical, though, to the healthiness and effectiveness of a proper vegetarian diet, he made clear, was raw food. "Those who adopt a vegetarian diet must remember that it is in their raw state that vegetables have their greatest nutritive value," Hitler proclaimed. "Science has proved, too, that cooking destroys the Vitamins," he continued. Along with scientific tests, the laws of nature demonstrated the rational superiority of raw foods: "the fly feeds on fresh leaves, the frog swallows the fly as it is, and the stork eats the living frog. Nature thus teaches us that a rational diet should be based on eating things in their raw state."[328] Hitler's endorsement of raw foods was clear.

The healthfulness of raw foods, in his opinion, were proving to have positive effects on the youngest generation of Germans. "Our children to-day are much healthier than those of the Imperial and Weimar Republic periods because mothers now realize that they contribute far more to the health of their children if they give them raw vegetables and roots."[329] The new generations had implemented more rational dietary habits; children needed the rough fiber of uncooked roots. A nutritional-cultural movement was thriving: "People are again finding room for a naturistic diet. It's a revolution," Hitler declared.[330]

Hitler believed that Germany was waking up, out of its cooked food stupor, and moving away from the public health collapse of the World War I age. But ignorant elements of the population still stuck to the old ways and threatened to drag down the nation's productivity with early-onset aging and death. And cooked food was to blame. "Country folk spend fourteen hours a day in the fresh air. Yet by the age of forty-five they're old, and the mortality amongst them is enormous. That's the result of an error in their diet. They eat only cooked

---

[324] Ibid., 443.

[325] Ibid., 26.

[326] Ibid., 231.

[327] Ibid., 572.

[328] Ibid., 443.

[329] Ibid.

[330] Ibid., 115.

foods . . ."[331] These rapidly-aged cooked-food loving peasants were not much use to their people, the economy, and the Nazi state if they were decrepit and plagued with diseases. All that food that was "cooked and re-cooked, and thus deprived of all its virtues" was ruining Germans.[332] These stupid people's ignorance of the value of raw food was killing them. They stuck stubbornly to their pernicious tradition of cooking their food to death and suffered their diet's "harmful consequences."

Connected with the productivity of his citizens, was, obviously, their survival. Hitler worried that cooked food could be linked with some of the most feared diseases that threatened the German people, like cancer. "It's not impossible that one of the causes of cancer lies in the harmfulness of cooked foods," he said plainly. "It's possible that the causes that provoke it [cancer] find a terrain that suits them in in-correctly nourished organisms."[333] Cooked foods sullied the landscape, the environment within the body, he believed. They set the foundation, the terrain, for disease to thrive.

As further evidence for the danger of cooked foods, dogs, he ar-gued, were plagued by the "maladies of civilization" like cancer. "50 percent of dogs die of cancer, there must be an explanation for that. Nature has predisposed the dog to feed on raw meat . . . To-day the dog feeds almost exclusively on mixed bread and cooked meat."[334] Too much cooked food—unnaturally and irrationally altered food—had destroyed yet another species.

But the Führer himself did eat some cooked food on his vegetarian diet, whether for taste or convenience. Later in life, he apparently liked junk food like white bread and cake. He may not have walked the walk but he talked the talk, constantly. If he didn't follow through in his own habits, he at least dreamed that the German nation would do so.

THE PHILOSOPHY BEHIND HITLER'S RAW FOODISM

Hitler's interest in raw food was connected to his interpretation of Darwinism and likely Nietzsche's philosophy.

In reference to Darwinism, raw food helped one survive. With re-gard to Nietzsche, Hitler had a similar idea to the famed philosopher, of escaping the "slave morality" of Judeo-Christianity, with its de-em-phasis on worldliness, strength, coercion, and the body. The Aryan race

---

[331]   Ibid., 81.

[332]   Ibid., 231.

[333]   Ibid. 115.

[334]   Ibid. 152.

could regain its original vigor if it embraced the importance of physical health, along with dumping counterproductive ideas of virtuous meekness and hatred of one's own flesh.

The ascetic negation of the body was out of vogue. Now, under the Nazis, as one historian put it, the "love of the body had to break with centuries of Christian alienation."[335] Leadership attempted to return the country to a pre-Christian classical affirmation of the flesh and a modern science-based meticulous care for it. Hitler summed up his classically-influenced vision for Nazi Germany when he praised the famous ancient Greek statue of a discus-thrower, the Discobolus: "You will see how splendid man used to be in the beauty of his body and you will realize that we can speak of progress only when we have not only attained such beauty but even, if possible, when we have surpassed it."[336]

Social progress and health were intertwined. A focus on athletics as well as abstention from smoke, drink, and drugs accompanied the dietary recommendations of the regime.

EMBRACING THE EARTH, REVERING THE FLESH

Part of reclaiming the German body from poisonous influences demanded a philosophical readjustment in addition to a "hygienic" crusade.

Although Hitler made use of Christian institutions in Germany and adapted them to Nazi ends, Hitler believed that Germany, through the centuries, had been weakened by what he called Judeo-Christian values. The nation had lost a natural respect for the human body and its instincts. Hitler associated Jewish ideological influence (and connected Christian values) with a "sad victory of spirit over flesh," in that it derided anything worldly.[337] Hitler also denounced certain Christian values as "poverty-stricken rubbish" that elevated worldly weakness and perversely subdued the instincts of the flesh.[338] The intimations of meekness, nonviolence, and condemnations of financial riches and various kinds of sexuality—values that appear in scripture and later Christian writings, were to him, the enemy of excellence, beauty, strength, and power.

---

[335]   Johann Chapoutot. "The Nazis and Nature: Protectors or Predators?" *Vingtième iècle. Revue D'histoire*, vol. 113, no. 1, 2024, 29–39,

[336]   Sooke, Alastair. "The Discobolus: Greeks, Nazis and the Body Beautiful." www.bbc.com, 24 Mar. 2015, www.bbc.com/culture/article/20150324-hitlers-idea-of-the-perfect-body.

[337]   Linge, Heinz. With Hitler to the End. New York: Simon and Schuster, 2009, 183.

[338]   Hitler, Adolf, et al. *Hitler's Table Talk, 1941-1944 : His Private Conversations*. New York, Enigma Books, 2008. 78.

It's not too hard to see that Christianity has indeed had strongly ascetic and at times world-hating tendencies throughout its history, as seen with the Desert Fathers. Hitler despised the philosophy that those monks lived by and their attempted negation of their own nature and carnality. Hitler sought to embrace and celebrate the body and the visceral instincts of life, including violent hatred. He sought health, strength, and worldly power for Germany. He wanted to vigorously kill and conquer, not physically waste away like a desert monk nibbling on raw cabbage, nor was the crowd-loving dictator the type of man to spend life praying in an isolated cell.

NIETZSCHE, THE NAZIS, AND THE BODY

"It was the Jews," Friedrich Nietzsche wrote, "who dared to invert the aristocratic value-equation (good=noble=powerful)."[339] "The wretched alone are the good; the suffering deprived, sick, ugly alone, are pious, alone are blessed by God," as Nietzsche described the mindset.[340] Christianity that grew out of Judaism, he wrote, is "a rebellion of everything that crawls on the ground against that which has height."[341] It is a perverted celebration of weakness, he felt, and an expression of bitter resentment against natural strength. It's a resentment like the conquered would feel toward the conqueror.

There is much debate about the ultimate meaning of Nietzsche's philosophy (or plural *philosophies* or whether he even had a cohesive philosophy) and its relationship to Nazi ideology or even culpability in Nazi atrocities. But one thing is certain—many Nazis formulated interpretations of Nietzsche's work in efforts to justify their actions and worldview.

Nietzsche was famous for his disdain of the "slave morality" of Christian beliefs and their supposed resentment towards worldly power and success. The Christian tradition had inverted classical paradigms of revering strength, wealth, and violent coercion in "an act of . . . spiritual revenge" against those who are naturally strong.[342]

Before this moral inversion, pre-Christian civilizations like those of Greece and Rome thrived on and celebrated worldly strength: "For the Romans were the strong and the noble, and nobody stronger and

---

[339]   Solomon, Robert C., and Kathleen M. Higgins. *What Nietzsche Really Said.* Schocken Books, 2000, 111.

[340]   ibid., 112.

[341]   Hicks, Stephen R. C. *Nietzsche and the Nazis: A Personal View.* Ockham's Razor publishing, 2010, 80.

[342]   Solomon, Robert C., and Kathleen M. Higgins. *What Nietzsche Really Said.* Schocken Books, 2000, 12.

nobler has yet existed on earth," Nietzsche gushed.[343] But the ethic of Judea had conquered Rome and Christianity had weakened Europe over the last millennia, and restrained natural healthy instincts and appetites.

Roman and Greek philosophies did sometimes advocate strict discipline but with the ascendency of the new "slave morality," a paradigm shift of rigid contempt for the flesh, took hold on a wide scale. One can read in the following quote, Nietzsche's disdain for the likes of the ascetic Desert Fathers: "the soul looked contemptuously on the body, and then that contempt was the supreme thing—the soul wishes the body meagre, ghastly and famished"—exactly what some of the Desert Fathers *did* wish upon the body. Centuries had passed under this life-denying asceticism: Europe had undergone a "self-crucifixion and self-violation" of man, according to Nietzsche.[344]

The philosopher wanted to replace these values with a return to a physical ethic that revered the earth and the instincts of the human body above all else. "There is a mighty lord . . . it is called Self . . . it is thy body," Nietzsche declared through his fictional prophet Zarathustra. For the body, whose instincts promoted survival and vitality was far more wise than anti-life slave morality. "There is more sagacity in thy body," Nietzsche's Zarathustra said, than in the moralities of the past. The flesh—not the Christian "hatred of one's own life," that Jesus referred to, was to be the new source of knowledge and wisdom. The body was the very essence of what it is to be a human. In fact, that's all a human is: "the awakened one, the knowing one, saith: 'Body am I entirely, and nothing more,'" Nietzsche wrote.

Our bodies grew out of the earth and are connected to its physical wisdom, thus the earth and its natural law should be the guiding morality of life, Nietzsche's Zarathustra argued: "remain true to the earth and believe not those who speak unto you of super earthly hopes." All of the promoters of life-defeating anti-worldliness and haters of body, "despisers of life are they, decaying ones, and poisoned ones." Instead of blaspheming the supernatural, "to blaspheme the earth is now the most dreadful sin, and to rate the heart of the unknowable higher than the meaning of the earth." One can almost sense a reverence for raw food growing out of the fertile ground of an ethic like this. What way to get closer to the sacred earth than to imbibe its inherent wisdom by eating its vegetation raw.

---

[343]   Hicks, Stephen R. C., 147.
[344]   Solomon, Robert C., and Kathleen M. Higgins, 27.

The Nazi Appropriation of Nietzsche

Hitler attempted to inaugurate this return of the reverence for the body and a naturalistic ethic. Like Nietzsche (but with much different and very sinister aims), Hitler wanted to banish the weak and unnatural ethic of so-called Judeo-Christian morality. He also wanted to banish the people, the Jews, that he connected to the inception of this morality. "A people that is rid of its Jews returns spontaneously to the natural order," he believed. [345] And to embrace the natural order was to create a domineering nation that was unafraid of subjugating neighboring states and winning the continuous natural violent struggle for dominion. It should also include a return to a "natural" diet, Hitler felt.

Hitler and other Nazis felt, for instance, a kinship with a sentiment expressed in Nietzsche's *Beyond Good and Evil*: "Life itself is essentially appropriation, injury, conquest of the strange and weak, suppression, severity, and at the least, putting it mildest, exploitation." As one historian summarized, in his opinion, "the Nazis can and did find inspiration in Nietzsche." Many of them read Nietzsche "avidly during their formative years and incorporated themes and sayings from Nietzsche into their own writings, speeches, and policies."[346]

Hitler had certainly absorbed an idea about the body and Christian morality very similar to Nietzsche's.

Nietzsche felt that excellence depended on a "physiological condition" which he called a "Great Healthiness." And Hitler certainly sought to bring a "Great Healthiness" to the Germanic people. Raw food was the way to do so, in the Führer's mind.

Dreams Die: A Ruined Nation and a Ruined Body

"When a man grows old, his tissues lose their elasticity. The normal man feels a revulsion at the sight of death."
—Adolf Hitler[347]

Hitler's mass-killing schemes and unwinnable war ruined his hopes for Germany, wreaked havoc all over the word, and destroyed his own

---

[345] Hitler, Adolf, et al. *Hitler's Table Talk, 1941-1944 : His Private Conversations*. New York, Enigma Books, 2008, 314.

[346] Hicks, Stephen R. C. *Nietzsche and the Nazis: A Personal View*. Ockham's Razor Publishing, 2010, 74.

[347] Hitler, Adolf, et al. *Hitler's Table Talk, 1941-1944 : His Private Conversations*. New York, Enigma Books, 2008. 85.

health. Regardless of his interest in diet and physiology, Hitler himself had no chance to thrive with the constant stress he was under. As World War II dragged on, intestinal cramps, involuntary trembling, and various other disorders forced him to languish in the beds of stuffy bunkers much of the time.

One of Hitler's doctors commented on the discrepancy between Hitler's uncommon interest in health and his own poor health, saying, "The Führer talks to me like a medical specialist about problems of nutrition . . . but he never considers that he should put his knowledge into practice with himself."[348] Hitler's health proclamations were more theoretical than practicable for himself and many Germans. As he became more stressed, depressed, drug-addled, and overwhelmed by the inevitable defeat of his Reich, his own dietary ideas would've seemed an unapplicable and ever more distant dream.

During this period of rapid deterioration—as Germany succumbed to defeat and its leader succumbed to illness, Hitler's valet constantly witnessed the "painfully distorted [facial] features" of the suffering mass-murderer.[349] The führer's "fear of dying before he had completed his work," his valet noted, was becoming a reality. Hitler increasingly soothed his mental anguish and bodily suffering with a powerful cocktail of drugs. His addiction to opiates and usage of methamphetamine, barbiturates, and cocaine fed alive a faint delusion of possible military victory, gnawed away at his vitality, and overshadowed his hopes for a "naturistic" health "revolution."

Before the war, a more lively and abstemious Hitler enjoyed tea and plant-based treats during fresh-aired countryside picnics.[350] During the war, he decayed in bunkers, projecting death and misery onto the world whilst getting injected with toxic drugs, sometimes desperately pleading with doctors for more oxycodone and cocaine.[351] Towards the end of the war, Hitler's valet lamented that this "now old, graying, bent, and degenerating" man and his world were so different from the hopeful "epoch of our picnic excursions."[352] Similarly, Hitler's doctor was shocked by how rapidly he had deteriorated, his lifeless complexion, and his involuntary trembling. Hitler looked like "a man absolutely exhausted and absent," said his valet.[353] "Like the Reich which he had aimed to bring into an era of unparalleled brilliance

---

[348]   Linge, Heinz. *With Hitler to the End.* New York: Simon and Schuster, 2009, 169.

[349]   Ibid., 185.

[350]   Ibid., 59.

[351]   Ohler, Norman, and Shaun Whiteside, *Blitzed : Drugs in the Third Reich.* Boston, Houghton Mifflin Harcourt, 2017, 181.

[352]   Linge, Heinz. With Hitler to the End. New York: Simon and Schuster, 2009, 185.

[353]   Ibid., 175.

and opulence and had become a heap of rubble, he was the disfigured embodiment of his earlier self."[354]

But even in the final two years of his life and the war, his now seemingly ridiculous raw food reveries continued—his familiar "song" as his inner circle called his dietary monologues.[355] These dietary musings seemed more and more pointless and insane considering the death and chaos surrounding him. While he denounced the cooked foods that were causing early "mortality," he himself was causing early mortality for people all across Europe. As German and other European cities were being bombed away, his plan to "keep our cities supplied with vegetables and fresh fruit" seemed laughable.[356] Regardless, amazingly, he preached his raw food ideas until nearly the end. On the day that the allied powers stormed the beaches of Normandy in 1944 and German defeat looked increasingly assured, he was still ranting about raw vegetarian foods and the dangers of smoking, whilst dazed in an opiate stupor at lunch.[357]

In some of the darkest moments, the power-hungry madman did not give up on his hope that raw plant food could empower the German people, as disconnected from reality as that belief seemed.

---

[354] Ibid., 2.

[355] Ibid. 36.

[356] Hitler, Adolf, et al. *Hitler's Table Talk, 1941-1944: His Private Conversations.* New York, Enigma Books, 2008, 26.

[357] Ohler, Norman, and Shaun Whiteside, *Blitzed : Drugs in the Third Reich.* Boston, Houghton Mifflin Harcourt, 2017, 142.

8.
Gandhi: Raw Food and the Happiness of India

"Queer food he eats; only fruit and nuts . . . [He feels that] no fire should be necessary in the making of food, fire being unnatural."
—An unknown contemporary of Gandhi, commenting on Gandhi's diet

"The life of all living beings is food. Complexity, clarity, good voice, long life, understanding, happiness, satisfaction, growth, strength and intelligence are all established in food."
—Charaka, a primary ancient figure in Ayurvedic medicine

Mohandes "Mahatma" Gandhi, the nonviolent activist who played a key role in helping India gain its independence from British rule, was obsessed with diet. Historian Nico Slate noted that Gandhi continuously "thought about food, talked about food, and experimented with food." Dietary theory was one of his "greatest passions" and he's even been accused of "dietary anxiety" and an "excessive concern with food."[358]

The gaunt-looking man, who famously wore a loincloth in late life to identify with India's poor, and whose image is etched in the world's historical consciousness, would spend months or weeks at a time eating only raw food. Why?

As the visionary in India's quest for independence, Gandhi's dietary concerns were wrapped up in political, economic, and spiritual motives. He tested minimalism and raw foodism with these aims in mind. He wanted India to thrive as a nation and he felt at times that raw food could play a critical role in accomplishing this. His focus was

---

[358]   Slate, Nico. *Gandhi's Search for the Perfect Diet.* University of Washington Press, 28 Feb. 2019. 7.

often on the welfare of his fellow countrymen as he experimented with different diets.

Gandhi even felt that dietary practices were at the core of ethics. What a person chose to eat, Gandhi believed, affected his spiritual state, the economy, the political landscape, and ultimately communities all over the world. Diet, he felt, mattered in nearly every facet of life and he was obsessed with using it to affect the things that he cared about. Gandhi and the venerated ancient Indian teachers of Ayurveda agreed. The effects of what you consume are potent.

Gandhi's intense curiosity about the effects of nutrition seemed to match his dedication to his better-known political activities. His interest, especially in raw foods, is apparent in his letters to Western friends. In one 1927 letter, he asked an American friend, the philosopher Richard Gregg, "At what point are vitamins destroyed when you boil leafy vegetables?" And more generally, "What is the virtue of vitamins?" Later, after conducting some research, Gandhi seemed to be on the path of embracing raw foodism and confidently proclaimed, "We get from uncooked vegetables the nutrients that we require. They are known as 'vitamins' in English, and . . . vitamins are destroyed as a result of cooking."[359] Facts like these, he felt, could empower Indians to get optimal nutrition.

Gandhi's interest in raw foods spanned his lifetime and he continuously conducted experiments on himself to see what dietary practices were most beneficial.

FOOD AS THE CORNERSTONE OF SPIRITUAL AND POLITICAL MORALITY

> *"The seeker has to have complete control over his diet.*
> *Whatever he eats he should eat as medicine, for the*
> *preservation of the body, never to pamper the palate."*
> **—Gandhi**

Our dietary choices reflect our character, Gandhi believed. In fact, they are at the core of our ethics. Moral failures, Gandhi declared, like "lying, pleasure hunting, perjury, theft, and so on," were tied to being a "slave of the palate"—that is, unable to resist momentary pleasures.[360] Whether a person had self-control while eating served as a litmus test. The "failure to restrain a craving" led to immorality in daily life and

---

[359] Ibid., 103.
[360] Ibid., 38.

harmful behavior in society. If one didn't have the discipline to restrain the urges of the taste buds, one had little hope of controlling other pernicious urges.

Similar to the ancient Hindu ascetics, Gandhi also connected dietary discipline to the ultimate spiritual accomplishment of *moksha*, a central goal within Hinduism, which signified being released from the bondage of the karmic cycle of birth and death and freedom from ignorance. Controlling what types of food one consumed as well as one's appetite was crucial to spiritual health. That way, *moksha* would be satisfied and material desires and worldly limitations overcome. Controlling desire was crucial to achieving this spiritual maturity and the tongue was a testing ground for that maturity. To abstain from luxurious foods was the mark of strength. "He who has his tongue under control, being . . . moderate in his taste for good food, must be reckoned to have achieved a great conquest," Gandhi explained.

Certain foods could awaken temptations that would make or break spiritual health. Salt, chocolate, fried foods, or milk were "heating and stimulating" and could fuel sexual lust and sinful mindsets. "For controlling your mind," said Gandhi, "try giving up the extra salt in your food." Salt imperiled *brahmacharya*—the pursuit of god, self-control of the senses (a practice that supported moksha)—and hindered the ideal serene passionless state of consciousness. "For everyone who wants to cultivate self-control," Gandhi advised, again, this time more specifically, "give up salt for five or six months and afterwards, from time to time.[361]"

Another ancient Indian principle that was integrated into Gandhi's diet was that of ahimsa, or nonviolence toward all sentient creatures. His dedication to ahimsa made consuming animal flesh practically unthinkable. His family's ties to Jainism, some of the most extreme practitioners of ahimsa, and his readings of the ethical arguments of British vegetarians contributed to his dedication to the nonviolent principle.

Gandhi's vegetarianism was not aimed primarily at physical health. "A moral basis" and an "altruistic purpose" were themes of this diet. For instance, he knew that health was "by no means the monopoly of vegetarians." Omnivores could be healthy as well. Spiritual ends came first. He pointed out that many religions agreed that "nothing is more detrimental to the spiritual faculty of man than the gross feeding on flesh."[362] Meat eating and alcohol consumption, he mused, might even be responsible for the "materialism," "religious indifference," and "dis-

---

[361] Ibid., 23.
[362] Ibid., 54.

appearance. . . of the spiritual faculty" in the twentieth-century world (although, it should be pointed out, he also admitted that it is possible for a meat eater to have a healthier "fear of God" than a vegetarian).[363]

Vegetarianism, not primarily a health practice, was dharma, a spiritual duty, which is to be "followed at the cost of one's life," Gandhi believed. Moral duty took precedence over physical survival. But physical health was another interest of Gandhi's and, he felt, necessary to accomplish his moral aims.

This sense of the spiritual detriments of certain foods was remarkably similar to Bircher-Benner and Ehret's own sense of food being at the root of the world's moral issues. All three of these men thought that the physical was important in the genesis of people's mindsets. Bad food was responsible for sociological ills and our distance from God.

Gandhi's food choices (including fasting) were also intertwined with his political ethics. He routinely abstained from foods that he perceived to enable oppressive systems. He refrained from items that enriched the British government and rejected food grown on plantations under slave-like working conditions. His dietary choices, in the words of historian Nico Slate, were connected to the "social, political, and economic structures he strove to transform" and the food choices he made "linked questions of individual consumer choice with anticolonial social movements."[364]

Gandhi's moral quest hinged on "two of history's perennial questions: how to live and what to eat."

BODY, SPIRIT, AND PURITY

Connected to diet, Gandhi saw the body was a vessel to be respected; a life of service to others and god was acted out through it. You respected your creator by looking after the body's well-being. "All religions have looked upon this body as a place where one may meet and recognize god," Gandhi explained.[489] "The body is of some service only if it is well used, that is, made the abode of god." God had entrusted humans to upkeep our bodies: "The human body is a sacred trust . . . Its proper upkeep is a duty."[490] When it is kept pure, one will be "pure in mind too," ready to do one's duty.[491]

---

[363]   Ibid., 55.
[364]   Ibid., 11.

Gandhi was interested in raw food and simple food for servicing the body as well as purifying the mind. In his autobiography, Gandhi wrote, of sexual lust and errant desire, "I realized that the mind is at the root of all sensuality. I saw that [. . .] food should be limited, simple, spiceless, and, if possible, uncooked." Raw food, Gandhi felt, similarly to how the Desert Fathers perceived it, was a tool to humble the body and chastise its unruliness. People ought to humble themselves and their bodies to attain spiritual mastery, Gandhi explained: "A man who wants to realize Truth must reduce himself to a cipher. He must become a voluntary pauper and live on the plainest food."[365] And food couldn't get much plainer than raw food.

Austerity was the mark of a spiritual person. One must nourish the spirit and not feed the lower carnal desires. This was why fasting was key to Gandhi's moral food choices. It helped break the attachment to food and starve the "animal" desires. "Fasting," wrote Gandhi, using Christian imagery, causes a "crucifixion of the flesh with a corresponding freedom of the spirit."[366] Stripping the flesh strengthened the spirit and Gandhi often used fasting as a test for his mental resolve. All his fasts, he said, were "undertaken for a moral purpose."[367]

When he was eating, he felt that simple, low-calorie foods were the next best thing to fasting. Gandhi felt that his dietary austerity helped him carry on his moral duties with vigor. This accounted for some of his interest in raw foods. Relatively light food like fruit, veggies, and the more dense but simpler food of nuts gave him energy for serving his community, he felt. Less food "clogged" his body on such a spartan diet. "I came to the conclusion," he said, "that to do full justice to service, I must reduce my wants and live a life of utmost simplicity."[368] By reducing his cravings for comfort and luxurious living, he was a more effective agent for change in the world. His spirit was purer and his body was lighter and less burdened in undertaking his moral and political work.

---

[365]   Mahatma Gandhi. *Story of My Experiments with Truth.* Popular Prakashan Ltd, In, 2013. Ch. 1.

[366]   Slate, Nico. *Gandhi's Search for the Perfect Diet.* University of Washington Press, 28 Feb. 2019. 147.

[367]   Ibid., 146.

[368]   Mahatma Gandhi. *Story of My Experiments with Truth.* Popular Prakashan Ltd, In, 2013. Ch. 1.

Swaraj: Personal and National Independence

"The word swaraj is a sacred word meaning self-rule and self-restraint."
—Gandhi

Throughout his life, Gandhi felt that raw food, abstention from certain foods, and fasting had potential to fan the flame of Indian independence and empower individuals in their daily lives. Dietary control was critical to accomplishing *swaraj*, a state of spiritual and political self-sufficiency that all Indians should attain to.

Political self-rule required *personal* self-rule. Each Indian, Gandhi felt, had to have mastery over his or her destructive passions. India's control over its own destiny depended on the ability of each individual to exert control over themselves. If they couldn't do that, there was little hope of dignified national sovereignty. And diet was a crucial testing ground for self-restraint.

Dietary self-control, in the service of *swaraj*, empowered a person spiritually and physically in the world. If Indians would "conquer the palate," their bodily "organs will be automatically under our control," Gandhi said.[369] And "one who has this body under control can subdue the world because such a one becomes god's heir, a part of him."[370] Disciplined food habits could prove one's resolve. Even if the British handed over power to the Indians, a type of immoral self-rule would take the place of colonization. Without self-control, Hindus and Muslim could be seized by tribal passion or hatred for one another, if they could be seized by their lust for sugar or chocolate, or general gluttony.

Diet was the daily way to prove the swaraj of the self and show care for the community. That's why Gandhi was, in his own words, "an ardent food reformer." Political morality was played out through diet.

Indians could fight British power by avoiding processed foods that were a source of income for the British. These easily preserved commercial foods could be packaged and shipped around the world for efficient profit. This association between junky commercial food and imperial power led Gandhi to seek whole food or raw food alternatives to such processed foods as margarine or white flour, which Gandhi lambasted as "insipid," "injurious to health," and "worthless as a food." He advised his colonized countrymen to make ghee from "undried

---

[369] Slate, Nico. *Gandhi's Search for the Perfect Diet.* University of Washington Press, 28 Feb. 2019. 44.
[370] Ibid., 26

coconut" instead of margarine.[371] The nation's landscape could provide politically correct raw foods.

Gandhi's public campaign to inspire Indians to abstain from monopolized British salt was another dietary tactic to chip away at British power. Gandhi wrote that the salt tax should be immediately abolished. The poor suffered the most when the price of salt was inflated, as it was a crucial part of their diet. Along with protesting the salt tax, Gandhi sought to limit his personal salt intake so as to not support the British government's cruel tax on the commodity. He told followers that he had "lived without any salt for over six years" and that they could follow his example in an effort to boycott colonial power.

Through diet, Indians could transform unjust economic structures. Tea, coffee, hot chocolate, and processed sugar were to be avoided because they were produced "more or less in conditions of slavery" by greedy monopolists who "have their eyes only on profit," Gandhi wrote.[372] And people who consumed these luxurious and unnecessary foods, because of the existing structures of dominance, were "guilty of the crime of murder."

To dismantle systems of oppression, Indians had better eat simply, closer to home, and incorporate more raw foods into their diet. Eating in this way would also help the plight of India's poor.

RAW FOOD, EMPOWERING THE BODY, EMPOWERING THE POOR

"We can get swaraj only when we improve the
lot of these [impoverished] people."
—Gandhi

Gandhi was a relatively affluent lawyer. In his early life, he dressed in expensive suits, and ate sumptuous meals. But he later adopted the peasant aesthetic that he is remembered for. He made a point of dressing like India's poor by wearing a loincloth and even adapted his body to their plight by emaciating it with his sparing, low-calorie vegetarian diet, which, like his clothing, could embody the grim reality of the poor's "eternal compulsory fast," as he put it.[373]

---

[371] Ibid., 84.

[372] Ibid., 34.

[373] Ibid. 152.

In Gandhi's dietary experiments, he always had India's poor in mind. He contemplated how he could improve their health, quality of life, and economic conditions, as well as empower them in their fight for India's independence. This is why he sought out the simplest and healthiest foods available. He wanted to minimize the cost and labor spent on buying, gathering, and preparing food while ensuring the highest nutritional quality. Leading by example and experimenting on himself, Gandhi felt like he could ensure the feasibility of his dietary recommendations.

Realistic, economical, and healthy food options could, in his mind, secure "moral and physical advancement of the villages" because they would nourish the poor.[374] That is one reason why his focus was on accessible vegetarian foods. Plant foods were "within the means of an average villager."[375]

Raw plants were especially within reach, as nothing could be cheaper.

But the British colonial government had contributed to the difficulties that poor Indians faced in getting access to fresh produce. Fruits and vegetables were "considered to be delicacies meant for [richer] city people"; additionally, the regular famines that struck India under the British were no help.[376] To add insult to injury, colonial officials advocated diets high in meat and dairy, foods that Gandhi saw as physically and spiritually harmful.[377]

One step toward securing quality raw food for Indians was private gardening. Indians of any means could access the highest quality fruits and veggies that way. Gandhi gardened himself and urged Indians to "grow plenty of green vegetables" to satisfy their nutritional needs and without depending on outside sources of sustenance.[378] "The soil of India is so rich that it can produce any vegetable you like," he said optimistically.[379]

If Indians consumed more food in its raw state, they would save money, labor, and time. Raw food could be a powerful way to improve the lives of Gandhi's poor countrymen.[380] Perhaps people did not have to spend hours each day on preparing, cooking, and cleaning, and they could save money on cooking tools. The "extreme simplicity" of raw

---

374   Ibid., 139.
375   Ibid., 116.
376   Ibid., 125.
377   Ibid., 136.
378   Ibid., 126.
379   Ibid., 137.
380   Ibid., 79.

foods and the intriguing thought that, in his words, "I could dispense with cooking" captured his imagination.[381]

"Much of the time of our womenfolk . . . would be saved" by raw foodism, Gandhi predicted. He thought that "Women will be set free from the prison-house of the kitchen" by dramatically reducing the time needed to prepare meals. Gandhi also supposed that less attention would have to be paid to questions of sanitation that that were involved in the cooking process—"his own version of fast food."[382] But unlike the conventional definition of "fast food," Gandhi's project saw a return to primordial naturalness.

Seeking to make use of the most rudimentary foods, for the use of the poor, Gandhi made uncooked "fruit" the core of his diet, although he had an expansive definition of fruit that included almonds, walnuts, peanuts, and coconuts. "Fruit" contained "all the elements necessary for health and energy" in his view. In justifying such a minimalistic diet, he cited scientists and argued that "chemists have shown by experiment that fruits contain all the elements necessary for the maintenance of human life."[383]

Gandhi spent many days eating only "purely uncooked fruitarian food." In the winter of 1912–13, he ate only this "fruit" (and nuts). He observed that even despite such severe dietary limitation, his physical and mental energy was "little short of miraculous," he claimed.[384] It was an exciting prospect that such a simple, uncooked diet could ensure physical stamina and heightened mental performance. These were the sort of findings that Gandhi had hoped for. So throughout his life, in the interest of empowering the poor as well as furthering the fight for political and economic justice and Indian self-sufficiency, Gandhi conducted many experiments on the usefulness of raw food. Unfortunately, some of the experiments weren't as successful as the 1912–13 fruitarian winter.

---

[381]   Ibid., 75
[382]   Ibid. 79.
[383]   Ibid., 93.
[384]   Ibid., 94.

Raw Food Experiments

"If it succeeds, it enables serious men and women to make revolutionary changes in their mode of living. It frees women from drudgery . . . the ethical value of uncooked food is incomparable."
—**Gandhi** [385]

In 1914, Gandhi spent a few months in London, where he hoped to discuss the rights of Indians with British authorities and support the diasporic community. But he became bedridden with a brief illness, pleurisy (inflammation of the membranes around the lungs). An English vegetarian doctor friend advised him to eat "brown bread, raw vegetables, fresh fruit, [and get] oil massages" and take walks outdoors. Taking up the advice, Gandi ate mostly raw food for a short period—carrots, cabbage, turnips, and figs. He also ate banana chips that had been dried in the sun.[386]

He felt that raw food played a role in his recovery and that he learned that it was unnecessary to cook certain foods. He noted later that "it is a waste of money and 'good' taste to cook" turnips, radishes, and carrots.[387] Their "natural good taste" could be "destroyed by cooking." After all, he had seen them function as part of a balanced diet for many of his vegetarian friends in London—uncooked vegetables were a "staple" for them.

By the time of this 1914 health episode, Gandhi was already amenable to raw foods. Previously, he had conducted numerous experiments with "vital food" as he called it. In 1893, he ate exclusively raw for twelve days. This was his first experiment. Later in life he would eat raw for months at a time.[388]

For this initial 1893 experiment, he tested what it was like to eat what would now be considered very odd raw foods, for modern day raw vegans. He ate wheat, peas, rice—foods that are usually cooked. Gandhi soaked these items overnight in water but never heated them. They were accompanied by raw nuts and fruit.

He recorded how his body felt on this unique menu. Unfortunately, he noted negative effects like low mood, headaches, bad taste in mouth, and indigestion. Perhaps anti-nutrients like phytates, lec-

---

[385]   Gandhi, Mahatma. *Collected Works of Mahatma Gandhi. LXXXV, July 16, 1946-October 20, 1946.* New Delhi, The Publications Division, Ministry Of Information And Broadcasting, Govt. Of India, 1982.

[386]   Ibid., 77.

[387]   Ibid.

[388]   Ibid., 74.

tins, or indigestible fibers had caused these symptoms. Despite this disappointment, he still thought that "vital food may have its grand possibilities in store." He hoped to refine a regimen, so that at some future point, he could "replace cooked items with uncooked articles and wheat by nuts."[389]

Much later in life, in 1929, he launched a "public experiment with raw food." He ate almonds, grated coconut, raisins, lemons, green leafy vegetables, and honey along with sprouted wheat and beans. This experiment accomplished a healthier blood pressure but made him too thin, perhaps due to its low calorie content, so he returned to eating some cooked food.[390]

The unfortunate side effects of eating raw precluded his public endorsement of a completely raw diet. Despite the theoretical sociological benefits of raw food, Gandhi noted an unpleasant digestive "feeling of emptiness" that accompanied an uncooked diet. He also thought that since most people were adapted to cooked food diets, it would be difficult to convince the masses to adopt an uncooked diet. The stomach of the average Indian, for instance, he thought, had become distended, overly enlarged from the "ill-usage" of heavy cooked foods. In Gandhi's own experience on these raw stints, the "temptation to take cooked fruit was great" for whatever reason and it was difficult to overcome the craving.[391] Humans yearned for cooked food, unfortunately, he found by personal experience.

Gandhi would have preferred to have succeeded on a completely raw diet and found that eating this way was superior, for the sake of India's poor, for the simplicity and cost-saving attributes of raw foods. But "eating raw food was … a dietary ideal Gandhi never fully realized." In practice, Gandhi ate as high a percentage of raw food as he felt he could, and it actually formed the core of his diet. His often-saltless fare consisted largely of fruit, goat's milk, and some nuts.[392] And Gandhi always maintained an intellectual interest in the potential of raw foods and the "the hidden possibilities of the innumerable seeds, leaves, and fruits for giving the fullest possible nutrition to mankind."[393]

Obviously raw food wasn't the principal aim of Gandhi's activism. His interest in raw food supported his larger aims of spiritual and political autonomy from Britain. His interest in raw diets ended

---

[389]   Ibid., 78.

[390]   Ibid.

[391]   Ibid., 81.

[392]   Ibid., 80.

[393]   Gavaravarapu, SubbaRaoM, and R Hemalatha. 2019. "Thought for Food: Mahatma's Views on Nutrition, Controlled and Balanced Diets." *Indian Journal of Medical Research* 149 (7): 119. https://doi.org/10.4103/0971-5916.251668.

where it did not benefit the poor of India. He aborted several raw food experiments because fruit proved to be too expensive for poor Indians to afford. "The price of fruitarian food is prohibitive here," he noted, disappointed.[394]

"While he strove to increase the percentage of foods he ate uncooked," Slate wrote, "he rarely approached raw food with the obsessive anxiety" with which he struggled with forgoing sweets or dairy.[395] First and foremost, Gandhi sought to end his consumption of foods that would enable harsh labor conditions or trigger unproductive passions within him like lust.

Although he was unable to consistently implement complete raw foodism, Gandhi did encourage Indians to include some raw foods in their diet for the sake of health and economics. He pointed out that "many people take raw vegetables, pulses, wheat, etc., which have sprouted after being soaked in water" in order to boost vitamin intake—vitamins that he believed were destroyed by cooking. He encouraged poor Indians to consume more green leafy vegetables.[396] Leafy greens, he thought, were some of the "simplest and cheapest foods that would enable villagers to regain lost health."[397] Conveniently, many could be eaten raw and required little preparation or energy to prepare while filling nutritional gaps in the eater.

Eating more raw food could help impoverished rural Indians break away from bread and salt, foods that Gandhi lamented were "heavily taxed." Raw food could target political and economic justice. The poor suffered greatly because this government-imposed inflated price of salt. Many Indians had to work and sweat in the heat of the day, so they especially needed salt in their diet. Gandhi called the salt tax "blood sucking" because of this. Achieving "equality" was at the core of what he ate and advocated for.

"Dieticians are of the opinion," Gandhi said, "that the inclusion of a small quantity of raw vegetables like cucumber, vegetable marrow, pumpkin, gourd, etc., in one's menu is more beneficial to health than the eating of large quantities of the same cooked."[398] Raw food, "vital food," was the most nutritionally dense food there was, and thus essential for the nourishment of the poor. "An ounce or two of salads

---

[394]   Slate, Nico. *Gandhi's Search for the Perfect Diet.* University of Washington Press, 28 Feb. 2019. 118.

[395]   Ibid.

[396]   Ibid.,76.

[397]   Ibid., 97.

[398]   Gandhi, Mahatma. *Collected Works of Mahatma Gandhi. LXXXV, July 16, 1946-October 20, 1946.* New Delhi, The Publications Division, Ministry Of Information And Broadcasting, Govt. Of India, 1982.

serve the purpose of eight ounces of cooked vegetables," he believed. "Among fresh vegetables," he instructed, "a fair amount of leafy vegetables must be taken every day . . . The vitamins contained in these vegetables are wholly or partially lost in cooking."[399]

THE RAW HALF-DREAM

In the end, Gandhi did think that incorporating raw foods into one's diet was a useful tool to accomplish spiritual discipline, Indian self-rule, and improved quality of life for India's poor. For Gandhi, raw food had moral, political, and economic value. Though, Gandhi had hoped that this value would be more overwhelmingly powerful than he found it to be. He couldn't recommend it as a way of life due to the limitations that he experienced on such diets. The dream of a widely-applied raw diet fascinated him but he knew that he couldn't pragmatically recommend it for his countrymen.

Gandhi had spiritual motives for his interest in raw food that were similar to the ancient Hindu and Christian ascetics but unlike them, he also tied the potential spiritual effects of uncooked food to the political and sociological improvement of his country. In later raw foodism, especially New Age raw foodism, this holistic blueprint of connecting spiritual and sociological aims would become more explicit.

---

[399] Gandhi, Mahatma. *A Guide to Health*. Translated by A. Rama Iyer, S. Ganesan, 1921.

9.
Eugene Christian: The Maligned "Food Scientist"

"We may live without poetry, music and art, We may live without conscience, and live without heart; We may live without friends, we may live without books, And civilized man can live without cooks."
—Eugene Christian

In 1930, a charismatic raw foodist vegetarian died of pneumonia in New York state. He was only sixty-nine years old—a fact that would've satisfied his critics who labeled him as a quack, as he claimed his regimen could secure an extremely long lifespan.

The man, Eugene Christian, had certainly made enemies. In 1905, the year after the release of his best-known book, *Uncooked Foods and How to Use Them,* he was arrested in New York for practicing medicine without a license. Medical journals criticized his "pseudo-science buncombe" and some labeled him the "dean of American food faddists."[400] For the American medical establishment, Christian became a symbol of a "quack," a practitioner of fake medicine who makes misleading claims to his patients. In his case, he also had no medical license to back him up. That did not stop him, however, from winning a Supreme Court case that decided that he could prescribe dietary changes to clients as he was not a doctor but a self-described "food scientist."

Christian was a starry-eyed dreamer whose hopes for not only the physical and spiritual betterment of man, as well as the liberation of women, overshot the course that reality would take. But Christian made a name for himself.

Born right before the American Civil War, in 1860, in Tennessee, Christian would absorb, in adulthood, some of the ethos of the New

---

400   Cramp, Arthur J. (1936). *Nostrums and Quackery and Pseudo-Medicine, Volume 3.* Press of American Medical Association, 57-59; Anonymous. (1923). *El Zair: Quackery's Latest Offer of an Elimir of Life. Journal of the American Medical Association* 81: 768.

Thought movement by the end of the century. New Thought was a philosophy of radically empowering the individual; a philosophy that claimed everyone had the power to attract whatever circumstances they wanted in their lives, including perfect health. Raw food, Christian thought, was the means by which to materialize the aims of New Thought. He made this sentiment public when he published his 1904 *Uncooked Foods* book.

HOPE AND TRAGEDY

Christian's friend, WRC Latson, wrote an introduction to Christian's 1904 *Uncooked* book. "Of all the problems of practical life," Latson emphasized, "the question of feeding is the most important."[401] Christian and Latson both believed that a change in diet would usher in the next revolutionary changes in history and the betterment of humanity.

In 1904, Latson believed that humanity was entering an age of great awakening and new potentialities. "It is only of recent years that the intelligence of mankind has been directed towards finding out the really useful things in life," he claimed.[402] Man was beginning to have "great, shining dreams of what he would be and know and do. He would work harder, think deeper, aspire higher than his forefathers."

Those "great, shining dreams" involved curing all the ills of society. But a change in biology had to precede societal improvement. "I firmly believe," Latson proclaimed, in one doctor's claim that "in diet lies the key to nine-tenths of those social and political problems that vex our age and time."[403] "Up to the present, the best solution of these problems," Latson declared dramatically, "is found in the use of the uncooked foods."

Despite these high hopes and his faith in the global transformative power of raw food, neither vegetarianism nor uncooked foods could save Latson from the gloom of the world and his own untimely death. Seven years after his words were published in *Uncooked Foods*, in 1911, Latson was found dead in his Manhattan apartment, at age forty-four. There was a gunshot wound to his head and reportedly he had ingested chloroform. Although competing coroners' reports disputed the nature of his death, it was generally believed to be a suicide.

---

[401]   Christian, E., & Christian, M. G. (1904). *Uncooked foods and how to use them: A treatise on how to get the highest form of animal energy from food, with recipes for preparation, healthful combinations and menus.* The Health-Culture Co. 8

[402]   Ibid., 10.

[403]   Ibid., 8

Perhaps the burden of a scandal involving an alleged affair with his secretary or public criticism of his work had made him feel hopeless.

Nevertheless, in 1904, he and Christian had hope for a rosy future. Christian, for his part, wrote that in the past, humans were only semi-conscious, they dragged through life like zombies. "The brain was a useless lump of clay; but in this decade, the people are thinking."[404] Awareness was building. The "food question" was nagging on the human consciousness. "Why do we find so many specimens of perfect health and development in all other forms of life," Christian asked, "and so few among mankind—the king [species]?" The future will be very bright when people "learn the true relations between food, energy and health."[405] Humans had fallen short of their physical potential—and much more.

The effects of raw food transcended the physical; they would change the spirit of humanity. Eugene and others were looking into what "kind of [edible] material will bring mankind to the highest state of mental, moral and physical development."[406]

Food and Natural Law

The average individual who eats everything in sight, who accepts as correct anything that is jumbled together and dished up by cunning Chinamen, greasy Africans and uneducated foreigners, knowing as little of the chemistry of foods and their nutritive value."
—**Eugene Christian**

The appeal to "natural law" was a common refrain in the early twentieth century, an era in the shadow of Darwinism and the beginnings of the naturopathy medical movement. In Christian's mind, it was the place to start in considering what habits led to health.

"Disease is merely the outward expression or penalty for violated laws. Health is nature's reward for conformity to her laws," Christian put it plainly.[407] Cooking was one of the most basic transgressions of such laws. Humans must give up this artificial preparation of food if they'd like to be healthy. We'd do "well to remember" that uncooked foods have already "been prepared once by a supreme intelligence." And uncooked foods' "chemical properties have not been changed"

---

404   Ibid., 10

405   Ibid., 18

406   Ibid., 22

407   Ibid., 10

for the worse.[408,409] Cooked foods, of course, have been pathologically changed and the results of consuming such "artificialism," such "violation of natural law," is, bleakly, "extermination."[410] The perverting, the cooking, and the artificializing of food, also foments "abnormal desires" for "stimulants" like tobacco, tea, or alcohol.[411] Cooked food dulls the human mind and body and we seek a way out of the malaise.

Raw food, conversely, led to the total elimination of all health problems, Christian claimed. The raw diet was perfectly designed for humans. That's why Christian didn't prefer to name this original diet "raw." He thought the term was offensive; it didn't capture the majesty of nourishment in its ideal state. "Foods that have ripened and been brought to a state of maturity by nature," prepared by the perfect processes of the sun and the soil, should not merely be called 'raw,'" he argued.[412] He turned the tables on our perceptions—cooked food, in a sense, was the true "raw" or unfinished and inadequate food—it's "hopelessly raw," in fact, he charged. "Elementary foods" signifying the basic foods of life, was his preferred term for uncooked edibles.

Raw food was the food of the past as well as the future. This seemingly "new diet," was not really new after all, Christian pointed out. It was "the oldest of all diets readopted."[413] It was a return to the necessity of natural law.

Man "originated in the tropics, or the warmer belts of the earth's surface. His primitive food was plants," Christian explained.[414] "Primitive man was active, nimble and agile. Fruits left no deposits in his veins and arteries to age and stiffen them. Fruits made for him pure blood, and breathing the open air kept it pure."[415] Primitive man was apparently in perfect health.

In eating like primitive man, all raw food was included. Christian was not a raw food vegan like many raw foodists before and after him. Vegetarianism was his protocol. Milk was allowed and so were raw eggs. Raw cheese was also mentioned in numerous recipes. He consumed little greens it seems. The menu was mostly fruit, nuts, and milk.

---

[408] Ibid., 31

[409] Ibid., 20

[410] Ibid., 31

[411] Ibid., 39

[412] Ibid., 17

[413] Ibid., 8

[414] Ibid., 15

[415] Ibid., 42

Christian described nuts as such an "excellent article of food" that contains perfectly proportioned amounts of water, proteins, carbohydrates, mineral salts, and fat to sustain people.[416]

Spiritual Values of Raw Vegetarianism

*"To live rightly is to live simply, with foods untouched by fire,
as they are the truest sustenance for body and spirit."*
—**Eugene Christian**

America, in the early twentieth century, was beginning to spiritually awaken, Christian and other naturalistic hygienists like Latson believed. And spiritual awakening was a result of investigating and knowing what to eat. "The best talent in America, that throne and home of genius whose light and literature have encircled the world, is beginning to turn toward this question," *Uncooked Foods* proclaimed.

What did it take, conscious minds asked themselves, "to create a living thing, what gives it form, color and intelligence?" What was responsible for the quality of a person's body and mind? Food, of course, said Christian.

Unfortunately, nutritional science had hardly made any progress as of 1904: "All these things are as deeply buried in the realm of the unknown as they were a million years ago," Christian lamented. Nevertheless, one could begin on the right path towards nutritional truth by following basic principles of the universe. "All we know is that all life must comply with certain natural laws in order to be free."

It's amazing, he thought, that the fundamental question of diet, and its relation to physical and mental optimization, had been ignored for so long. The wealthiest people of every civilization throughout time had spent a fortune on grand monuments for posterity but nothing, "absolutely no thought or attention to the selection of the material out of which the body and brain are made."[417] The most critical facets of human existence were shamefully ignored.

But Christian had found that by addressing such questions, not only the human body, but perhaps most importantly, the human spirit would be taken to a higher level of prosperity. Humanity, fed with the right "elemental" raw foods, could experience "more sympathy, more affection and more love." Nutrition would bleed into the soul. Ele-

---

[416]   Ibid., 59

[417]   Ibid., 13.

mental foods would give people "higher senses of Mercy and Justice," which, Christian believed, "flow more freely from a fountain of robust health." A "higher civilization" is attainable when the physical well-being of people is attended to. The "body is a temple of the soul," after all, Christian said, a familiar argument throughout the history of raw foodism. A quality temple is the groundwork for a quality soul.

Elemental food facilitated high caliber and clear thinking. "Cooked foods clog the system and dull the mind," Christian said, while raw foods keep the faculties "clear and receptive." Cooked food is like a drug that stupefies the eater; raw food is like a soft inflow of caffeine, conducive to lucidity. And along with clarity comes a feeling of unity with existence. "When we eat foods as nature provides them, we align ourselves with the universal order, fostering harmony within." We stop fighting reality. We take it raw, without trying to transmute life in the cooking pan. We are at one with the way things are.

Latson, in the introduction to *Uncooked Foods*, had the same vision as Christian. With proper dietary practice, "the kingdom of self-knowledge, self-control and self-development" was at hand. Elemental foods were the foundation of virtue.

THE BODY AND THE NEW THOUGHT MOVEMENT

The interest in self-knowledge and self-development came to a cultural fever-pitch in the American New Thought movement of the nineteenth and twentieth century. The self-improvement focus of Christian and Latson fit right in with this movement.

The notion that people had power over their destiny, including their health and lifespan, affected Christian deeply, and was articulated in the American New Thought movement of the nineteenth and twentieth century. This would also influence future raw foodist Ann Wigmore, along with others, as we'll see later.

We could have total power over our bodies, raw foodists who were influenced by New Thought believed, if we had the right diet along with the right thinking, if we made use of uncooked food, affirmations and visualization techniques.

Non-raw-foodist New Thought representatives proclaimed that the mind had the power to create the material conditions of a person's life—outward circumstances as well as bodily health, New Thought apostles claimed that thought was practically the only thing that created one's reality. "Consciousness is the one and only reality," and an individual's thoughts and feelings were "the mechanism used in the production of the visible world," claimed New Thought writer Neville

Goddard. Even more clearly, "Nothing comes from without," he said. "All things come from within." The entire physical reality of your life came from only your thoughts.

New Thought gave its readers hope that they could accomplish anything if they implemented the right methods of positive thinking. Humans were cast as psychic co-creators with God. As a nineteenth-century New Thought pamphlet said, God is a spirit which "finds its highest expression through and as the mind of man." We are little gods, it taught. "We teach men," the pamphlet outlined, "the unity of themselves and God so that . . . they may say as the Master, 'I and the Father are one,'" as Jesus said.[418]

Along with the general circumstances of one's life, New Thought especially focused its positive thinking on empowering the health of the body. Thoughts were to be directed daily toward reinforcing a belief in one's healthiness. Thoughts had the power to alter or even conjure the surrounding material world, so how could they not affect your own body?

New Thought confidently heralded a new era of corporeal possibilities. Disease could be a thing of the past, as it's all in one's mental state. Many New Thought writers, including Prentice Mulford, Neville Goddard, Wallace Wattles, Warren Felt Evans, Phineas Quimby, and numerous others wrote with deep conviction about the mental origins of nearly all disease and the ability of the mind, once corrected, to heal the body. Physical health had earned a worshipful status in the works of New Thought-ers.

"Why comes so much of pain, grief, and disappointment in the physical life?" writer Prentice Mulford lamented. "Why do we seem born to suffer and decay?" Luckily, he felt, his right mental practices could fix the problems of the body and solve the painful realities of disease, aging, and suffering.

As Wallace Wattles wrote in 1910's "The Science of Being Well," it wasn't the medicines of allopathy or its opposite, homeopathy, or the shrines of saints' bones that healed people. It was the "principle of health" within them—in their beliefs. Mulford wrote near the end of the nineteenth century that your thoughts "shape your face . . . and the shape of your whole body" and that "beauty" and "perfect health . . . depend entirely on the state of your mind."

---

[418]   Braden, C. (1963). *Spirits in Rebellion; the Rise and Development of New Thought.* Southern Methodist Univ Pr, 14.

But New Thought-influenced raw foodists didn't believe that everything was purely metaphysical. They obviously thought that correct eating was a crucial part of determining one's health.

Raw food advocates like Christian and Latson believed that the tenets of New Thought had opened the minds of people to eat in new ways. Scanning history, Latson proclaimed, "In the early times [humanity] was a blind instrument in the hands of the Great Father. Blindly he worked and rested and slept." But now "man has graduated from the dull life of the flesh," from the unthinking life of reflexive instinct.[419] In these new times, "he would work harder, think deeper, aspire higher than his forefathers." In the process of remaking its mind and aspiring to loftier ways of living, new ways of thinking about nutrition were inevitable.

Those who were believed in the power of diet, like Christian and Latson, believed that raw food was the perfect accompaniment of this increased awareness.

But most people still wallowed in the low-awareness cooked-food mindset. Most of humanity was not living up nearly to its potential. "If man's present condition is imperfect and unnatural," asked Christian, "to what must it be attributed?"[420] Cooked food most certainly.

The state of women, Christian believed, was especially imperfect. Elemental foods, he was adamant, could liberate them from the constrictive bonds that society imposed on them.

Women's Liberation

"The stomach is a veritable gehenna, and the appetite its grizzly
gorgon that holds millions of women in a worse bondage
than the negro suffered in the South before the war."
—Eugene Christian

One of the spiritual and cultural transformations that Eugene Christian and his wife, Mollie Griswold Christian, sought to inspire was the liberation of women from the bondage of the time-consuming labor of cooking food.

"There is nothing more complicated—more laborious and more nerve-destroying, than the preparation of the alleged good dinner,"

---

[419]   Christian, E., & Christian, M. G. (1904). *Uncooked foods and how to use them: A treatise on how to get the highest form of animal energy from food, with recipes for preparation, healthful combinations and menus.* The Health-Culture Co. 8
[420]   Ibid., 10.

Christian pointed out.[421] Cooking was keeping American women (and women the world over) "imprisoned vassals" of tedious labor. They had no time or energy left over for any other pursuit; they were in a state of "slavery" to the ravenous and artificial desires of modern stomachs.[422] If people gave up the perverted desire for cooked food, this suffering of womanhood could be ended.

Cooking is extremely complicated and expensive, Christian noted.[423] Women were forced to cook "for an hour in the morning and breathe the poisonous odor of broiling flesh, and spend another hour among the grease and slime of pots and dishes, instead of occupying that time walking in the life-giving sunlight and drinking in nature's purifying air." They were confined in darkness and detached from nature. This confinement and labor is "little lighter than that which society puts upon the criminal."[424] Women were practically in prison.

Wives spend six or seven hours of each day preparing food, Christian estimated. The "mark" of this burdensome labor is "nervous exhaustion and premature old age."[425] Cooking is a torturous weight, "laid upon the delicate shoulders of woman," and society does nothing to alleviate this injustice.[426]

By eliminating cooking, we give "the wife enough mental and physical freedom to allow her to preserve her youthful charms, which is her solemn duty."[427] There's no need for worn-out, demoralized, and prematurely aged wives who've lost their beauty. If a family instead decides to eat raw, the wife can remain fresh and charming, not worn out by eating cooked food in addition to slaving over it. One of the great pleasures of life for a man, Christian says, is to have a wife that looks pretty, after all.

A sweet temperament is also a crown of a good wife. The quality of the food she makes and eats, beyond the question of the labor involved, creates the quality of her spirit. It is "impossible for a woman to construct her body, her brain and her heart with all their varied sympathies, desires and emotions out of such material as the flesh of dead animals, fermented fruit (wine), fermented bread and the innumerable narcotics and cooked or devitalized foods with which the average table is laden, and think beautiful thoughts and keep her sympathies." Dead

----

[421]   Ibid., 18.
[422]   Ibid., 22.
[423]   Ibid., 18.
[424]   Ibid., 22.
[425]   Ibid., 23.
[426]   Ibid., 33.
[427]   Ibid., 23.

food, dead spirit. "Making a perfect woman" with healthy emotions and graces, "lies in the selection of the food material."[428] Having a healthy spirit is not possible on a devitalized diet.

Christian and his wife said that if their book on uncooked food "contributes one degree to the elevation and freedom of woman, if it gives her one hour more of pure air and sunshine, if it gives her new thoughts, new dreams, new hopes . . . if in all the world it changes one hour of suffering to an hour of peace or pleasure," then their work has been "repaid."[429] Elemental food can change the whole emotional and aesthetic experience of women: pleasure, nature, and color are on the other side of the dark cooking dungeon. If Christian's book "shifts the scene from four dark walls hung with pots and bones to gardens and fields," the authors are satisfied—they have helped relieve the civilizational burden of women.[430]

DREAMER AFTER ALL

Along with the suffering imposed on the cooks, cooking causes the degeneration of our health. There's truly no purpose to cooking, Christian believed. But of course, his warnings did not make much of a dent in the American habits of the kitchen. His own premature death in his sixties would not have endeared his ideas to most people, especially since he promised his lifestyle would result in living to 100 or older. *Why Die?* he cheekily titled a 1928 book. Well, why did he choose to do so himself, one might wonder.

In the end, Christian did not accomplish the power he sought from raw foods, and succumbed to a common illness. Raw food, of course, also didn't save the mind of his friend Latson, who was in all likelihood demoralized when he passed. Neither of them stood out as shining examples of elementary food's powers. No great paradigm shift in longevity or social change happened. Nor were women the world over liberated from the cooking kitchen. But Christian's Supreme Court case freeing him as having specific agency to treat patients as a "food scientist" instead of a doctor helped pave the way for nutritionists and naturopaths to practice their distinctive forms of therapy without being strictly classified as medical practitioners. The one thing he did accomplish was giving future alternative practitioners more legal leeway in their unique methods.

---

428   Ibid., 23.

429   Ibid., 5.

430   Ibid., 6.

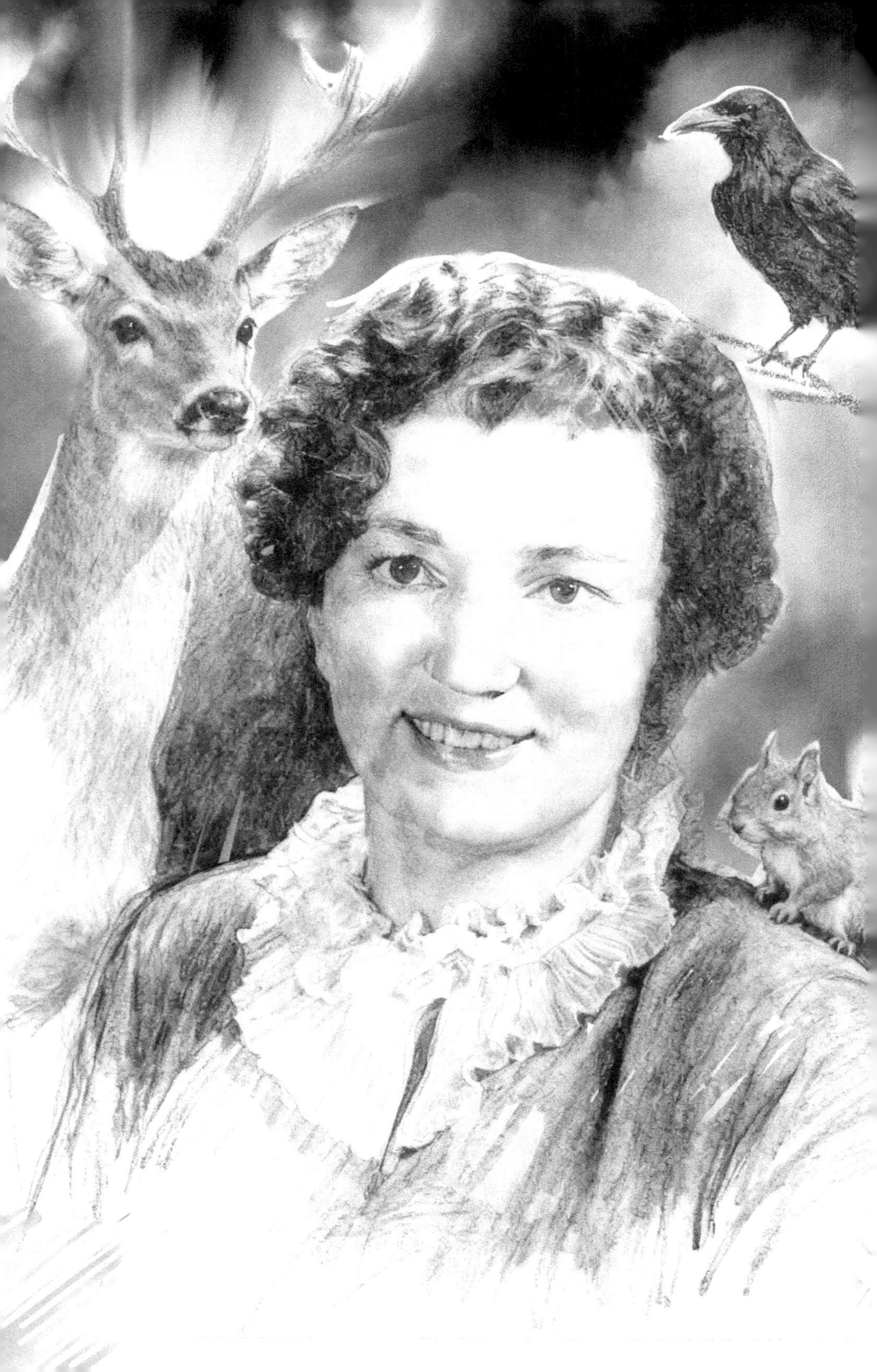

10.
Ann Wigmore:
The Faith-Filled Juicer

"As far back as I can recall, I was conscious of the comfort that only strong religious convictions can bring," Ann Wigmore wrote in her 1964 autobiography.[431] Throughout her life, she certainly had a strong conviction that raw food could heal the planet.

Wigmore must've had a feeling of comfort throughout her life, as a result of her distinct worldview and sense of her own moral clarity. Throughout her many trials, in war and peace, in experiences of deadly disease and vigorous health, in experiences of cruelty and natural hardship, Ann's faith in the benevolence of God helped her survive and stay on her mission.

"I learned that with faith, mountains of obstacles and doubt vanished," she said.[432] Her faith intensified as she survived a slew of challenges throughout the years: World War I-ravaged childhood in her native Lithuania, a treacherous immigration to America in the 1920s, hard labor, gangrene in her legs, and colon cancer.

Early on, her beloved grandmother instilled in her not only a faith in God but also beliefs about nature and food and their connection with God, that would guide her through the rest of her life.

AIDS AND OPPOSITION

In the 1980s, toward the end of her life, Ann was applying her strong religious convictions to a seemingly insurmountable obstacle: the AIDS crisis. In 1988, seven years after the first cases of AIDS were reported in the United States, the state of Massachusetts sued Wig-

---

431   Wigmore, Ann. *Why Suffer?* Book Publishing Company, 18 Jan. 2013, 7.

432   Ibid., 6.

more. The *Boston Globe* reported, "State Sues to Stop Woman Offering Remedies for AIDS." Her confident convictions got her into trouble.

The Massachusetts attorney general was targeting the dramatically optimistic health claims of this raw food advocate and pioneer of the use of wheatgrass juice. Wigmore had been distributing a booklet entitled, "Overcoming AIDS and other 'Incurable Diseases' the Attunitive Way Through Nature."[433] Wigmore was claiming that raw foodism and positive thinking could cure AIDS. The provocative title and shocking implications triggered the ire of government officials and healthcare professionals.

The state argued that the book, with its unsubstantiated health claims, was dangerous. It was also a problem that Wigmore did not have any commonly recognized medical credentials. Massachusetts sought to halt the the book's distribution. The state felt that people could die as a result of being duped by Wigmore's extreme bullishness.

AIDS only takes hold, Wigmore claimed, in vulnerable people with unhealthy immune systems. "I personally do not believe that AIDS is incurable," Wigmore wrote, "nor any other disease." "The AIDS virus," she boldly claimed, "would cause no problem in a detoxified, highly energized body that had adopted the living foods lifestyle." In an energized raw-fed body, the "self-protective mechanisms" fended off problems when the "laws of nature" were adhered to.[434] Doctors who said that the body couldn't repair an AIDS-damaged immune system, didn't understand the body's capabilities for self-healing, she declared.

AIDS was as serious as illnesses come, especially in 1988, and considered incurable. The year previous, 1987, saw the release of the first partially effective AIDS drug, AZT. But AZT could only slow down viral replication and delay AIDS progression, not halt it completely, and it was associated with significant side effects. It wasn't until 1995, and the introduction of protease inhibitors that effectively stop viral replication, that dramatic improvements in quality of life and survival were accomplished for AIDS sufferers.

But it was still 1988, and Ann was claiming she possessed a path to complete healing that didn't involve pharmaceutical drugs. By living according to the laws of nature, she argued, the body could heal from

---

[433]   Quill, Ed. "STATE SUES to STOP WOMAN OFFERING REMEDIES for AIDS." *Archive.org*, The Boston Globe (Boston, MA), 2015, web.archive.org/web/20150924200656/ www.highbeam.com/doc/1P2-8045670.html. Accessed 4 Mar. 2025; The Boston Globe. "JUDGE SAYS WOMAN CAN CLAIM AIDS CURE." *Archive.org*, 2025, web.archive.org/ web/20150810033341/www.highbeam.com/doc/1P2-8050504.html. Accessed 4 Mar. 2025.
[434]   Ibid., 25.

just about anything. Such a claim must've shocked and offended many people who had witnessed the abnormally virulent, cruel, and deadly effects of HIV and the resulting AIDS. Evidently, the attorney general of Massachusetts was one of those people.

Wigmore wrote of her childhood that the "physical helplessness" of sick adults in her village made a deep impression on her and that she was inspired by her caring grandmother's healing remedies that alleviated much of their suffering. Perhaps in the 1980s, she was inspired by a sympathy for AIDS sufferers along with her belief that it was her mission, as her grandmother instructed her before she emigrated to America, to help people there.[435] But the way she was going about that mission was potentially very dangerous for her HIV-positive readers and full of legal woes for herself.

She shocked society, including authorities, when she wrote that raw foodism could heal and prevent AIDS. A war was triggered. Officials would not stand for such childlike faith in the all-healing wisdom of nature, when it didn't seem realistic.

FALL OF EDEN: REBELLION AGAINST THE LAWS OF GOD'S NATURE

So what led Wigmore to develop such controversial beliefs about the power of raw foods?

As just noted, her faith in God pervaded her worldview and healing endeavors. It also gave her firm convictions that could get her into trouble. This faith could be considered unorthodox by some Christians, as it was influenced greatly by the New Thought movement and pantheistic thinking, as we'll see later. Nevertheless, Wigmore viewed God as a benevolent creator and caretaker, who gave humans, through nature, everything they need for a thriving and healthy life. Many raw foodists subscribe to a similar type of faith. It was only when humans, she felt, rebelled against nature and lived unnatural lives that they developed problems like mental and physical illness.

Rebellion against the laws of Mother Nature is a sin that would reap judgement. And in 1988 America, Ann perceived many unnatural sins. "We have abandoned Mother Nature and will pay the price for our folly," she claimed and cited the letter to Galatians from the New Testament: that "whatever a man sows, he will also reap, good or

---

[435] Wigmore, Ann. *Why Suffer?* Book Publishing Company, 18 Jan. 2013, 49.

evil."[436] This was not good news for most people, since "most people do not follow or understand the spiritual laws of Nature or God, and as a result they are lacking in . . . health, joy, or prosperity."[437] In our rebellion of ignorance and artificial lifestyles, "We have wandered away like sheep from our shepherd, (Nature, God)," she warned.[438] And as a result, the whole of our life suffered. Being ignorant, an average non-raw-foodist American would struggle to have joy and would also have an increased susceptibility to diseases like AIDS.

Americans were paying in pain and ill health, for their unnatural lives—their pollution of the air, consumption of processed and cooked food, their lack of sunlight exposure, and other "wanderings" from God's natural law. Spiritual toxicity accompanied physical toxicity. And the addiction to television helped ruin peoples' minds. TV was a "crime against the Divine God's intention for our lives" because of its portrayal of humans as naturally having uncontrollable sexual and violent appetites.[439] America was sick in mind and body.

Echoing Bircher-Benner's criticisms of civilization's effect on health, she proclaimed that "we cannot continue to live a synthetic lifestyle while inhabiting an organic body."[440] Wigmore's second half of the twentieth century, as compared to Bircher-Benner's first half, had become even more industrialized and technologized. Because of this "synthetic lifestyle," people were severely limiting their health potentials.

Earlier in life, Wigmore had "learned something about health: that the wild animal, unhampered by civilized restrictions . . . possesses energy and stamina even in times of want."[441] Not only is sickness banished when the laws of nature are properly followed, incredible endurance, that could little be imagined by people living artificially, would follow. This was the case in her own life, as when she was writing her AIDS book, Wigmore claimed that her raw food diet enabled her to work long hours on a tight self-imposed deadline, with only one hour of sleep each night, and at that point, she was in her seventies.[442]

By that age, she had proven to herself the merits of a raw "living foods" diet. She had, as a doctor friend said of her, returned to the

---

[436] Wigmore, Ann. 1987. *Overcoming AIDS and Other "Incurable Diseases": The Attunitive Way through Nature*. Boston: A. Wigmore, 25.

[437] *Ibid., 33.*

[438] Ibid., 31.

[439] Ibid., 32.

[440] Ibid., 40.

[441] Wigmore, Ann. *Why Suffer?* Book Publishing Company, 18 Jan. 2013, 5.

[442] Wigmore, Ann. 1987. *Overcoming AIDS and Other "Incurable Diseases": The Attunitive Way through Nature*. Boston: A. Wigmore, 1.

Biblical injunction that "every herb-bearing seed and fruit of the tree, shall be for you as meat," as stated in Genesis. She was living out the divinely instructed ideal. "She was given the responsibility to choose between life and death," the doctor said, "between living in accordance with the truths of nature, or the untruths of modern misguided man. And thus was born the living foods lifestyle." Raw foodism was the truth and the way.[443]

And so she tried to get others to live out the same truth. People could thrive in every way and no illness, including HIV, was beyond remedy if someone lived out the proper tenants of a living foods lifestyle.

THE LIVING FOODS LIFESTYLE

"The timeless truths of nature" that Wigmore and her followers revered were to be lived out through "the living food lifestyle"—a "total way of being" to which she dedicated her life.[444] Embracing nature and God required sustaining oneself with "simple, uncooked foods . . . vegetables, greens, fruit, sprouted seeds, grains, beans, and nuts, along with . . . vegetable juices."[445] Through these unadulterated uncooked foods, you imbibe the energetic power of God's nature.

Living foods were "the only solution to physical and mental problems," that plagued unnatural societies.[446] Combined with a proper mental attitude, raw foods were a panacea because they solved the twin causes of ill health, according to Wigmore—"toxemia" and nutrient deficiency. They were non-toxic and full of nutrients. They eliminated the issue of poor digestion and the inability to assimilate nutrition and thus solved the physical and emotional degeneration from which 80% of our population is suffering.[447]

The drug addiction that the Raegan administration fought in its War on Drugs, Wigmore pointed out, was the result of this widespread nutritional and emotional degeneration. Toxemia and deficiency were the root causes of the cravings for drugs and only raw food thoroughly solved these deep-seated issues. The nutritional science was still opaque as to why raw food was the only answer, Wigmore noted, but intuitively, she agreed with theories similar to Bircher-Ben-

---

[443]   Ibid., 4.

[444]   Ibid., 11.

[445]   Wigmore, Ann. *Why Suffer?* Book Publishing Company, 18 Jan. 2013, 149.

[446]   Wigmore, Ann. 1987. *Overcoming AIDS and Other "Incurable Diseases": The Attunitive Way through Nature*. Boston: A. Wigmore, 56.

[447]   Ibid., 11.

ner's—like his theory that raw foods transmitted the sun's perfectly organized energy to eaters.

Vitamins are "superior" and more absorbable in raw foods, as compared to supplements and other foods, because natural foods contain the high levels of sunlight energy, she claimed confidently, despite the fact that "little is known" about the particulars.[448] The "living forces" in raw foods are "separate and apart from materialistic concepts"—there were energetic realities within living foods that couldn't be understood by our current scientific paradigms. As an admiring doctor from Switzerland testified in Ann's AIDS book, "conventional nutritional scientists . . . neither search for nor discover the most important ingredient [in food]—life energy . . . weightless . . . shapeless" that raw foods contain. Vitamins in bottles are like "dead" batteries that can't compare to those in living foods that are energetically organized in just the right way so as to pass on their vitality to the eater.[449]

Because of their nearly mystical power, living foods energetically transform a person's life along with their body. Humans, the "most incredible electrical machine[s]," receive life giving electrical power into themselves and increase their "life energy."[450] The energy, the "living forces," in raw foods, such as solar energy and enzymes, are the "depository of the cosmic life forces," the vitality of the universe, Wigmore claimed vaguely.[451] Even though the science of materialism couldn't quantify these forces yet, more people were realizing by direct experience of their healing power that there was something special about living foods.

As mainstream science supposedly lagged behind, dietary pioneers were finding success in experimenting with a "diet for the new age" and finding nourishing solutions to fortify the body against the "increasing pressures of a space age society." Raw plant food was as old as time yet the food for the future. Meat, she dismissed as simply an antiquated obstruction to the body. Seeds and sprouts were superior forms of protein. They were more assimilable, devoid of the "toxins" in meat, and require less energy to digest. Meat, milk, eggs, and processed sugar "cannot be digested, due to their lack of enzymes." Space-aged humans should fill up on easily assimilated chlorophyll-rich foods instead, foods that capture the sun's energy and "cleanse the blood and rejuvenate new cells" while supplying adequate protein. Nutritional pioneers had also realized that human teeth, made for chewing for-

---

[448] Ibid., 14.

[449] Ibid., 5.

[450] Ibid., 19.

[451] Ibid., 47.

wards or backwards, unlike the carnivorous up and down motion of other creatures, were most suitable for "grains, seeds, vegetables, and fruits."[452] Get with the times and wake up, Wigmore implied.

Workaholic modern Americans, after all, could have more energy and be more productive on a raw diet. The energy usage (of electricity, natural gas, and human effort) and time spent on long cooked-food meal preparation could be done away with. Raw foodists would save money and their time.[453] Many meals would be made from quickly-blended smoothies and raw soups that would make people feel better, need less sleep, and allow them to accomplish more in life.

NATURE

"You cannot cheat Mother Nature. There are no shortcuts to health."
—Ann Wigmore

Wigmore's faith in raw foods and striking claims about the self-healing power of the human body, even when it came to the most fearful diseases, like AIDS, were actuated in large part by her early life experiences in Lithuania, which gave her an extraordinarily deep belief in the sentience of nature and its benevolence towards humans.

Wigmore was born in the "small, isolated village" of Cropos in Lithuania in 1909, on the eve of World War One. Her youth in this war-torn, impoverished rural landscape was full of trials—hard farm labor, marauding bands of raiders and soldiers, and later, financial despondency when the German marks she collected inflated beyond usefulness. But within this maelstrom and, at times, seeming hopelessness, Wigmore developed a symbiotic relationship with the natural landscape and claimed a striking intimacy, a "long association," with certain wild animals. She learned to revere the natural world, which was under the watchful care of God, who used nature as an outgrowth of his own love and care towards humans who were receptive to its power.

Stories of trusting relationships with squirrels, birds, mice, skunks, and other creatures filled Wigmore's account of her own childhood. The critters would gather comfortably on her own picnic cloth, sharing crumbs of rye bread. The providence of nature or "something seemed to bring the little animals, unafraid, to my side," she explained.[454] In

---

452   Ibid., 15.
453   Ibid., 68.
454   Wigmore, Ann. *Why Suffer?* Book Publishing Company, 18 Jan. 2013, 4.

one instance, a mother skunk rested on the girl and nursed her skunk babies, unthreatened by the close proximity of the human.[455] Wigmore also claimed to have had a friendship with a crow, who impressively turned from a "mere friend into an actual protector," warning her of threats and discriminating between suspect strangers and unthreatening familiar village acquaintances.[456]

In these harmonious intimacies with wildlife, Wigmore found "ample evidence that Mother Nature was kind, loving, and considerate."[457] Wildlife and the Earth itself were consciously aware and conspiring daily to aid humans. As she led sheep through the countryside, she later wrote, she could feel a oneness with all of creation: "I could feel the close connection that joins all human beings, animals, and plants."[458] The feeling inspired a spiritual calling. "Studying Nature's plan for this earth became the pattern for my everyday life."[459] Her studies continued with experiences of the healing effects of nature, in addition to its kindliness.

The young Wigmore was subjected to nature-based therapies devised by her intuitive grandmother, who was revered as a healer in their home village. To treat ailments, the grandmother sent her granddaughter to soak, up to her neck, in black mud on the edge of a swamp. After being inundated in its "health-giving substances," Wigmore soon noticed improved bodily proportions and that her indigestion and constipation had ceased.[460] It really worked, they felt, as her grandmother would often recommend, with great success, these mud baths to elderly people for the alleviation of arthritic aches and pains.

The Earth's healing powers were evident. Another therapy devised by Wigmore's grandmother involved resting at the foot of a large oak tree. She would cover the girl with leaves and sometimes leave her to sleep there through the night.[461] No explanation was given of the supposed efficacy of this therapy but it demonstrates Ann and her grandmother's belief that physical intimacy with the Earth had wide-ranging healing effects. When one lived "in harmony with God" and God's nature, "few problems of the physical body were unsolvable."[462] Inundation in healing soils, or resting at the root of a tree, were representa-

---

[455]   Ibid., 9.

[456]   Ibid., 15.

[457]   Ibid., 15.

[458]   Ibid., 16.

[459]   Ibid., 16.

[460]   Ibid., 10.

[461]   Ibid., 138.

[462]   Ibid., 6.

tions of embracing a natural lifestyle and the "the infinite wisdom of nature."[463]

Nature freely extended that wisdom to Wigmore, through plants and animals. During one of the mud baths that she took a frog leaped onto her face offering the young girl a warning, she and her grandma believed, of an incoming storm that wreaked havoc on the village. If Wigmore would've stayed in the mud, she could've been crushed by trees. She and her grandma were convinced that the frog functioned as an "angel" to warn her and save her life. As the Earth's mud healed her, the Earth's creature, the frog, had intelligently saved her life from a deadly situation. "There are angels everywhere to aid in time of need," her grandmother proclaimed—angels embodied in the animals that God created, like frogs and crows.[464]

During the AIDS crisis, later in her life, Wigmore would still believe her grandmother's notion that angels existed everywhere in nature, waiting to help those who were open to their influence. "A society," she would say, "which trusted Nature more than technology . . . would not be a victim to AIDS."[465] Instead of trusting the "modern day idol" of "scientific method" and waiting for pharmaceutical drugs to be developed, she wrote in her AIDS book, Americans should trust the ". . . the timeless truths of Nature" and heal themselves with raw food immediately.[466]

Considering her early life experiences, it makes sense that later in life, Wigmore realized that an even more powerful way to experience the healing effects of nature, as compared to mud bathing and other therapies, would be to consume its raw life force directly through living foods. Each unadulterated plant, after all, contained God's power or was like a little god in itself.

PANTHEISM AND PANENTHEISM

This "inspirational faith in nature" that an admirer later credited Wigmore for, had echoes of a pantheism and panentheism of which one can find instances throughout history.

Pantheism is the belief that "God is everything and that everything is God." The physical universe is God. Some pantheists say the statement "Nature is my god" is the simplest way of summarizing the

---

[463] Ibid., 16.

[464] Ibid., 10.

[465] Ibid., 27.

[466] Ibid., 5.

belief.[467] The Irish writer John Toland was the first to use the word *pantheist* in 1705, and he defined it as the belief that there is "no other eternal being but the universe."[468] The German philosopher Arthur Schopenhauer once remarked that pantheism was just polite atheism. This can be true to a degree since many pantheists do not believe in supernatural gods as entities with distinct personalities.

In Wigmore's case, she did believe in a supernatural creator—one whose power was expressed in nature and was constantly working out its purposes through nature. That's why Wigmore could be considered not quite a pantheist but a *panentheist*.

Panentheism is similar to pantheism in that it holds that God's presence pervades all of nature—but distinct from pantheism in that it holds that ultimately God exists superior to nature. It is a belief "in a personal creator God who transcends the world, but is also intimately present and active in the world."[469] Both pantheistic and panentheistic views have been expressed in the writings of the Stoics, Hindus, Daoists, Zen Buddhist monks, Romantic era poets, as well as Christian, Jewish, and Muslim mystics and Wigmore followed suit.

She detailed her religious framework—"All is under the supervision of our Father, whose divine energy acts through nature in constructive or destructive forms."[470] Every form in nature, whether seemingly scary or inviting, comes from God's design. As fellow pantheist/panentheist Marcus Aurelius said, there is "delight" in "the brow of a lion, the froth of a foaming wild boar" just as there should be delight in the "hanging down of grapes," because they both emanate from the "ruler and governor of all things." Delicious raw food, Wigmore would agree, is just as much a part of the Creator's power as a threatening lion.

"The most precious truth and the only reality are God's ways as expressed through Nature," Wigmore wrote.[471] Nature is the outpouring of God to us. "The tiny spear of grass [that] bursts its way through the earth . . . is an expression of God's energy in action," she wrote. God is alive in and through nature. He intelligently designed the laws of the universe and oversees their constant fulfillment. "God is the father, the law, energy and electricity . . . the law that governs all nature."[472] Just as

---

[467]   Harrison, Paul. *Elements of Pantheism : A Spirituality of Nature and the Universe*. Colorado (Colo.), 2013, 1.

[468]   Ibid., 28.

[469]   Ibid., 2.

[470]   Wigmore, Ann. 1987. *Overcoming AIDS and Other "Incurable Diseases": The Attunitive Way through Nature*. Boston: A. Wigmore, 84.

[471]   Wigmore, Ann. *Why Suffer?* Book Publishing Company, 18 Jan. 2013.. 61.

[472]   Ibid., 84.

Isaiah 6:3 and Jeremiah 23:24 proclaimed in the Bible, God's presence fills the whole universe.

Being infused with God's presence, the universe, and its planets, rocks, and vegetation is not just some lifeless backdrop for human life, meant to be ignored or exploited. It's alive. "Mother Earth . . . she is alive. Our planet is a living organism," Wigmore declared plainly. "The universe is one vast whole, all composed of Living Consciousness."[473] Plotinus, a philosopher in third-century Roman Egypt, similarly declared, "This universe is a single living being . . . possessing a single Soul that permeates all its parts."[474] Marcus Aurelius, before Plotinus, held the universe as "one living being, having one substance and soul." Wigmore was keeping the panentheism end up.

By revering the universe and living in harmony with it, Wigmore said, we return to a "faith in nature and God, which are one."[475] We evolve to a higher consciousness, leaving behind an ignorance about the meaning of nature, or at worst, the brutal exploitation of nature. By "respecting all lifeforms" and seeing God in them, we feel a unity with and love for them. Since we and every life form are expressions of God, we should "focus on our oneness with all life," including the Earth itself and know that a narrow, egoic "separated existence" that sees nature as expendable, "is not the truth."[476]

Not only is the panentheistic universe alive and infused with God; its "Living Consciousness" is active in engaging with the lives of humans, with guiding specially chosen people to fulfill its purposes. As a doctor admirer of Wigmore's said, Nature chooses "favorites" throughout history to pursue "preordained goals" by way of "providential guidance." These individuals are infused with "knowledge more profound than that which is ever contained in all . . . books."[477]

In Wigmore's case, that profound knowledge was the knowledge of raw food. God's nature had chosen her to reveal the truth of "living" nourishment to the world.

---

[473] Ibid., 92.

[474] Harrison, Paul. *Elements of Pantheism : A Spirituality of Nature and the Universe*. Colorado (Colo.), 2013, 20.

[475] Wigmore, Ann. 1987. *Overcoming AIDS and Other "Incurable Diseases": The Attunitive Way through Nature*. Boston: A. Wigmore, 85.

[476] Ibid., 129.

[477] Ibid., 17.

PANENTHEISTIC PHYSIOLOGY AND SUNRISE CHRISTIANITY

*"One of the reasons I joined the religious school . . .
was to bring about this healing in my body."*
—Ann Wigmore

Raw Foodism was a natural consequence of Wigmore's panentheism and early life immersion in nature.

If nature was infused with supernatural intelligence, and if God designed and oversaw the workings of nature, then nature would surely supply humans with perfectly nourishing food infused with all the complex qualities of an intelligent creator.

Wigmore's raw foodism was based on this panentheistic assumption that nature contained the highest wisdom imaginable. A blade of grass, a leaf, a flower, and a "weed" take on a deeper meaning, and a wholly different nutritional meaning, when they're seen as containing the complex design and loving intentions of a creator God. Rather than only being seen as pretty things, ignored aspects of a landscape, or pesky weeds that threaten a garden's health, these plants are perceived as cosmic keys to healing and empowerment.

People who are ignorant of panentheistic truth have no reverence for nature and are bound to make their meals of adulterated things like refined grains, that are stripped of their natural fibers, or diced up animal flesh fried in a pan. It makes a quick meal of expedient slop and condensed calories, good a few moments of cheap pleasure. A conscious mind that has reverence for God's universe, on the other hand, yearns for a direct intimacy with nature's unadulterated, unprocessed, uncooked perfection. It seeks plant food raw, plucked right from the ground or the tree. Food full of "living" enzymes, chlorophyll, undamaged nutrients, and most importantly of all, intricate energy patterns that nourish the body and mind.

By eating raw, one would follow Wigmore's suggestion to "trust nature to take its natural course within you." One imbibes the theological significance that "Nature and God are one," and feels the effects of this truth in one's body. You trust God and benefit from his care and power "by choosing the . . . living food lifestyle," Wigmore said.

This mindset also facilitates a brand new view of the body, in addition to the universe. It is not just a machine meant to be used and abused for a few decades. It is a sacred temple that houses a piece of God—your soul. Wigmore says that, "by taking responsibility for our body, as a temple of the God within, all the evidence indicates that we will be protected [from disease]." When we care for our body like we would a beautiful temple, keeping it clean, pure, and tending to the hallowed objects or organs within, "we live as the Creator intended—in communion with the divine God-self within each of us."[478] We wouldn't seek to house God, or a "God-self" in a filthy or structurally unsound building—so neither should we house ourselves in a body filled and built with corrupted cooked food.

It was this taking of stock of the sacredness of the universe and the natural physical objects within it—plants, animals, and humans—that convinced Wigmore to adjust her Christian faith to include a care for the body and not just the soul.

She had an epiphany when her friend, a Doctor Shadman, whom Wigmore considered to be an impressively progressive medical doctor who practiced homeopathy, argued to her that "churches, as we know them, fall short of their possibilities. They seem to [only] concentrate on the development of the soul." What the churches forgot, Shadman added, is that "spiritual needs" and "physical natural laws" are intertwined. "A minister of the gospel should have a dual capacity. He should watch over his congregation, both spiritually and physically," he argued.[479] The body, wedded to the soul, was important for its spiritual prospering.

Wigmore took these words to heart and realized that a reverence for the sacredness of the physical aspects of existence had been forgotten in modern Christianity. Wigmore found herself "overwhelmed" at Shadman's wisdom, when he pronounced, "I have hoped that those might come along who would appreciate the necessity of each human being housing his or her spark of God in a temple worthy of the preciousness of life," that is, that we honor God with our bodies.[480] Wigmore felt a thrill of excitement as she believed she was the person for such a task.

Enlightened by Dr. Shadman, Wigmore had awakened to a new form of Christianity that she called "rising Sun Christianity," which "uniquely emphasized the importance of healing the whole person, physically . . . and spiritually."[481] She had a new understanding of the Biblical phrase about "building" God's "temples"— "instead of structures of brick and stone, it meant bodies of flesh and blood," she declared.

---

[478] Ibid., 27.

[479] Wigmore, Ann. *Why Suffer?* Book Publishing Company, 18 Jan. 2013, 82.

[480] Ibid.

[481] Ibid., 85.

"Only through healing the body was spiritual unfoldment possible," she said of her newly defined beliefs.[482] She set out to wake the world up to the importance of the body and God's presence in material things by explaining to them the panentheist Christianity of what Ann called a "New Age."

Through this supposedly more conscious lens, Wigmore uncovered new interpretations of Biblical texts. A story in the Old Testament Book of Nehemiah caught her attention. The Israelites had wandered into the Arabian desert where farming was impossible, yet somehow God "sustained" the Israelites for forty years. Wigmore concluded that it was nutrient-dense raw wild vegetation that had supplied their sustenance. The Israelites realized that plants that humans had previously ignored and regarded as "useless" helped their stranded tribe thrive in a desolate landscape. From interpretations like this, Wigmore had realized in the 1960s that "slavery to the kitchen stove" and "greasy pans"—the world of cooked food—could be "cast aside forever."[483] Even weeds, raw weeds, could provide vitamins, minerals, and trace elements that would give us "health, strength, and youthfulness."[484] The uncooked grass and other plant foods were all that was needed.

A similarly unorthodox interpretation of the Book of Daniel's story of the Babylonian king Nebuchadnezzar, who lost, in her words, his "mentality and his physical well-being" along with his throne and was instructed by God to live in the wilderness and "eat grass as did the oxen."[485] A traditional interpretation of this story holds that eating grass was a shameful punishment for the king's excessive pride and his challenging of God's supreme authority. But Ann focused on the therapeutic effects of Nebuchadnezzar's grass diet, as if it were a healing dietary regimen prescribed by God. After a period of eating grass, the king does regain his throne and mental health. Eating grass, to Wigmore, was a cure and almost a privilege, and not primarily a shameful punishment of exile and subhuman existence.

These interpretations occured alongside Wigmore's personal experimentation with nutrition. After studying the nutritional potential of different kinds of grasses and being the most impressed with wheat grass, the first leaves of the wheat plant, she was surprised that more attention had not been previously given to this superfood.[486] She started juicing the grass for herself, believing it to be the most easily digest-

---

[482]   Ibid.

[483]   Ibd., 92.

[484]   Ibid., 94.

[485]   Ibd., 100.

[486]   Ibid., 101.

ible way of consuming it and then decided to test wheatgrass's healing properties on ailing seniors. She witnessed numerous improvements in health among these frail elderly people. After a few weeks of serving them wheatgrass juice, to get dense raw nutrition into their systems, bedridden "incurables" at least had the strength to be more active, get out of bed, and feel better than they had in years.[487] In more dramatic cases, cancers were allegedly cured after just a few weeks of wheatgrass juice. Some animals even healed from her juice. Wigmore was convinced, by study and experience, that wheat grass juice was "the richest nutritional liquid known to man" and that the Bible had given us a clue to this fact.[488]

Soon, Wigmore found that adding a raw vegetable salad, including buckwheat lettuce, sunflower greens, carrots, and sprouts, with a dressing made of seed or nuts, was particularly effective at healing people.[489] By trusting the foods of nature and what she interpreted as God's instructions to eat raw, Wigmore found that raw foods could provide all the nutrients that the body needed—plenty of vitamins, minerals, and even protein. And she didn't even have to buy dairy salad dressing—the plant world provided nuts and seeds to add creaminess to her leafy greens.

Ann would go on to implement her panentheist raw foodist regimen on many and fulfill her physiological-religious quest. One patient, a frail Syrian Catholic bishop, found that his strength improved on raw plant foods and his description of his healing, which blurred the lines between the physical and spiritual, affirmed the outlook of Wigmore's "sunrise Christianity." "My constipation," he testified, "has almost been eliminated and new life, new ambition, new hope is rising in me. It is almost like being born again."[490] Eating raw seemed like a spiritual experience; it seemed like salvation.

New Thought, New Spirit, New Lifespan

This spiritual health quest stood on the foundation created by the New Thought movement. Just like Eugene Christian before her, Wigmore was intrigued by the enormous possibilities that such a movement brought to mind. To have control over one's destiny, including disease and lifespan, was a seductive idea that she embraced.

---

487   Ibid., 107.
488   Ibid., 104.
489   Ibid., 113.
490   Ibid., 121.

The New Thought movement that preceded Wigmore heralded a new paradigm about the human lifespan. Eternity was the limit. Prentice Mulford, for instance, was not talking about a disembodied afterlife or a traditional Christian resurrection upon the eventual return of Christ when he proclaimed that our lifespans are indefinite. "We believe that immortality in the flesh is a possibility . . . that the physical body can be retained so long as the spirit desires its use." Mulford's claims were shocking and explicit. The human body, in its current form, could live on forever so long as the spirit wanted it to. "The body is always an external correspondence of your mind or spirit." The only thing that caused people to be "bowed down by age" was that they believed in this "perishable" state—they had "faith in weakness and decay." They expected it, so it happened. As time went on, Mulford believed, and humans became more aware of their spiritual power and the "God within," more people will be able to "spiritualize" their bodies, make them ever more correspondent to their timeless soul, and materialize a limitless lifespan. The unspiritual "carnal" mind, noted Mulford, "says we must accept a standard" of disease and aging made by others of the past. But the New Thought consciousness was shattering those old standards.

Wigmore held similar views on lifespan but raw food, of course, played a big role in achieving a long life. From what she wrote, there's little reason to believe that she did *not* think that lifespan was practically indefinite. In her AIDS book, she wrote that "once we consume only living food . . . the cells can regenerate themselves, perpetually, and indefinitely keep us free from sickness and old age, if we wish to take the responsibility."[491] It was a choice. It was up to us. We could live raw forever, she seems to say; with regard to health in general, she said, "You make the choice to live or not to live." "You determine your destiny . . . you are the Master"—words that almost read as if extracted from a New Thought text.[492]

Being true to her viewpoint, in her own life, she didn't absolve herself of culpability in her own health troubles. Her AIDS book states that "in her early fifties, she contracted colon cancer, as a consequence of her irresponsibility."[493]

If a person did take responsibility and lived the way nature intended, human lifespan should be at least 250 years. She put her unique Biblical interpretation skills to the task of describing a verse in the

---

[491] Wigmore, Ann. 1987. *Overcoming AIDS and Other "Incurable Diseases": The Attunitive Way through Nature*. Boston: A. Wigmore, 20.

[492] Ibid., 74.

[493] Ibid., 4.

Book of Psalms by saying, "It is predicted in the scriptures, that 'He shall renew his youth like the eagle.'"The eagle lives 250 years, she said, therefore, this means the "body can renew itself as long as we wish," or at least up to that point.

While infused with an extreme optimism and belief in self-empowerment similar to New Thought, Wigmore differed from them in believing diet, as opposed to just thought, to be the most important guarantor of a long life. The quality of your food, and most importantly whether it was cooked or raw, was the foundation of health and disease.

Also, in her outline of health, the body and mind were a dual-feedback system. The mind could affect the body tremendously but the physical toxicity and malnutrition that plagued people on unhealthy cooked-food diets hugely affected their minds. Without raw "living" food, the "proper fuel" for humans, it could be difficult to conjure the energy, good mood, or high quality awareness needed for New Thought-type productive positive thinking. It was raw food that fed the "extremely delicate" nervous system and thus consciousness.[494] Living food with material nutrients and solar energy were keys to building a powerful mentality, motivation, and spiritual intuition. "Light eating is the key to energy. Living Food is a new, dynamic way to approach your whole life," Wigmore claimed.[495] Raw food was key, in her scheme, for "Expanded awareness and personal growth." Food became spirit.

To accomplish our goals, Wigmore believed, we need intuition to decipher the right paths to follow—ideal routes given to us by God. "People who eat heavy foods get soot on their antennas and thus cannot receive the messages coming from the Universal God Mind," she stated in *Overcoming AIDS . . .*[496] If deluged with cooked foods, we might fail to conjure the right feelings or "creative process" needed for the "manifestation" of our goals, as New Thought author Neville Goddard described.

To achieve "self-expression" was the primary goal in life, Wigmore believed, because God wished to express himself through humans and He created us to be "co-creators" with him. Your ability to be a co-creator would be greatly diminished if there was "soot" on your spiritual signal receivers—your "antennas." "God has created all things for self-expression," and has given us a guiding voice of "what we are and

---

[494]   Ibid., 19.

[495]   Ibid., 30.

[496]   Ibid., 34

why we are here," according to her.[497] But cooked foods risked us not being able to even receive that guiding voice. Our fleshly machinery had to be fed by living foods.

The life extension that New Thought leaders touted, as well as our ability to creatively shape our destinies, were only possible "once we consume only living food," Wigmore made plain.[498] Cooked "poison" was not permissible. Nutrition was the foundation for actualization, both physical and spiritual.

BECOMING A MASTER OF LIFE AND BODY

"Health is what one makes of it."
—**Ann Wigmore**

"It is the one thing impossible for man to take this quality out of his own spirit—the quality of ever rising toward more power and happiness."
—**Prentice Mulford,** *Thoughts are Things*

Both Wigmore and the New Thought philosophers were fixated on personal empowerment. Both sought an entirely new degree of control over personal health and destiny in general.

What was the purpose of life? Besides happiness through self-expression, it was to make the "temples of God," which Wigmore and Prentice Mulford both imagined human bodies to be, "rise superior to sickness or pain." It was "to command the body, through the power of the spirit," according to Mulford.

"Each individual is the engineer and guardian of his own body and mind. We have great responsibility for our own bodies," Wigmore claimed.[499] Prentice Mulford concurred that there was "power" available to us "greater than men and women now possess and enjoy." You had to take charge. You had to admit that you, in a sense, created your body and were responsible for its destiny. You had to eat raw, warned Wigmore, and complement that with New Thought-like positive thinking.

The meaning and success of our lives, though, in Wigmore's mind, were derived from more than just the state of our body—we had life to live, tasks and journeys to undertake, relationships to build. But our body and its health were the foundation from which we built our

---

497   Ibid., 84.
498   Ibid., 56.
499   Ibid., 38.

spirits and the other parts of our lives. "The better we understand our own bodily needs," she said straightforwardly, the better "we are truly fulfilling the purpose of life on this planet."[500] Our bodies determined how we felt, how we perceived the world, the quality of the energy that we put out into the world, and how we received divine instructions for our lives. The state of our bodies was connected to our purposes.

"Our bodies and our minds are priceless" because we are "human beings, whose destiny has always been God's co-creators," she said, echoing New Thought (as Neville Goddard wrote, "man has control over creation").[501] To become a co-creator, and a "free agent in control of one's life," in Wigmore's words, we need to be fed with the right beliefs and living food. We have to have strong minds and bodies to act with near-divine powers of creation. Those who fail to achieve personal power in life and bodily health have "not enough of a sense of selfhood or self-esteem, to experience any power in life, or to find satisfaction in life and thus they are motivated to escape from self-awareness."[502] Spiritual qualities like self-awareness, in Wigmore's mind, were deeply tied to one's diet and one's ability to exert agency over personal habits. People who rejected living foods and their spiritual responsibilities as co-creators with God, are apt to escape from the painful feelings of their disempowerment by taking drugs or numbing themselves with cooked food.

But for those who chose to adopt their true responsibilities in life and enact positive change in the world, they must add spiritual values to the right diet. They must build their self-esteem to be worthy of god-like power. They must, Wigmore told them, "become the person you want to be" and conquer "low self-esteem." Along with banishing toxic food, people must banish limiting beliefs and emotions. "BANISH self-defeating guilt," she told readers.[503]

Wigmore's faith in God, Nature, her self-esteem, and sense of purpose helped her gain some level of this "power in life." She overcame a stifling marriage with an overbearing husband as well as conservative religious leaders who wouldn't allow her, as a woman, to hold any institutional authority in Christian circles she was involved in.

Wigmore believed that we could manifest our desires if we successfully visualized their reality. This could happen if humans realized what she called "the full potential of our brainpower," the "divine en-

---

[500] Ibid., 84.
[501] Ibid.
[502] Ibid., 29.
[503] Ibid.

ergy" within, or "our true nature as expressions of God."[504] Neville Goddard believed similarly that the "creative process" of "imagining and then believing the state imagined could make dreams come true." Similarly, Wigmore claimed that "the true function of the will is to act upon the ... subconscious ... that can produce the desired effects."[505]

As part of a raw foods lifestyle and in the service of healing ailments, Wigmore discussed achieving "relaxation of body and mind" to "visualize and thereby manifest." Relax and visualize your body in a healed state, she instructed. Goddard wrote decades earlier, "To yield successfully to the wish as an accomplished fact, you must create a passive state, a kind of reverie" in which you are "assuming the feeling of the wish fulfilled."

Not by forcing things to happen, Wigmore guided, but by "relaxing and allowing the possibilities that already exist to manifest" will the healing process be materialized.[506] "The divine energy must radiate brightly" and it will do so if we guard over the "kinds of vibrations we are allowing into our lives and consciousness"—vibrations of both thoughts and food.[507]

There was no tragic situation that was insurmountable. She was passionate about implementing the power of living foods and optimistic visualization techniques even in the context of HIV. "My solution to AIDS," Wigmore declared boldly, is to teach AIDS victims the following: They must believe in their body's ability to heal itself."[508] Hold tight to the mast, even after the direst diagnosis, she instructed. Only in taking "responsibility" for one's diet and quality of thoughts could an AIDS patient achieve full healing. She urged them to impress upon their conscious and subconscious mind the affirmation, which some might take as cruel: "I take full responsibility for my life and for what I create through my thoughts and actions."[509] It shocked many, as noted earlier, to see that Wigmore was attributing one of the most extreme and fast-progressing illnesses, AIDS, to one's thoughts and diet. A long-term degenerative disease like atherosclerosis could be more closely connected to one's habits but connecting diet and thoughts with a virus, HIV, that took the lives of young people just a couple years after contraction, was quite an unpopular framing. But Wigmore held very firm in

---

504   Ibid., 31.
505   Ibid., 217.
506   Ibid., 33.
507   Ibid., 128.
508   Ibid., 71.
509   Ibid., 68.

her belief that thoughts create reality and that raw foodism could build such a powerful immune system that no virus could survive.

Her belief in God's perfect design of nature and the healing power of its food, along with the power of our minds, could not be shaken by the most daunting of illnesses.

DEATH BY FIRE

At age eighty-four, in 1994, Ann Wigmore was said to be in "remarkable" and "peak" health.[510] Nevertheless, tragedy struck. Somehow, as she was sleeping at her foundation headquarters in Boston on the third floor, a fire broke out. Some escaped the building where she taught her raw doctrine, but Ann was trapped. She died in the early morning hours from smoke inhalation.

Ironically, the effects of fire and heat—those enemies of Wigmore's system of raw living, those forces that corrupted natural food, had taken her life. Some trapping of modern life, perhaps an electrical heating system, had killed her, despite her embrace of the most ancient way of eating. No doubt that she planned on living for decades to come and continue her work.

Her work lived on though, through the Ann Wigmore Foundation and the Hippocrates Health Institute (a raw vegan spa retreat in Florida)—two entities she built. Her teachings on wheatgrass therapy and living foods would live on into the following decades. Wheatgrass became a popular drink in juice bars, smoothie shops, and wellness stores.

---

[510] "Ann Wigmore." *Vegetarian Times,* Apr. 1994, 18.

Modern and New Age Raw Foodism

The Industrial Age raw foodism of the 1800s and 1900s was promoted largely by earnest physicians like Benner-Bircher or political figures like Gandhi and Hitler. Nearly all of these people believed that raw food had spiritual implications.

The supposed spiritual implications of raw food would be detailed in more expansive ways in the internet age—the 1990s until the present moment. A New Age raw foodism arose, especially in the early 2000s and had its roots in the hippy era of the 1960s and 70s.

We will also explore the beliefs, unrelated to the New Age, of fringe Christians who have attempted to wed their Biblical beliefs with a strict adherence to uncooked food.

Raw food advocacy in the modern age would also take on a more intense focus on aesthetic effects of the diet. Occasionally, new concerns, like ecology, would also factor into raw foodists' motivations. Even the aesthetics of gender entered the raw food conversation. Some advocates would note how raw food accentuated their masculinity or femininity.

In this latest age of raw foodism, advocates still believed that the diet would have phenomenal, far-reaching effects beyond the improvement of health. The spiritualization tradition of raw foodism lived on.

11.
Ecological and Evolutionary Raw Veganism

Eating for Ecology

Spirituality, personal health, and politics aren't the only motivations for the adoption of a raw food diet. Ecology was also in the mix.

Over 200 years after the Industrial Revolution, environmental destruction and toxicity has plagued the world. Noxious substances unleashed by human industry have tainted water systems, soil, and air. Worries about climate change and forecasts of planetary disaster have burdened the minds of many.

These concerns about environmental degradation have spawned a search for solutions from a vast array of professionals in various fields. Scientists, technologists, politicians, agronomists, engineers and even a raw foodist philosophy professor have chimed in on how we can avoid ecological catastrophe.

Carlo Alvaro, that philosophy professor, at New York City's College of Technology since 2011, published a book in 2020 on raw vegan diets and their relationship to personal and planetary health. He argued that our food choices can decelerate or accelerate climate change and are interconnected with the health of the earth. Specifically, both the consumption of animal products and cooked foods, he argues, contribute to environmental degradation and climate change.

Meat, Cooking, and the Environment

For Carlo Alvaro, veganism is the first step toward repairing the natural environment. It's long been a common argument that the livestock industry is one of the primary causes of environmental destruction. Proponents of this argument claim that the massive amount of deforestation that occurs to make room for raising livestock increases the amount of global-warming-causing carbon dioxide in the atmosphere. Two of the most important carbon dioxide-producing side effects of deforestation are that trees help absorb carbon dioxide from the air (so, removing the trees eliminates their beneficial carbon dioxide-sequestering effects) and that the carbon dioxide already stored in trees is released into the atmosphere when they're cut or burned. It's also noted that carbon dioxide and methane that livestock produce themselves from flatulence and manure also contributes to an excess of greenhouse gasses.

In setting the foundation for his raw vegan beliefs, Alvaro argues for lesser-known potential ecological dangers of livestock farming. Raising livestock means more water usage and more energy consumption from fossil fuels and electricity· The energy usage required in clear-cutting forests as well as feeding, transporting, and killing animals pollutes and warms the world, he argues.

The livestock industry uses and pollutes more freshwater than any other sector, Alvaro claims. The phosphorus fertilizers that livestock raisers apply to farmlands, in order to replenish the soil after intensive animal agriculture, seep into the world's water systems, causing the excessive growth of oxygen-stealing algae, which leads to low oxygen levels in rivers and seas, and causes the "suffocation of aquatic ecosystems."[511] Vegan diets, along with minimizing energy consumption and deforestation, cause less water consumption and help safeguard water quality.

But the kicker to Alvaro's ecological arguments for dietary change is that veganism, in itself, is not good enough. Alvaro believes that humans must go beyond just dumping animal products. Cooking should also be given up for the sake of the planet.

"Veganism," he clarifies, "is more ethical and more environmentally friendly than using animals for food." "Still it is not the most ethical and the most environmentally friendly approach," he says. Cooking itself still does harm to the planet. "After all, cooking requires the use of ovens, stovetops, microwave ovens, which use coal, wood, gas, and electricity," Alvaro points out.[512] The various forms of energy used during cooking emit greenhouse gasses. Cooking in homes, restaurants, and

---

[511]   Alvaro, Carlo. *Raw Veganism : The Philosophy of the Human Diet.* Abingdon, Oxon, Routledge, 2020, 92.

[512]   Ibid., 3.

food production factories all add to worldwide energy usage and its consequences.

Alvaro argues that raw vegan diets, compared to cooked vegan diets, require less dishwashing and the resulting water and detergent use. By using less detergents, we'd cut down on plastic waste and phosphorus, chlorine, and other compounds that are detrimental to the environment in excessive amounts.[513]

Other vegan advocates have joined Alvaro in lauding the especially environmentally-friendly aspects of uncooked diets. All-Creatures. org, a Biblically influenced animal rights and environmental advocacy group, notes the possibility of reducing the "tremendous destruction of the earth" caused by cooking.[514] Raw food diets could reduce the amount of pots, pans, stoves, microwaves, ovens, toasters, and other equipment that have to be manufactured to support cooked lifestyles. The "mining and production of metals and plastics" that occur from manufacturing of such instruments could be reduced. Shipping, like trucking, the plethora of cooked food products would also be reduced, All-Creatures.org claims: "The resources needed to manufacture, house, maintain, transport, distribute, promote and sell all of these enterprises and their products are incalculable."[515]

If someone is eating a raw food diet, they are likely getting some of their fresh produce locally, cutting down on transportation emissions and the industrial processes used to package some cooked food. A salad made from one's garden or a local farmer's market is surely cutting down on environmental destruction, compared to a cooked TV dinner or other packaged foods which require canning, freezing, and more plastic packing.

These other vegan advocates agree with Alvaro that raw veganism is the ultimate environmentally protective diet. Mere vegan diets—that is, cooked vegan diets, some of which are grain and soy based, still can contribute hugely to the brutal forms of agriculture in which all forms of life are "subjugated" to the expedient desires of the food industry and by which millions of tons of pesticides, herbicides, fungicides, and chemical fertilizers poison the earth.[516]

---

[513] Ibid.

[514] Miller, Rob . "Raw Vegan vs Cooked Vegan." *All-Creatures.org*, 2006, www.all-creatures. org/articles/rawvegan.html. Accessed 7 Mar. 2025.

[515] Ibid.

[516] Ibid.

Rawness Saves the Earth

Corporations often trick unwitting cooked-food vegans into taking part in expedient environmental destruction. Unlike raw veganism, cooked food veganism still destroys the environment.

By using "pop philosophy and ethics, pseudo-science, and fashion," Alvaro says, to portray cooked vegan junk food as "automatically healthful," food companies involve the consumer in their perpetuation of environmental degradation under a veneer of benevolence and implied healthiness.[517] Unfortunately, when cooked-food vegans purchase a vegan meal from a large food chain, they support businesses that perpetuate environmental destruction. Often, these large corporations manufacture or serve animal products as well, so vegans are reinforcing the companies' non-vegan profits and facilitating the livestock industry.

Many vegan meat-replacement products, frequently used by some who eat largely cooked vegan diets, mimic meat patties. Companies package them in a similar fashion to meat, use unhealthy cooking methods to replicate tastes and looks similar to actual meat, and even attempt to produce a "blood" dripping effect of the meat replacement by adding beet juice. This mimicry of actual meat is counterproductive for veganism in Alvaro's opinion and reinforces the "notion that eating animals is the norm" and that these meat replacements are freakish but fun replacements for the "the real deal"—actual meat.[518] The end result of this meat-mimicry and cynical marketing technique is a psychologized reinforcement of meat consumption, excessive plastic packaging, and the elevation of profit at the expense of the environment and human health.

These processed meat substitutes are, ecologically, similarly destructive as meat production, as research has shown—some cooked "plant-based meat substitutes in certain conditions could have a carbon footprint very similar to that of chicken meat, and in terms of resource demand (land, energy, and water), it could be even higher."[519] One recent study has shown that some processed meat replacements have "1.6–7 times higher environmental impact" than less processed,

---

[517]   Alvaro, Carlo. *Raw Veganism : The Philosophy of the Human Diet*. Abingdon, Oxon, Routledge, 2020, 84.

[518]   Ibid., 85.

[519]   Smetana, Sergiy, et al. "Meat Substitutes: Resource Demands and Environmental Footprints." *Resources, Conservation and Recycling*, vol. 190, no. 106831, Mar. 2023, 106831, https://doi.org/10.1016/j.resconrec.2022.106831.

more traditional plant protein sources like tofu, pulses, and peas.[520] And raw plant foods, of course, are less environmentally damaging than even traditional cooked plant proteins because there is less energy used in preparing them.

Cooking and the livestock industry, according to Alvaro, are also not conducive to human health. The micro-ecosystem of the human body can be poisoned by cooking as well as by the environmental impacts of animal agriculture.

THE CONNECTION BETWEEN THE BODILY AND PLANETARY ECOSYSTEMS

The environment doesn't stand alone. It provides the context for, is connected to, and even seeps into every living thing on the planet. The landscape of the planet affects, to some degree, each individual's inner physiological landscape. The trillions of cells inside your body, as well as the trillions of foreign (but symbiotic) bacteria in our intestines respond to the air we breathe, the water we drink, and the pollutants in our food.

This interconnectivity between the human body and the surrounding landscape is one of the reasons advocates like Alvaro are concerned with the connection between our eating habits and both the external environment and our internal environments.

The World Health Organization estimates that 99% of the world's population breathes polluted air that exceeds the organization's guideline limits. Soil and water are similarly vulnerable as they can be poisoned by just about anything. Crops grown in tainted soil suck up the embedded pollutants and can be unfit for consumption. Pollutants from our air, water, and food like toxic metals, plastics, synthetic pesticides, and a multitude of other toxic byproducts of industrial processes can accumulate in our tissues over time in a process called bioaccumulation.[521] Most people have some degree of toxic pollutants including heavy metals, flame retardants, and pesticide residues within their bodies.[522] And both cooking and the consumption of animal products

---

[520]   Ibid.

[521]   McLachlan, Michael S., et al. "Bioaccumulation of Organic Contaminants in Humans: A Multimedia Perspective and the Importance of Biotransformation." *Environmental Science & Technology*, vol. 45, no. 1, 11 Aug. 2010, 197–202, https://doi.org/10.1021/es101000w. Accessed 14 Feb. 2025.

[522]   Genuis, Stephen J., and Kasie L. Kelln. "Toxicant Exposure and Bioaccumulation: A Common and Potentially Reversible Cause of Cognitive Dysfunction and Dementia." *Be-*

increase not only the pollutants in the environment, but the accumulation of these noxious chemicals inside our body.

Besides nutritional arguments for raw foodism, like keeping crucial vitamins and minerals intact and undamaged from heat, along with avoiding toxic compounds generated by cooking, Alvaro discusses the effects of negligent agriculture's effects on the landscape. Our dietary choices, Alvaro makes clear, affect not only synthetic chemical release into the environment and our bodies but also generate harmful viruses and bacteria. This is why a raw vegan diet, he argues, is the most effective diet at protecting the entire world in addition to our bodies.

The "carnist values" of the non-raw-vegan world, especially the livestock industry, poison the environment in ways that threaten all life on the planet, including, sadly, even raw vegans, albeit indirectly.[523] The food choices of some people, can affect everyone and that is why it's so important that more people, and eventually everyone, would eat a nearly completely raw vegan diet—to safeguard the health of people, animals, and the planet.

"In affluent societies, consumption of animal products endangers the environment and human health unjustifiably—even the health of those who do not consume animal products," Alvaro argues.[524] The livestock industry is the biggest contributor to "zoonotic" diseases: infectious diseases that spread between animals and people. A plethora of potentially deadly viruses, bacteria, parasites, and fungi are passed from animals to humans and Alvaro argues that by consuming animal products, people contribute much to deadly illnesses.[525] Tuberculosis, listeria, salmonella, rabies, bird flu, West-Nile virus, Ebola, monkeypox, giardia, ringworm are just a few of the zoonotic diseases that threaten humans but are released into the environment by animals. Added to this concern, the overuse of antibiotics to control livestock diseases, promotes drug-resistant strains of bacteria that threatens human health.

"Vector-borne" diseases—transferred between insects and humans—also become more problematic because of carnist habits. Such diseases became more virulent as a result of the environmental changes that resulted from the practices of animal agriculture, such as defor-

---

haviioural Neurology, vol. 2015, 2015, 1–10, https://doi.org/10.1155/2015/620143. Accessed 20 Apr. 2022.

[523]   Alvaro, Carlo. *Raw Veganism : The Philosophy of the Human Diet.* Abingdon, Oxon, Routledge, 2020, 85.

[524]   Ibid., 89.

[525]   Ibid.,91.

estation and reduction of biodiversity.[526] Most diseases, Alvaro points out, are vector-borne (HIV, influenza, etc.).

Additionally, land is wasted by the livestock industry. That land could be used to grow and feed people ideal raw vegan food (or at least plant based food). Instead, the space is squandered on growing massive amounts of food to feed livestock. Alvaro argues that more humans could be fed properly if we gave up livestock projects. Vegetarian diets generally require five times less arable land than meat-based diets, he writes.[527] Less land could be used to feed more people.

Saving Earth, Legislating Rawness

Because the planet is so imperiled and because of the threat that animal agriculture and cooking poses to the environment and human health, Alvaro argues that we need legislation and re-education to turn things around.

To save the health of the planet and the human body, we need a return to a raw vegan diet or the "human diet," as Alvaro calls it. Both the "right to have a healthy environment" and the "right to healthcare" demand action—we must target animal-based foods by "increasing prices and applying heavier taxes to animal based products."[528]

Alvaro advocates for gradually increasing taxes on animal products so that they become less desirable and affordable to consumers. Eventually, governments would squash the ecological and health threat posed by the livestock industry by a "total ban" on animal products and more people would become aware that raw vegan food should be the foundation of their diet.[529]

Alvaro argues that the need for legislation is urgent. But he admits that a legal ban on animal products is an "enormously complicated goal to accomplish." It would require widespread education reform to reorientate the minds of the masses into substantially changing their dietary habits. There would be new laws as well, that steer people towards raw veganism. Cultural values would have to change—the pro-meat "carnist values" pervasive in many cultures, and pernicious corporate marketing, along with the civilizational habit of cooking, would have to be expunged for there to be widespread support for serious legal measures against meat consumption as well as the environmental

---

[526] Ibid.

[527] Ibid.

[528] Ibid., 90.

[529] Ibid.

damage that cooking causes. But if that were accomplished, perhaps we could prevent total environmental catastrophe.

EVOLUTIONARY RAW VEGANISM

Alvaro's stance about the environmental need for raw vegan diets is clear. But can people, from all over the world, really be convinced to drop the tradition of cooking and the comfort it brings, and go raw? There are many obstacles to Alvaro's plan. Cooked food tastes better to many people. Even Alvaro notes that animals often prefer to eat cooked food over their usual raw fare if given the choice.[530]

In order to overcome the short-term gratification of the taste buds, people have to truly value health a deeper understanding of what is actually good for them. We have to know for certain what kind of food our bodies are best adapted for.

The guiding light for many in the secular twenty-first century is the scientific theory of evolution. Ever since nineteenth-century British naturalists developed the theory of evolution, it's been considered a key insight into the origins and physical history of human beings. An optimal diet, surely, according to believers in theory of evolution, like Carlo Alvaro, should be compatible with our evolutionary history and acquired traits.

"Out of all the species of animals, humans are . . . the only ones who suffer from obesity, cardiovascular disease, atherosclerosis, diabetes, and more," Alvaro claims.[531] Why? Because our diets are out of sync with our natural propensities. Humans are primates, he notes. And we have primate digestive traits, formed by our habits over millions of years. Our extinct ancestors, the species *Homo erectus*, emerged almost two million years ago; *Homo sapiens* emerged 300,000 years ago. For most of this evolutionary history, Alvaro argues, our ancestors consumed primarily raw fruits and tender leafy greens. Cooking has only emerged in the last 20,000 years—a fraction of our whole evolutionary timeline.

"There is an optimal diet for every species of animals on earth, and humans are just animals," Alvaro summarizes. A diet based largely on raw fruits and greens is what he calls the "human diet" because it "aligns with our biological needs" and history. A diet made of cooked food and animal products is a far cry from our ancestral diet of raw colorful fruit and veggies. "Squirrels can eat fries . . . and other hu-

---

[530]   Ibid., 77.
[531]   Ibid. 69.

man junk food. However, neither of those foods is optimal for squirrel health," he illustrates.[532] The same applies to humans. Squirrels evolved to eat nuts and fruits; humans, fruits and leaves. Of the approximately nine million different species on the planet, humans are the only ones who cook their food. We are also the only animals who don't stick to their "specific diet"—the uniquely fitting and limited diet that we adapted to over eons.

The human body, evolutionary biologists point out, has *not* undergone significant change in tens of thousands of years. There's been no biological change in humans in 40,000 to 50,000 years, Alvaro notes. Thus, our bodily needs are not all that different from even our monkey-like ancestors who ate largely fruits and leaves. Additionally, our closest relatives, bonobos and chimpanzees, eat mainly fruits and leafy greens to this day. "Our anatomy is similar to theirs," and that is why we are "indubitably frugivores."[533]

In Alvaro's view, clinical studies in the modern age have justified the hypothesis that a plant-based diet is most healthful for humans: "There are no studies that show that fruits and vegetables can be deleterious for human health," he notes. The clinical reputation of meat, on the other hand, is, at best, ambiguous, as there is plenty of evidence that animal products are not beneficial for human health, he says.[534]

RAW OR COOKED BRAIN: THE EVOLUTIONARY DEBATE

But did raw foods actually make humans what we are today: the most intelligent creatures on the planet? Gradual cognitive enhancement and enlargement of the human brain are only possible because of cooked foods, according to one theory of human evolution. Alvaro discusses this argument in detail and argues otherwise.

Some researchers, he notes, have claimed that cooking may have been a driving force to the rapid increase in brain size because it facilitated higher calorie consumption, more free time due to less foraging demands, and a larger number of brain neurons.[535] However, Alvaro points out, this is a speculative area of research, and other researchers have supplied evidence that the cooked-food brain enhancement theory is groundless.

Alvaro discusses this theory despite the fact that it "concerns a period of time so remote that it precludes researchers from clearly un-

---

[532] Ibid., 75.
[533] Ibid., 77.
[534] Ibid.
[535] Ibid., 70.

derstanding what was in fact the case."[536] But the line of reasoning is important to him because his conception of evolution plays a foundational role in his advocacy for a raw diet.

Luckily for him, numerous researchers have countered the cooked food theory of evolutionary cognitive enhancement. It's argued that the increase in human brain size occurred millions of years *prior* to the time when humans began cooking food.[537] The researchers state that "thermal food processing" was not responsible for brain development and that "early hominids are likely to have obtained enough energy to sustain a large brain on a raw-food diet."[538]

The researchers do stipulate that this raw food diet wasn't strictly vegan since it did include a little bit of raw meat, but they still believe that a diet based on raw fruits and veggies was fuel enough for brain development of our intelligent species.

Longer hours foraging for raw foods, and not the introduction of the practice of cooking, the researchers argue, is one of the main causes of hominid brain development.[539] These explorations and longer walking distances meant that our ancestors had to remember routes and landscape patterns and therefore "develop memory and other such cognitive skills required to improve foraging efficiency." Raw fruit was enough to increase brain size in humans because unlike raw meat, it was easier to chew, easier to digest, and caused less energy expenditure to gather compared to hunting animals. Researchers who support this hypothesis note that the chewing physiology of hominids is and was more easily adapted to food "requiring fewer, less forceful chews" like fruits and leaves.[540] It follows that since fruit is "the most efficient and optimal food for humans," easy to come by, and high in glucose, raw food was the "principal" promoter of brain growth, in conjunction with more complicated foraging habits. Alvaro claims that in sum, current scientific literature does not support the idea that cooked food was the "catalyst" factor that enhanced brain expansion during evolution. Thus, there is all the more reason to continue eating raw, even to the present day.

---

[536]   Ibid.

[537]   Cornélio, Alianda M., et al. "Human Brain Expansion during Evolution Is Independent of Fire Control and Cooking." *Frontiers in Neuroscience*, vol. 10, 25 Apr. 2016, https://doi.org/10.3389/fnins.2016.00167. Accessed 19 Feb. 2020.

[538]   Ibid.

[539]   Ibid.

[540]   Alvaro, Carlo. *Raw Veganism : The Philosophy of the Human Diet*. Abingdon, Oxon, Routledge, 2020, 72.

PLANETARY AWARENESS

Carlo Alvaro's arguments for raw foodism are unique. Ecological and evolutionary arguments are less common than those focusing on health and spirituality. Most raw foodists have not been primarily motivated by the well-being of the non-human aspects of the planet nor living in line with our evolutionary past. But raw veganism, in Alvaro's mind, fits perfectly into our health aims, as well as saving the planet. Uncooked eating, it's claimed, can help clean up Earth's current toxicity and blunt the climate catastrophe, in addition to being ideally compatible with the human body and our hominid ancestor's habits over millions of years. The most ancient way of eating can be the cure for our modern woes.

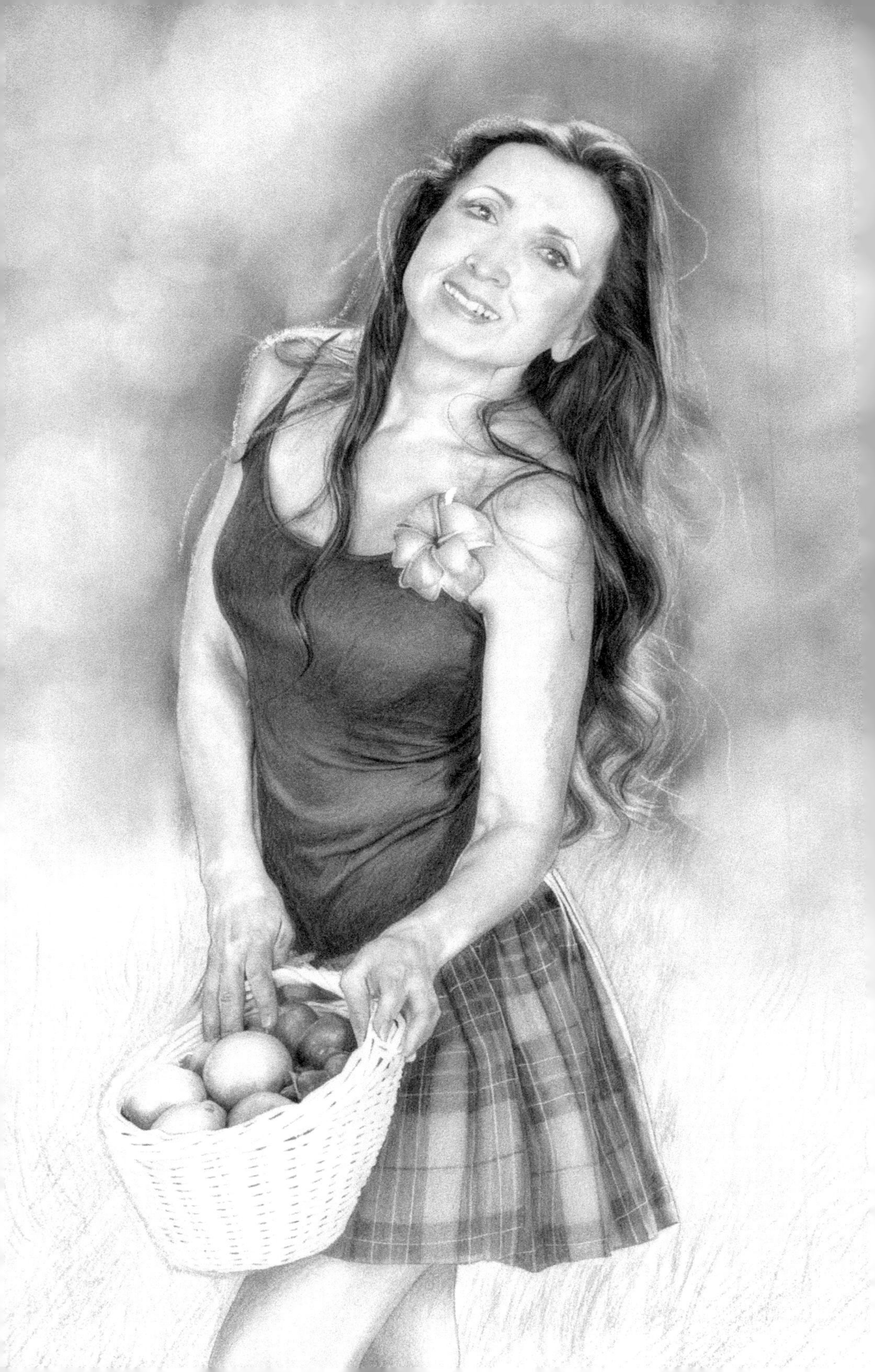

12.
The Aesthetics of the Body:
Tonya Zavasta and David Wolfe

Eating to optimize the appearance of the body is another important aim of modern raw foodists. The importance of personal appearance can be underestimated, when it comes to what motivates some raw dieters. Health concerns seem to take second place to aesthetics in these cases.

"What a woman won't do for health, she will do for beauty," writes Tonya Zavasta, one such raw foodist who focuses primarily on raw food's supposed beautifying effects.

The possibility of increasing one's beauty, sex appeal, youthfulness, and thus charisma through raw foodism is powerful idea and numerous raw foodists have felt that there's a receptive audience for it. Tonya Zavasta and David Wolfe, whom we'll discuss in this chapter, exemplify such approaches. Relatedly, Markus Rothkranz, whose aesthetics, spirituality, and views on health intertwine, will be discussed in the next chapter.

This largely new aesthetic way of approaching raw foodism, grew in prominence in the 2000s. Nevertheless, the common motivation of eating for health was not forgotten in this paradigm, nor did it have to be sacrificed to attain visual attractiveness. Internal health, as we'll see in detail, is reflected in external appearance. The outside of the body mirrors the inside of the body, in the worldview of David Wolfe, Tonya Zavasta and other raw foodists.

Spirituality, interestingly, was also part of the cosmetic quest and is often intertwined with beauty concerns.

To many, appearance is a more exciting realm to focus on, compared to the often invisible realm of internal health. People see your exterior, not often your interior. Your exterior affects how you're perceived, how attractive you are. It's how you relate to the world. It's visible, public, interactive, and powerful. People will often spend more effort, time, and money on what others see of them as opposed to what's hidden.

The appeal of aesthetics and the social, erotic, and artistic aspects that accompany it, are just what David Wolfe, Tonya Zavasta, and Markus Rothkranz tap into, rather than a potentially less inspiring focus on the health effects of nutrition.

For these raw proponents, if a state of health, gained from the adherence to a raw food diet, isn't observably beautiful and if it doesn't increase one's sex appeal, then it isn't exciting. Life is meant to be magical, they preach, full of fun and beauty. Every day is supposed to be "the best day ever"—a trademark phrase of Wolfe's. If you didn't at least *look* good as a result of adhering to a raw food lifestyle, perhaps it wouldn't even be worth forgoing the pleasures of cooked food.

Tonya Zavasta

> "*The Rawsome Diet [will] transform them from plain-looking to beautiful. What a woman won't do for health, she will do for beauty. This is the first time beauty asks no sacrifice from health.*"
> —Tonya Zavasta[541]

Zavasta, born 1958, experienced a pivotal moment in her early life in Soviet Russia, a moment that set the course of the rest of her life. In junior high, she and her friend found themselves staring at their reflections in a restroom mirror. This friend, Helena, who possessed a "breathtaking beauty" and "cold vanity," savored her own reflection for a moment and then, as if to ruthlessly enhance her sense of her own beauty, fired an insult at Tonya. "If I looked like you, I would not even want to live." The cruel teenage barb made a deep impression on Zavasta, plain by birth, and encumbered with a congenital hip dislocation that gave her a limp. "I got the message: 'to live I must be beautiful,'" Zavasta noted with despair. There entered into her an awareness that she had been denied something essential for existence. This realization became a grievance but also a mission statement. "Justice had to be served," she remembered. "I clenched my fists, and swore: 'As God is my witness, I will be beautiful.'"[542]

---

[541] Zavasta, Tonya. *Your Right to Be Beautiful : How to Halt the Train of Aging & Meet the Most Beautiful You.* Memphis, Tenn., Br Pub, 2003. 11.
[542] Ibid.

"Beauty became my lifetime ambition," she recalls, "a matter of justice . . . a passion bordering on obsession."[543]

At first, in her quest for aesthetic power, she experimented with imitating the gestures and postures of supermodels but this wasn't effective. Zavasta knew that she needed "leverage to level up with so-called normal people." She wondered if there was a better way than performative gestures to be seen as good-looking—if there was, as she put it, "a way to bring beauty into the realm of personal control."[544]

Later in life, she found that leverage: the key to physical beauty—raw food. Despite what she felt was congenital homeliness, she eventually believed that she had achieved an uncommon beauty in her forties, metamorphosing from a disadvantaged youth into an eye-catching mature woman. "If there has ever been such a thing as a self-made beauty, I am it," she declared of her early limitations and subsequent transformation.[545]

Zavasta feels pride in this self-directed improvement of her body.[546] Therefore, she feels, she has earned the right to turn a deaf ear to the excuses that others make "for not becoming beautiful" themselves. Having said that, she concedes that raw foodism does require a great deal of discipline to adhere to. If it were easy, we would see beautiful people everywhere. Nevertheless, the choice is there for all to enhance their appearance by eating the ideal diet. Most people have potential but their beauty is unclaimed, she believes. But luckily, it is "biologically possible" to look beautiful at any age.[547] "Between you and beauty lies only your effort," she urges readers. "So take responsibility for your looks."[548] In a world that often sees attractiveness as pure luck by birth, Zavasta had proven that you can nutritionally reclaim this prize as your birthright.

Because of her self-made transformation, Zavasta feels that she is the best person to teach others how to achieve good looks. Any person not born to beauty, like herself, can show others how to actually build beauty and not just restore or preserve the luck you received at birth. That's what makes her advice so compelling, she feels, compared to a person born with exceptional symmetry of features or a nice bone structure.

---

[543] Ibd., 14.

[544] Ibd., 16.

[545] Ibd., 319.

[546] Ibd.

[547] Ibid., 10.

[548] Ibid.

She helps people realize they can eat their way to supermodel status. Their full beauty potential can be realized by abandoning cooked food. Most people don't have a glow because of their "failure to live up to your body's potential," Zavasta says.[549]

The body is a record book so we'd better log good habits. "The older we get, the more truly our appearance reflects who we really are. The lifestyle we choose, the discipline we demand of ourselves … all of this information is carved on our faces." One's aesthetic destiny hinges either on raw victory or cooked defeat. In time, the body will testify to the work you've put in or shunned. Looking beautiful at age twenty, when a body is often still intact, regardless of habits, is not special. But "if you look beautiful after forty, people think of you as special," Zavasta reminds, because you've achieved something rare.[550]

Aesthetic achievement—natural, holistic, and authentic—looking beautiful in a wholesome and natural way—comes only from eating raw food. Plastic surgery is not a convincing fix for ugly, unhealthy bodies. Natural beauty, built from raw food, is the only type of beauty that people subconsciously accept. People will notice when the face looks artificially altered (odd and forced tightening or too much plumpness and puffiness) or when it does not match the characteristics of the rest of the body. The face doesn't look real and the arms and neck look comparatively decrepit. Anyway, as plastic surgery becomes more popular, true natural beauty will become more coveted, and more valuable because of its increasing scarcity, Zavasta argues.[551] Surgery forfeits your "unique identity" by smothering your distinctive features and the "opportunity to see yourself as God intended."[552] You can only eat your way to respectable and convincing beauty.

Edenic Beauty

"Beauty is God's handwriting; welcome it in every fair face."
—Ralph Waldo Emerson, as quoted by Zavasta

There is a theological underpinning to Zavasta's beliefs about raw food and its cosmetic effects. Her ideas about the meaning of the Bible's creation story are central to her belief that raw plant foods heal and beautify.

---

[549]   Ibd., 21.
[550]   Ibd., 56.
[551]   Ibd., 60.
[552]   Ibd., 61.

Zavasta did not always believe in God nor hold Scripture in high esteem. In early life, she was by default an atheist, like many who grew up in Soviet Russia or other religion-averse communist governments. She scoffed at friends who believed "naive" Bible stories. But after adopting the "rawsome" lifestyle, as she calls it, and perceiving a new beauty in the world and her body, her mind was opened up to the divine. "This lifestyle gave me lucid proof of the existence of God," she says, and she is convinced that you cannot follow the raw diet for long, and see its effects on yourself, "without coming to the revelation that a Creator has to be behind this wonderful body."[553]

Having experienced a profound awareness of the divine through a nutritionally altered perception of reality and her own transformation, diet became a critical part of Tonya's Biblical worldview. She came to believe not only in a Creator but also that God designed humans to flourish on raw plant food.

Before humans were cursed out of the garden of Eden, Zavasta believes, they thrived on colorful raw plants and enjoyed perfect health and practically unlimited lifespan.[554] Genesis 1:29 endorses this diet, in her view. It's a line often cited by vegetarians and cannabis advocates, in addition to being used by raw foodists: "Behold," God says, "I have given you every herb bearing seed, which is upon the face of all the earth, and every tree, in the which is the fruit of a tree yielding seed; to you it shall be for meat." In this paradise, there was no need to cook food and humans could simply pluck the perfectly designed fruits and leaves surrounding them and start chewing.

On this raw vegan diet, "The body had the resilience of God, Himself," Zavasta boldly claims. The body was meant to renew itself continually, according to God's original creation plan. "When God created . . . human beings, He did not intend for them to die, much less to age," says Zavasta. "Maybe that is why" the loss of beauty that comes from aging is so "difficult psychologically," she wonders.[555] But fortunately even today, we can reclaim some of the ever-renewing effects of the original Edenic dietary plan, she believes. This diet will "allow you to ripen, not to decay," and "old age will lose its sting," as you realize that you can be beautiful at any age.[556] And it is an exciting realization that beauty at advanced ages is even more admirable than the attrac-

---

[553] Ibd., 39.
[554] Ibid., 264.
[555] Ibid.
[556] Ibd., 266.

tiveness that comes easily with extreme youth. "A beautiful young girl is a delight, but a beautiful mature woman is magic."[557]

Zavasta, however, is not claiming that all of the original health attributes of the first humans, like immortality, can be achieved in contemporary times on a raw diet. After humans were banished from Eden for sinning, the genetic inheritance for everlasting life was revoked. "After the first people left the Garden of Eden, God knew that their wonderfully made bodies would get sick," she says. Today, although our ancestors had forfeited their immortality, we can still be healthy and beautiful until just about the end of our natural lifespan. To "live as long as God intended and to look as He envisioned you" is the point of the "rawsome" lifestyle. Now, on a raw food diet, "aging comes a week or two before death" and "deterioration takes place rapidly" at the end of well-lived life. This sudden and natural type of death, which physical beauty preserved until nearly the end, "is the way it should be," Zavasta feels, instead of a gradual, miserable decline in function and appearance.[558]

After leaving God's all-protective presence and the raw fruits and leaves of his Edenic garden, man's beauty waned. In the Old Testament, Zavasta argues, the word "beautiful" occurs forty-five times, in the New Testament, only eight and none of those references refer to humans. Human bodies degenerated and fell shorter and shorter of their original ideal as centuries passed. At the time of creation, according to Zavasta, "man's body was God's pride" in its visible loveliness and perfect health. As our flesh deteriorated after the Fall, "the average human body must have become repulsive to our Creator." By the time of the New Testament, hopelessly, all dietary injunctions that would've preserved health and beauty were dropped, as the focus turned almost entirely to the afterlife since humans became so ugly and were reduced to relatively miniscule earthly lifespans.[559]

Part of the punishment for man's original disobedience, God forced strange dietary compulsions on humans. He clouded the minds of people and steered them toward life-destroying nutritional habits. "The deviation from the original diet of raw fruits, vegetables, nuts, and seeds, was one of the channels God used to shorten man's lifespan." Noah and Methuselah lived over 900 years on "a diet close to God's original menu." But then "after the flood, meat was introduced." Bread was also an omen and cause of man's reduced lifespan and beauty—at least what we think of as bread in the modern world, that is,

---

[557]   Ibd., 267.

[558]   Ibid., 275.

[559]   Ibid., 37.

cooked bread. Zavasta claims that the bread in the Old Testament, being more in line with God's original plan, was raw. The true Biblical bread, she claims, which sometimes symbolized God's provision, was the bread of the Essenes, made from uncooked wheat kernels that had been sprouted and dried in the sun instead of baked, as Edmond Bordeaux Szekely claimed.[560]

Despite man's fallen condition, there were clues in the Old Testament as to God's meal plan for man. Hints about proper dietary practices can be found in the Book of Daniel, Zavasta notes. Daniel rejects the rich food of the Babylonian king, subsisting on vegetables and water. His appearance improved for the better on this cleansing vegan diet, Scripture notes. Clues of nutritional truth were subtle in the sacred text and were there for perceptive minds to notice, but the vast majority of humans had been misled.

Exiled from the Garden, Exiled from Beauty

"All of God's children are not beautiful. Most of God's
children are, in fact, barely presentable."
—Fran Lebowitz, as quoted by Zavasta

To reclaim our aesthetic birthright, we need to be aware of our fall from Edenic perfection and the causes behind it. We need to know the "cause of so much ugliness" in the world.[561]

"Double chins, protruding stomachs, stooping shoulders, and sallow complexions are seen everywhere, even in young people. What went wrong?" Zavasta asks. "Did God himself, the great aesthete of all, create beings that are capable of depressing him in all their naked humanity?" How far we have fallen from grace. Even "common looking people were meant to be beautiful."[562] But our fallenness and diet have destroyed our appearances.

Physical flaws are natural for post-Eden humans, Zavasta admits. They are inherited. But ugliness is acquired by nutrition and lifestyle. Ugliness reveals that our bodies are not healthy nor following God's injunctions.[563] Ugliness "proclaims the stupidity of our habits," she says. Your "hands, neck, hair, eyes, elbows . . . cry out" whether you are heeding or rejecting a raw food diet. The purity or impurity of your

---

[560]   Ibid.
[561]   Ibid., 49.
[562]   Ibid., 34.
[563]   Ibid., 50.

diet will be reflected on the most visible parts of your body: "The truth will be written on your face. It speaks louder than words."[564] Health and beauty are two sides of the same coin. Good habits and the inner health that results from them are testified to in our outer beauty.[565]

"Why do plants and animals often display a greater visual beauty than God's favorite creation, man?" Zavasta laments.[566] Because they live closer to God's natural plan. In the case of animals, they eat uncooked food. Humans, on the other hand, because of their perverted ways, are aesthetically shamed by these less-sentient but more intuitive creatures.

Humanity must make an overhaul in its diet if it is to experience the appearance that God had in mind for it. The naive and even dangerous notion of "accepting our bodies" in whatever state they're in might be even "more damaging than an extreme obsession with beauty," Zavasta warns. "Desire for beauty," after all, "is a self-protective drive" since it will push us into healthy habits. We will "make concessions for beauty that we won't make for health."[567]

The Ugly Sinfulness of Cooked Foods and the Beautifying Virtue of Raw Foods

In Zavasta's layout of existence, ugliness and sinfulness are intertwined; conversely, beauty and goodness are linked. Every day that humans eat cooked food, they are becoming uglier and sinning against God. Zavasta describes how this sin mars us physically and what it signifies spiritually.

Most humans gradually become "de-beautified" throughout their lives by consuming "devitalized foods," mainly cooked food and animal products, Zavasta declares.[568] This is the karma they deserve from transgressing God's diet stipulations. Animal flesh, for instance, was intended for burnt offerings to God, not to "be put into our beautiful bodies, which are designed entirely for plant eating."[569] Eat animal products and you'll experience a "puffy moon face," double chin,"

---

[564]   Ibid., 29.
[565]   Ibid., 57.
[566]   Ibid., 50.
[567]   Ibid.
[568]   Ibid., 39.
[569]   Ibid., 81.

rough skin, moles, and even excessive body hair. Dairy, processed sugar, and table salt also ruin our skin collagen, and cause inflammation.[570]

Cooked food is an insult to God's design of the universe and a sign of humankind's sinful rebellion. "To process food is an arrogant notion—we seem to be saying God's menu needs improvement," instead of trusting "the Creator of human life with food."[571] To "fry it, bake it, refine it" is to kill the life in the food. We "mutilate and manipulate" raw produce, not recognizing the "divine food" that it is. The "rainbow of colors" in raw food, that could become a part of us if we ate them, "fade like old laundry" after cooking.[572] We are desecrating the sacred gifts of our Creator. "Cooking," Zavasta proclaims starkly, "is the most profound abuse of food."[573] "There is no food after fire; what is left is only fabrication."[574] Raw food is the only actual food and cooking is akin to vain and spiteful corruption of what the Creator designed.

This sin becomes justly etched in our flesh. The cheap, transient pleasure gained from consuming devitalized foods accelerates the death of the body and bereaves it of looks. Decrepit slaves to cooked food invert the values we're supposed to live by. They "depend on food for pleasure" instead of deriving pleasure "from living." and so they give into shallow temptation. [575] Even Christians, who should be more attuned, compared to non-believers, to God's design for their lives, often indulge in "perverse eating as the only pleasure available to them."[576] They proudly abstain from drinking, smoking, and other sins only to pollute themselves unapologetically by eating cooked and processed foods. We should find joy in more wholesome aspects of life, not cake or casserole— not from perverting God's creation.

We can put an end to this slavery to devitalized cooked food by exercising some discipline. Your tastebuds can be restored once you've spent a while on a raw diet. A "simple salad will be divine" and the sins of cooked food will no longer seem appealing.[577] Damaging desires are purged and the remaining desires are oriented toward healthfulness. The raw eater will have a newfound respect for God's miraculous plant life and a newfound disgust for perverted edibles. For Zavasta,

---

570   Ibid., 83.
571   Ibid., 86.
572   Ibid., 90
573   Ibid., 89.
574   Ibid., 91.
575   Ibid., 92.
576   Ibid., 93.
577   Ibid., 96.

the smell of cooked food became "offensive, even repugnant," sensually distasteful and seen as immoral [578]

The "utter absurdity" of non-nutritious cooked food will "amplify with each day" in the consciousness of someone adhering to a raw food diet. It's not only unnecessary, it's destructive. The eater will ask herself whether she wants to be beautiful and full of fresh plants or cultivate ugliness through a regretful slavery to corrupted desires. The choice is to be virtuous and good-looking or decaying and sinful; to be raw or cooked.

Purity is key for total transformation. "Eating an abundance of fruits and vegetables is not enough," and you will never see the optimal "natural you," the peak of your beauty, unless you're eating "100 percent natural [raw] food."[579] Even a little cooked or unhealthy food can thwart one's aesthetics: "Between a beautiful face and an average one lies a very thin line. Take any cover girl picture and add eye bags and a little puffiness here and there and the magic is gone," explains Zavasta.[580] Dietary cleanliness is the only way to be truly sexy.

The face reveals the truth about the body. It is so telling of inner health that Zavasta stipulates, "When a health expert gives advice, I want to see her face." If that person doesn't "look 10 to 20 years younger than her age," Zavasta doesn't care what they have to say because that person is evidently not eating raw.[581]

The only way to have an appealing face is to let raw foods heal your body from the inside out. On the raw diet, the "artistic ability of your body" will be unleashed as it remolds the texture, color, and symmetry of your bodily tissues.[582]

No matter your age, raw food can make you beautiful. Conversely, a cooked food diet continually degrades beauty. "While your non-raw-eating peers discover new blemishes, blotches, and moles on a nearly daily basis, you will see your own skin irregularities gradually fade or disappear." Skin around your eyes will lose puffiness and natural collagen production improves. More collagen will fill in the places where it is needed. Raw food will fill in your hollow cheeks."[583] The body will continually re-balance and re-beautify and "clarify and refine your

---

[578]   Ibid., 97.

[579]   Ibid., 134.

[580]   Ibid., 136.

[581]   Ibid., 68.

[582]   Ibid., 138.

[583]   Ibid.

features."[584] "Raw food will work magic for you without the surgical knife," Zavasta promises.[585]

The divine intelligence of the body, fueled by divine-endorsed food, will correct imperfections when toxicity is removed and true nourishment replaces it. The "intelligent body" will "work out" to "co-operate" what previously seemed like exaggerated features—a "nose you thought didn't belong on your face" will end up being molded more fittingly with other features.[586] "Texture, hues, and shape will be harmoniously arranged into a genteel whole."[587]

In one year, 99 percent of our cells will be replaced by new ones, Zavasta claims, which is why the raw diet can reform your appearance.[588] Even the structure of our bones can be refashioned for the better, as they are replaced within two years.[589]

Additionally, the hydration from raw plant foods will preserve the youthful, moisturized plumpness of bodily tissues (which are made mostly of water). You can't just drink water and eat cooked food to achieve that plumpness. That may have the opposite effect, as it washes away nutrients needed for skin beauty.[590] You can eat or juice raw vegetables, however, to nourish your "glowing complexion."[591] Moisture-filled raw plant foods have minerals, vitamins, sugars, and antioxidants holistically integrated into them, which can help water be easily absorbed by our tissues, she claims.

Skin isn't the only body part to profit from raw foodism. If your diet "predominantly consists of vegetables, nuts, and seeds, you will have firm, thick hair."[592] Animal products and fried food are a detriment to hair growth and ideal texture and dandruff is an attempt of the body to get rid of excess fat and protein.[593] Gray hair, according to Zavasta, results from toxicity, especially from animal fats and proteins.[594]

Raw food will also correct the scent of your body. "The need for deodorant is a forerunner of many degenerative processes."[595] "After

---

[584]   Zavasta, 138.
[585]   Zavasta, 138.
[586]   Zavasta, 139.
[587]   Zavasta, 139.
[588]   Zavasta, 146.
[589]   Zavasta, 146.
[590]   Zavasta, 325.
[591]   Zavasta, 325.
[592]   Zavasta, 243.
[593]   Zavasta, 243.
[594]   Zavasta, 243.
[595]   Zavasta, 147.

several months on the raw food diet . . . one's body will emanate a pleasant, sweet scent."[596]

You reap what you sow. Raw food beautifies you with its purity and cooked food transmits its moral ugliness onto your flesh.

Metaphysical Effects of Raw Food Aesthetics

The aesthetic consequences of one's diet transcend the material. They impact psychology and spirituality. "Dissatisfaction" with one's looks arises, not from onerous cultural beauty standards but from the "subconscious awareness that we haven't achieved our optimal look."[597]

Cooked food severs your emotional connection to your body. On such a devitalized diet, "the body is experienced as alien, an imposter, or a non-self." This disastrous feeling of alienation from one's own body triggers a "lack of self-esteem," as one is ashamed to present one's appearance to the world. We are designed to desire to be beautiful and can't escape it. Only the raw food diet can prevent this disastrous mind-body suffering complex.[598] "Satisfaction," comes from "being pure, clean, and healthy inside and beautiful and serene on the outside."[599] And cooked food isn't going to give you cleanliness or serenity.

Our bodies, Zavasta claims, also project spiritual meaning into the minds of others. Others sense our "physical integrity," in a way that transcends purely material structural observation. The moral meaning of raw foods shines through. We actually can signal the appearance of a pure moral character to others, Zavasta claims: raw food becomes character. "Goodness in one's food summons up goodness in one's appearance and character," in her words. Raw food transmits a spiritual quality to your "aura," a "transcendent nobility and complacent dignity." The aesthetic consequences of the "rawsome diet" also give the beautiful person a mental high: they "lift the limitations of one's spirit and release . . . tensions in both your mind and body."[600] They are a salve for body and spirit.

Having confidence in your outer beauty calms inner spiritual turmoil and nurtures a harmonious vibe within. And without, it transmits meaning to others. After all, "there is such a thing as physical morali-

---

[596]   Zavasta, 147.
[597]   Ibid., 142.
[598]   Ibid., 144.
[599]   Ibid., 285.
[600]   Ibid., 182.

ty," she claims.[601] The visible can signify spiritual qualities and healthy cells and bodily structures could be thought of as having material virtue or integrity if there are in their optimal state.

The moral meaning that people perceive, consciously or subconsciously, in your beauty or ugliness affects how they intuit your character and how they treat you. "A beautiful person is perceived as gentle and kind," Zavasta claims. Ugly people are "expected to be evil, rude, sneaky."[602] We're even perceived as more competent if we're beautiful. Perhaps because it signifies conscientiousness of self-care.

In Greek, Latin, and Russian, she points out, *beautiful* and *good* are often used interchangeably; the concepts are yoked. Nevertheless, there exists an opposing ethos: there are people who "believe only the ugly can be moral and good. But these are ugly wives' tales," Zavasta quips.[603] These people are living in denial of the aesthetic-moral truths of the universe.

Along with affecting how we transmit moral meaning to others, raw food affects how we perceive everything around us as well. Eating in such a way sensitizes our aesthetic awareness of the world and other people's bodies. "You begin to see how much people's appearance differs from their optimal one." You will see how far people have eaten themselves from the way God meant them to look, how far their current cooked-food ugliness diverges from their potential raw food-fed attractiveness.[604]

Beauty and Empowerment; Ugliness and Despair

"I am sure that nothing has such a decisive influence upon a man's course as his personal appearance, and not so much his appearance as his belief in its attractiveness or unattractiveness."
—Tolstoy, as quoted by Zavasta

"How many husbands find themselves tied down to a fat, dowdy woman who bears no resemblance to the beautiful girl they married? How many wives see a balding and pot-bellied male who was once a handsome man?"
—Tonya Zavasta

---

[601]   Ibid.

[602]   Ibid., 31

[603]   Ibid.

[604]   Ibid., 138.

The far-reaching consequences of beauty and ugliness—of choosing raw food or cooked food—affect not only your spirit but your place in the world as well.

Far divorced from the aphorisms of "don't judge a book by its cover" and the like, Zavasta acknowledges that personal appearance can affect your life prospects in a multitude of ways. She embraces this fact, which other people would prefer to discard. "I cannot think of anything as empowering as being beautiful," she says. "Beauty generates positive energy and arouses excitement within us when we see it . . . It influences your effectiveness in whatever you are doing."[605] Other people will be stimulated by your presence and will be more likely to be kindly disposed to you and conspire with your desires. It can propel your professional or relational goals.

Looking your best infuses you with a feeling of power. You have more boldness and courage. Beauty gives us the freedom to express ourselves more confidently, Zavasta says. Aesthetic pride and comfort in one's skin lends us more belief in attaining our aims. "The fewer qualms we have about our appearance and health, the more we can let go of the subconscious clamps that suppress our talents and restrict our initiative."[606] Vocational and general self-doubt fades as the flesh gets prettier.

Beauty influences others. "Beauty is a trump card. It is an advantage in every encounter with others . . . and causes one's personal success to soar." Attractiveness can bolster your career or other opportunities because it "empowers you with the ability to influence people."[607] Zavasta quotes Aristotle: "Beauty is a greater recommendation than any letter of introduction . . . People cater to beauty" and are more likely to indulge you.[608]

Being ugly and disempowered is another story. Year by year, the destruction of bodily beauty can be psychologically devastating and leave women especially feeling demoralized, Zavasta claims. "As a woman loses her looks, she feels her opportunities slipping away." She quotes with approval another author who says, "Failure to achieve beauty or to retain it contributes to women's sense of helplessness." A woman's attractiveness is a near superpower in its ability to influence others and it's quite painful to see that power eroded. People cater to her much less. Let's face it, Zavasta argues, "Life is more beautiful if you are."[609]

---

[605] Ibid., 26.
[606] Ibid.
[607] Ibid.
[608] Ibid., 24.
[609] Ibid.

"There is no immunity to the craving for physical attractiveness," Zavasta warns.[610] It's irrevocably written upon the human heart. It is a desire that cannot be exorcised, so we all might as well embrace the need to be beautiful and do all we can to look our best. It will always break your heart when prettiness is destroyed.

Rebellious art, made in an effort to "reject and defy beauty" is futile. The desire for beauty, including that of the human body, is inescapable, it's "here to stay."[611] The short sighted effort to "re-educate" culture to not judge by appearance will fail. Zavasta is adamant that this is a true and universal law. There is no hope of comfortably rejecting the pursuit for physical beauty "as long as we have zest for life and the quest for truth."[612] To live is to desire beauty and its transcendent moral meaning.

First impressions matter and "no one" can prevent us from "evaluating people as they really are." That's right—as they really are, the deep reality of a person's being, visible in the quality of their flesh. Our "aesthetic nature," our sensitivity to the way things look and the meaning we gather from appearances, is not cultural; it is innate.[613] You cannot fight against the inescapable truths of the universe. The drive for beauty, in sum, is divinely ordained. Luckily the Creator also gave us a path to attain it—raw food. If we don't take this path we'll suffer the physical and psychic consequences of our spiritual and dietary rebellion.

DAVID WOLFE

"Every human population seems to commit regular transgressions
against the laws of raw nourishment and beauty."
—David Wolfe

The curly haired, smiley American raw food celebrity David Wolfe has been touting an unprocessed, organic, raw food diet since the 1990s. In the mid 2000s, Wolfe had risen in stature to become one of the most prominent advocates of uncooked food. He was selling books, attracting the acclaim of celebrities, and was involved in numerous health food businesses.

---

[610]   Ibid., 45.

[611]   Ibid.

[612]   Ibid., 49.

[613]   Ibid.

Wolfe represented a new generation of raw foodism. It was a break away from the earnest elder juicers of previous generations, those like Ann Wigmore, who extolled dietary discipline. Wolfe tried to focus more particularly on living a vivacious life filled with youthful fun and sexiness in addition to his New Age spiritual beliefs—as Wolfe's famous catch phrase goes, he was focused on "having the best day ever."

Raw foodism, he set out to prove, was not just about purity and discipline. It was about living a rock star life (the term "rawk star" has been used in the movement), writing new rules for living, rebelling against the oppressive systems of the past and present, and expanding human empowerment. And one way to empowerment was to enhance personal beauty.

Wolfe's prescription for improved bodily aesthetics is similar to Zavasta's, but he has his own explanations for the beautifying effects of raw food as well as a differing sources of inspiration for his philosophy of beauty.

Eating for Beauty

David Wolfe's third book, *Eating for Beauty* (2007), advocates for a raw food diet on the basis that it physically beautifies people.

The supposed health benefits of raw food are a given in Wolfe's dietary program and underlie the cosmetic benefits. But, uniquely, Wolfe's description of the health benefits of raw food are sometimes framed in erotic and experiential terms. For instance, he says, that when we eat "raw food that the body needs, it feels as if cells in various parts of the body are having orgasms!"[614]

Looking and feeling good are king in Wolfe's paradigm. The health benefits or detriments of every diet, after all, are evidenced by the cosmetic results. Surface appearances reveal the proof of a diet's healthfulness. Wolfe opines that "the authors of other diet books should be subject to public view in order to see . . . whose diet really produces results."[615] "Only results matter, not theories," he says. If the skin does not "radiate exquisite freshness, thus expressing the inner truth of excellent health," then any so-called health expert should not be listened to.[616]

---

[614]   Wolfe, David. *Eating for Beauty: For Women & Men.* Berkeley, Calif., North Atlantic Books, 2009, 14.

[615]   Ibid., 24.

[616]   Ibid., 63.

Inspired by Greek Beauty Ideals

*"The ancient Greeks truly tapped into a magical concept. We see, even
as far back as Homer's Iliad, that beauty was the motivating theme."*
—David Wolfe

*"The Earth gives enough nourishment from just its vegetable
realm, without the need for torture or violence."*
—Pythagoras, ancient Greek philosopher

David Wolfe was inspired by the beauty-revering culture of ancient
Greece, as he explicitly states: "Of all eras and cultures, the classical
Greek conception of beauty seems to resonate more powerfully than
any other," he writes in the first chapter of *Eating for Beauty*. He dedicated the book, which is about "recreating one's internal and external
appearance," to "the art, culture, and feeling of ancient Greece."[617]

The Greeks, as he noted, took beauty seriously. They praised their
gods for their aesthetic perfection and erotic lure. Their statues and
athletic contests celebrated proportionate and fit bodies. They would
also occasionally, as Wolfe notes, spare enemy combatants if they were
exceptionally beautiful. They worshiped beauty as a share of divini-
ty and connected it to moral good. The Greek word for beauty, *kalos*,
could denote nobility and goodness, as well as physical attractiveness.
"To the Greeks, beauty was a function of the divine," historian Edith
Hamilton said. It was the workings and language of the supernatural.

Wolfe relates to his ancient predecessors. "The desire for beauty is
not only good and natural but is in fact one of the most divine attributes" of humans, he proclaims. To desire to be beautiful, is to desire to
discover and draw out our dormant attributes of excellence.[618]

Inspired by the ancients, Wolfe's raw foodism encourages people
to "rejuvenate and surpass ancient beauty ideals" by building ever more
beautiful bodies in modern times. We can be better looking today than
those beautiful statue bodies of Grecian marble or bronze. Wolfe's aim
is to activate "the power of diet … to reshape and remake the body," to
make the best looking bodies ever.[619]

Beauty should be humankind's highest aspiration. "The enjoyment
and creation of beauty seems to be unmatched by any of life's quests,"
Wolfe believes. He "desires to create more beauty in the world," and in

---

[617]   Ibid., 1.

[618]   Ibid., 5.

[619]   Ibid., 2.

providing dietary guidance on beautification, by acting as a raw food artist of the flesh, Wolfe "aspires to the same type of drive that Michelangelo must have felt when he painted the Sistine Chapel."[620]

And those who follow his instructions and eat to become beautiful get to experience the reshaping power of uncooked food. The raw eater becomes "a work of art" as "Nature's paintbrush immediately sets about applying food-mineral cosmetics to the inner tissues, which become visible externally."[621] The eater is the artwork and artist at the same time. People choose their painting materials from the foods they eat. They will either be high quality or devoid of any beautification value—devoid of minerals, phytochemical antioxidants, vitamins, or other essential ingredients that mold the flesh to become picturesque.

"Creating an attractive state of physiology" and "poise," like that of an ancient Greek statue, "results from consistent actions."[622] The daily habit of eating raw foods "shape[s] our forms subtly, slowly," and "each meal becomes part of who we are at the deepest level," including our surface as it appears to others. Our physicality takes form and our most important features respond to each meal we eat: "The face is a canvas on which our food choices paint." The maxim "you are what you eat" is "cosmic law," Wolfe notes.[623]

Wolfe teaches readers how to turn Greek beauty standards into reality by eating raw food. Our proportions and coloring can be changed depending on the food we eat. We can become the Greek ideal if we stick to raw plants. "The symmetry of fruit imparts its pattern upon us," Wolfe claims. And symmetry is one of the classical determinants of beauty. We mirror the food we eat. When we eat fruit, we start to look, in a sense, "like a beautiful fruit tree," Wolfe claims. The "more profound symmetry" that the near-miraculous effects of raw food impart on us is not just a side effect of good health, it's "the purpose of eating raw foods."[624] He's clear: beauty, or lack thereof, are the most important results of our dietary choices.

Raw food is "symmetrical nutrition." The eating of "geometrically harmonious" raw foods "impart" their balancing pattern upon us. Kirlian photography—a technique that purports to show electromagnetic radiation or "auras of vibrant energy" around food—has proven the superior energetic geometry of raw food. Cooked foods, it has been

---

620   Ibid.
621   Ibid., 11.
622   Ibid.
623   Ibid., 2.
624   Ibid., 7.

shown, have the symmetry of their energetic output distorted, compared to the "luminescent patterns found in raw foods."[625]

Impart the energetic and chemical beautification on yourselves, the raw food guru tells his followers, as he waxes poetic: "The ancient beauty ideal/ Is one we still can feel/ One we can revive."[626]

The Beauty of Raw Food and the Ugliness of Cooked Food

"Remember: nutrition is an art—it is an art form. Every bite is a brush stroke. Every swallow is a new color. Each meal is . . . a piece of the painting that you are becoming. You are becoming an ever more attractive work of art."
—David Wolfe

"The first element of The Beauty Diet is to transition your body onto a living plant-food diet."
—David Wolfe

A main aspect of Wolfe's theory of the nutrition/beauty connection is the maintenance of the so-called "juiciness" of bodily tissues. Juiciness denotes fullness, moisturization, plumpness, and elasticity—typical characteristics of healthy or youthful flesh.

Wolfe sees the human body as "truly an advanced juicing machine.[627]

"Hydration is essential in keeping us clear, bright, and beautiful . . . the main factor that keeps one's tissues 'juicy.'" Proper hydration comes from organic raw plant foods and water that is free from environmental contaminants—"fresh spring water" or reverse-osmosis purified water.[628] Vegetable juice is another way to receive hydration. "Fresh juices filled with chlorophyll . . . maintain a beautiful body for a lifetime," Wolfe says.[629]

Cooked foods, as compared to raw plant foods, "contain no vital juices."[630] Water is sucked out of them by heat. Cooked food is "dead

---

625   Ibid.
626   Ibid.
627   Ibid., 18.
628   Ibid., 44.
629   Ibid., 50.
630   Ibid., 18.

solid."[631] Our tissues dry up and shrink from their ideal plumpness because of cooked food. "Heavy meals of cooked animal protein and fat make the tissues dense and coarse" and "detract from a beautiful complexion." Raw food, on the other hand, instead of stiffening your tissues and promoting "density," can restore elasticity, he maintains.[632]

Besides bequeathing moisture and flexibility, uncooked plant fats also play a critical role in juicifying tissues. In Wolfe's conception, there is a dramatic dichotomy between raw plant fats—avocados, nuts, seeds, and cold-pressed olive oils and other oils versus cooked fats and oils. Raw oils nourish us cosmetically. Cooked fats, oils, margarine, and fried foods "are absolutely detrimental to the complexion."[633] They lead to acne and skin disorders, he maintains.[634] Fats are "corrupted" by cooking, triggering inflammation and oxidative stress in the body, and losing beautifying nutrients like vitamins A, D, E, and K.

It's these same fat-soluble vitamins in raw fats, like coconut oil, olive oil, avocado, and hemp oil, that "promote the beautiful bone structure." Raw plant fats are also the "best foods" to "beautify the skin" and "lubricate" the inside of your body—your joints and intestines.[635] Unheated fats are also important for supplying your skin with visually plumping fat.

Cooked carbohydrates, like cooked fats, are also not cosmetically permissible, as "the abuse of cooked carbohydrate foods makes the skin pale-white and often puffy."[636] They're "energetically weak" and strip the body of minerals and B vitamins, leaving us with "chapped lips and wrinkles."[637] Wolfe even assails "beans and legumes" as "unfavorable to beauty," implying that their "coarse proteins" are not easily assimilable and thusly can't efficiently build healthy skin, hair, and nails.[638]

Minerals are a key beautifying aspect of raw organic foods, according to Wolfe. It's "internal food-mineral cosmetics that add color and hue to the face, skin, hair and nails."[639] He argues that cooked and processed foods are deficient in minerals and that the minerals from raw plants are most assimilable because they contain minerals in their "living state" and the co-factors that accompany them.[640] The effects of

---

[631]   Ibid., 44.

[632]   Ibid., 21.

[633]   Ibid., 19.

[634]   Ibid., 36.

[635]   Ibid.

[636]   Ibid., 38.

[637]   Ibid., 37.

[638]   Ibid., 41.

[639]   Ibid., 48.

[640]   Ibid., 61.

raw plant minerals, as opposed to cooked, are beyond what nutritional science can understand, he claims. He describes them as being sentient substances.[641]

Minerals build beauty. Their effects on the body are described in aesthetic terms. Sulfur, for instance, is described as the foundational mineral of all beauty. It produces a "flame-like tint in the skin."[642] It creates a subtle luster as delicate as the halo around the full moon on a clear desert evening."[643] The sulfur you eat from raw hemp seeds, arugula, onions, spirulina, kale, cabbage, and other greens and fruits is "truly . . . the best cosmetic in the world," as it is highly concentrated in the proteins in your hair, skin, and nails.[644] Other minerals like silicon, zinc, and manganese are critical for building the collagen that keeps skin plump and youthful.

Eating cooked food is akin to putting poison on a beautiful garden. Eating raw food, on the other hand, is like softly nourishing the soil of your body. Skin, hair, and nails are "grown from ideal raw foods."[645] "Nutrient-rich raw food" builds "luster in the hair, freshness in the skin, and herbal fragrance in the body."[646]

Lastly, general purity was a major beautifying advantage of a raw food diet. Toxemia, similarly to what Ann Wigmore talked about—the "accumulation of toxic substances in tissues" from the environment and from processed and cooked food—is the "primary cause of problem skin . . . , accelerated aging, and poor muscle quality."[647] Pesticides, heavy metals, corrupted cooked fat and protein, intestinal debris, and even "emotional residue" and "buried hurt" are gradually cleansed out of the body on a raw organic diet, he claims. By this physical and emotional "self-purification" we become "beings of pure essential beauty."[648]

In considering all of these benefits of raw food, Wolfe says, we come across a "startling truth: You can change your bone structure; you can greatly alter your appearance; you can change the mood of your flesh to suit your ideals."[649] You engage in an intelligent conversation with your body by choosing what food to eat. You build yourself. You form the personality of your body and its appearance. You are

---

[641]   Ibid., 63.
[642]   Ibid., 65.
[643]   Ibid., 65.
[644]   Ibid., 67.
[645]   Ibid., 3.
[646]   Ibid., 13.
[647]   Ibid., 51.
[648]   Ibid., 59.
[649]   Ibid.

the creative master and raw foods are the servants that carry out your wishes. You should feel, Wolfe tells us, empowered to create the body you want. "The raw food ideal . . . represents the highest aspirations of beauty in the human spirit," sings Wolfe.[650]

The Beautification of Body Parts

Wolfe believes that raw food nourishes all of our cosmetic assets, even beyond skin. He describes our hair as an agricultural crop that has its roots in the blood-enriched lymphatic soil beneath the skin. The consistent nutrition and blood flow that is fed to the hair when we adhere to raw diets prevents hair loss and premature greying. Animal protein, cooked fats, and demineralized foods on the other hand, clog blood vessels, inflame hair follicles, and destroy hair quality, Wolfe claims.[651]

Healthy teeth are maintained by highly mineralized "rich green foods" like leafy greens and silicon-rich herbs and grasses. Teeth are built from the inside out, so conventional toothpastes can be left aside. The only hygienic materials needed for teeth are hemp, mint, and neem oils to brush with.[652]

Eyes also take on a new vibrancy on a raw diet. They can even change color. "Typically on a raw diet, the eyes soften, lighten, become more luminescent, and show more gold, green, or blue." "Eye beauty," says Wolfe, "is a natural by-product of real and deep tissue cleansing caused by eating a raw-food-based diet."[653] Cooked oils assail the eyes by clogging "the tiny capillaries of the eyes and lead to cataracts." For the area surrounding the eyes, like dark circles underneath, they can be corrected and recolored by eating raw foods that contain sodium like celery, chard, kale, or spinach.[654]

Even the beauty of one's voice is affected by a raw diet. "Vocal beauty" increases and "takes on more pleasant tones in both the higher ranges and deeper baritone ranges."[655] Mucus and vocal cord inflammation from poor or cooked diets resolve.

---

650   Ibid., 15.
651   Ibid., 134.
652   Ibid., 136.
653   Ibid., 137.
654   Ibid., 138.
655   Ibid.

The Beautification of Life

Besides the body, raw food beautifies the experience of life as a whole, Wolfe believes.

"Different foods fuel different types of thoughts, different potentials for success, and different destinies." Raw foods bring positivity to the mind, put you on a higher vibrational frequency, enhance your destiny and fuel success in your endeavors. Raw food enables self-actualization. It enables you to be spiritual and healthy enough to "express one's mission on Earth."[656]

Expanding on his corporeal "juiciness" theory, Wolfe claims that raw foods not only make our tissues juicier, but they also "make you more juiced about life, and juice allows you to squeeze more juice out of every moment."[657] You'll be more alive to the beauty of life and its possibilities, and more enthusiastic.

Civilization as a whole suffers from not living out a raw foods lifestyle. Consuming toxic food, including cooked food, destroys our "art, architecture, cinema, music, literature" because these creations are made by people who are highly deficient in raw food —"devoid of the raw essence of beauty." They don't have the magical spirit of uncooked plant foods within them; they don't have the feeling of beauty in themselves and so are not able to conjure beauty in their work. The art that is created by people with toxified bodies and brains is just as unappealing as their unhealthy flesh and impoverished spiritual state. "Inner toxicity has created the dismal corporate cities we see on the outside." In life, "pollution and ugliness" go hand in hand, inside and outside the body.[658]

---

[656] Ibid., 2.
[657] Ibid., 14.
[658] Ibid., 23.

13.
Aesthetics Looking Outward:
Painting While Eating Raw

Joe Alexander

*"So I hope more painters will take up [a] raw food diet because
I'd like to see some more REAL painting in the world."*
—Joe Alexander

*"[The] raw food diet has great potential to enhance
the beauty and vitality of human culture."*
—Joe Alexander

As we've seen, raw foodist discussions of aesthetics are usually centered around how diet shapes our bodies. But a unique perspective on how raw food affects our experience of beauty in the world—the perceptions of our environment and art—comes from American painter Joe Alexander.

In the 1990s, Alexander wrote that his "major goal in life" was to fulfill van Gogh's prophecy that "the painter of the future will be a colorist such as has never been seen before." Nobody thus far, Alexander claimed, had been able to fulfill this prophecy.[659] In his mind, the reason there had been such an artistic shortfall on a wide scale is due to diet.

"All the painters pollute their sense of color with cooked food," Alexander claims—their visual sense is diminished by their diet. The vibrancy, coloring, and shape of the human body, in this view, was not the only thing that cooked food ruined. It ruined our sense of beauty,

---

[659] Ibid., 6.

as we perceived it in our surroundings. If we don't consume colorful uncooked plants, our brains and spirits would not perceive color correctly, out there in the external world. The raw food diet, Joe made clear, "is the way to liberate a painter's sense of color" to be able to fulfill van Gogh's prophecy and create especially vibrant art.[660]

But most painters are aesthetically subdued, like the modern world surrounding them. Nearly everyone has diminished aesthetic sense and most human-made things like buildings, films, etc. fall short of their potential because people have a corrupted sense of what is visually attractive. They have been lulled by cooked food.

Twentieth-century society, Alexander wrote, was in a "downward spiral" of spiritual and aesthetic "degeneration." "No longer feeling a unity with nature, people construct the debilitating artificial environments of . . . cities" in which they live. People were disconnected from the primary source of aesthetic inspiration, the natural world, because they were not eating natural things. Ugliness thus pervaded human-made environments and an ugly spirit infected people's souls. "People eat cooked food which depresses and irritates them thus leading to a depressed and angry emotional atmosphere."[661] The vibes are bad and the ugliness of cooked-food inspired architecture further "debilitates" the soul. Cooked food is at the genesis of darkness; it sets off the horrid chain reaction.

People who feel the depressing spiritual atmosphere caused by cooked food and are subjected to this ever-present visual ugliness, predictably create "ugly music and art." "Destructive technology" and anything that produces fumes or other pollution "further poisons the environment." Negative behavior grows out of this toxic atmosphere: alcoholism, drug addiction, crime, child abuse, abortions. Cooked food also generates a twisted sense of entertainment and beauty in peoples' morphed brains. They become "utterly fascinated with the . . . morbid, the horrible and terrifying, and have a sort of sneering contempt for what is normal, natural, healthy, and beautiful."[662] It disturbs the mind and creates perversity.

The "root cause" of why cooked food initiates all this misery is that it contains "dark, stagnant, negative anti-life energy, or DOR [deadly orgone radiation]," as New Age thinker William Reich named it.[663] This pathological energy, Reich posited, accumulates in environments and people due to unnatural pollution, emotional suppression,

---

[660] Ibid.
[661] Ibid., 72.
[662] Ibid., 74.
[663] Ibid.

and, as Alexander submits, cooked food consumption. "Cooked food poisoning" is blamed as "the most universal and widespread" cause of this DOR "pollution" of our "consciousness."[664] We must clean up this heavy energy in our diets because it is the source of our thwarted sense of aesthetics, among other miserable traits.

Alexander believed this to be true because he experienced both sides of this sensory binary. "As an artist, when I ate cooked foods I painted bleak, grotesque surrealist-type pictures with drab and dull, muddy colors," he explained. "But when I became a raw food eater, I began to paint instead vibrantly alive pictures with lush abundance of healthy shapes and brilliantly beautiful colors."[665] William Reich, Alexander pointed out, connected "the sort of lush jungle growth" that Alexander painted with the healthy orgone energy.

But many cooked-food artists had a "corruption of the life-force" or "deadly orgone" within them and couldn't connect to nor desire to paint lush natural beauty.[666] The eye, brain, and spirit on cooked food crave images of ugliness, of distortion and blunted colors.

On a raw diet, Alexander claimed, "My drawing became much more rhythmic." When eating cooked food, drawings "tended to be a tangled mess of chaotic lines." The improved drawing patterns "was of course an outgrowth . . . of a more properly and rhythmically aligned energy field," he believed, accomplished as a result of eating raw.[667] Inner energy from food ends up on the canvas.

Alexander made clear how the artistic improvements he experienced on a raw diet, and not just the physical benefits, were key to continuing the diet. When he wrote his book, cheekily titled *Blatant Raw Foodist Propaganda!*, He said that maintaining the "improved sense of color and visual rhythm" were some of the primary reasons for abandoning cooked food.[668] The energetic vibrations within this more alive food apparently changed even the "rhythm" of the painter to a healthier state.

"The raw food diet did wonders for my color sense," Alexander said. "I felt that a dark cloud had been swept from my mind, revealing an inner world of brilliant and beautiful color."[669] His description blurs the spiritual and artistic, as the change in sensory perception had enlivened his soul.

---

[664]   Ibid., 75.
[665]   Ibid.
[666]   Ibid., 75.
[667]   Ibid., 102.
[668]   Ibid., 105.
[669]   Ibid., 103.

People started to remark on his raw foodist paintings, saying that they'd never seen such strong and beautiful color in paintings before. Alexander concurred with their opinions—other artists rarely had such results. Most cooked-food artists painted as if they saw through a "smoky mirror," their vision obscured. His paintings, on the other hand, "have a clarity that is very seldom seen" and look as if "through a freshly washed, clear glass."[670] Colorful, pure, undistorted raw plant food had cleansed the vision.

The "lush and abundant life" of the raw foodist painter was a stark contrast to the "dull, dreary and desolate-looking" images of the cooked foodist. "Raw food put me back in touch with nature's force of creation," Alexander believes. The same force that "creates grass" and trees works through the raw foodist artist.[671] By eating food in its most natural state, the artist supposedly imbibes the powers that nature possesses.

RECONNECTING WITH NATURE THROUGH RAW FOOD

The aesthetic conversion brought about by raw food was confirmed by Alexander's "sudden renewed interest in Nature." By eating nature in its purest form, he now felt at one with it. Gardening and farming became enjoyable. Animals captured his attention as well. He started finding "squirrels, cats, birds, and dogs fascinating." He would stop and gawk. Cities "for the first time," seemed ugly and unnatural.[672] He eventually "couldn't stand" the lifeless concrete of the city and had to move out. Raw food had naturally generated aesthetic antipathies to artificiality in addition to the deepened enjoyment of natural objects.

On the diet, he said, "the world of Nature becomes far more interesting than artificial entertainments."[673] "I would rather go see a garden than a movie," Alexander explained.[674] Other people remained disconnected from nature and kept to their morbid movies and other diversions because, he reminds us, they "eat cooked food which depresses and irritates them."

The "anti-life and degenerative influence that is built into the very fabric of our common way of life," from cooked food, makes it difficult for an artist to appreciate the beauty of nature. Degenerative food gen-

---

[670] Ibid.

[671] Ibid.

[672] Ibid., 104.

[673] Ibid., 62.

[674] Ibid., 104.

erates a "pollution of consciousness," spawning a craving for degenerate landscapes.[675] But when diet is changed and the "dark, stagnant, negative anti-life energy" is purged from the body, the artist embraces the beauty of nature.[676] The "sneering contempt for what is natural, normal and healthy and beautiful," as he called it, vanishes.[677] The artist's "life-force" is replenished and energetic harmony prevails, thus he can appreciate nature. The raw food artist also absorbs the luscious and fertile qualities of the plants he eats and obtains the desire to express those qualities on canvas.

In appreciating nature and creating art, Alexander no longer needed chemical crutches to feel good or be inspired. "Recreational drugs lose their attraction because raw food diet is a better high than even LSD."[678]

The Future of a Beautiful Raw World

Beyond his art, Alexander hoped for a prettier, cleaner, and happier future for humanity, in which a utopian society, fueled by "fruits, nuts, vegetables and sprouted grains, all uncooked," builds renewable energy resources, breathes in fresh re-forested air, and practices "a high degree of very fine artistry and craftsmanship."[679] A renewed environment, better health, and a deep connection with beauty all came from raw food, he felt.

---

[675]   Ibid., 73.
[676]   Ibid., 72.
[677]   Ibid., 74.
[678]   Ibid., 103.
[679]   Ibid., 97.

Spirituality of New Age Raw Foodism

Health, aesthetics, and ecological benefits aren't the only perks praised by modern raw foodists. Enhanced spirituality is another supposed attraction of a raw food diet. In the worldview of spiritualist raw foodists, the body feeds into the spirit. What we feed the body seeps into the soul.

The health of the body and the spirit (or mind) are indeed often seen as intertwined. But in what might be called the New Age corners of the raw foodist movement, the connection between the body and spirit takes on new intricacies and depth and food is held to have especially far-reaching metaphysical influence.

New Age raw foodists don't just look at general physiological patterns and how they affect the brain. They look beyond the modern mechanistic-materialist facts such as that inflammation in the body, for example, affects the brain and thus our moods. There are more subtle effects on the spirit and consciousness from food, raw foodists claim.

Mainstream science is left behind because, raw foodists believe, it hasn't caught up with the knowledge they claim to have. Their supposed knowledge is gained by a mixture of intuition, historical tradition, and personal experience instead of relying on commonly valued peer-reviewed studies for insight into the human condition.

THE NEW AGE

The nutritional-spiritual paradigms of many late-twentieth-century and early-twenty-first-century raw foodists are saturated with influence from the New Age movement that preceded them, which initially came to prominence in the 1960s and 1970s.

The New Age movement comprises a wide ranging amalgamation of spiritual practices from different times and places. Traces of Buddhism, Daoism, Kabbalah, Christianity, Sufism, Indigenous spirituality of the Americas, and Hinduism have been infused in this eclectic movement. Author and expert Nevill Drury notes that the movement hankers for "experiences of higher consciousness and personal growth."[680] The New Age "argues for a spirituality without borders or confining dogmas," writes Drury.[681] "Behold the Age of Confluence," says raw foodist David Wolfe in regard to the "extraordinary vista" of possibilities that converge in this movement of trans-cultural spirituality.[682]

The New Age seeks, through a combination of mysticism and occasional science, to deepen human awareness while eroding superficial boundaries between religious traditions. It sees common core truths in all religious traditions. It also rejects the skeptical purely materialistic non-spirituality of some of the modern world.[683]

The movement seeks to reclaim a respect for the power of intuition as well. Intuition, the movement's proponents hold, can sometimes be well in advance of science in determining truth about our bodies and spiritual health. As raw foodist Joe Alexander said, "true science and intuitive understanding never contradict."[684] Intuition is considered almost a superpower that guides our food choices and other aspects of life.

The mind and the body, consciousness and health, the physical and the metaphysical, are all linked very closely together in the New Age paradigm. Our awareness and individual subjective experiences, it typically holds, can be changed for the better by not only spiritual practices but physical manipulation as well, like body work and diet. The body can be altered by our consciousness and vice versa—our consciousness can be substantially affected by our body and the food that we eat.

Food, New Age raw foodism holds, can either transport us into the upper levels of insight, happiness, and harmony with the universe or can slide us under a veil of ignorance and gloom. With our dietary choices, we can help usher in a new era for enlightenment and peace or continue patterns of oppression, destructive ego consciousness, suf-

---

[680]   Nevill Drury. *The New Age: A History of the Movement.* New York, Thames & Hudson, Inc., C, 2004, 8.

[681]   Ibid.

[682]   Wolfe, David, and Charles Nicholas Good. *Amazing Grace : The Nine Principles of Living in Natural Magic.* San Diego, Calif., Sunfood Pub.; Berkeley, Calif, 2008.

[683]   Nevill Drury. *The New Age: A History of the Movement.* New York, Thames & Hudson, Inc., C, 2004, 8.

[684]   Alexander, Joe. *Blatant Raw Foodist Propaganda!* Blue Dolphin Publishing, 1990, 63.

fering, and ignorance. Cooked food, in this paradigm, is darkness; raw food is light.

For our discussion on New Age raw foodism, we start with Johnny "Lovewisdom," a pioneer in intermingling eclectic New Age spirituality with raw foodism.

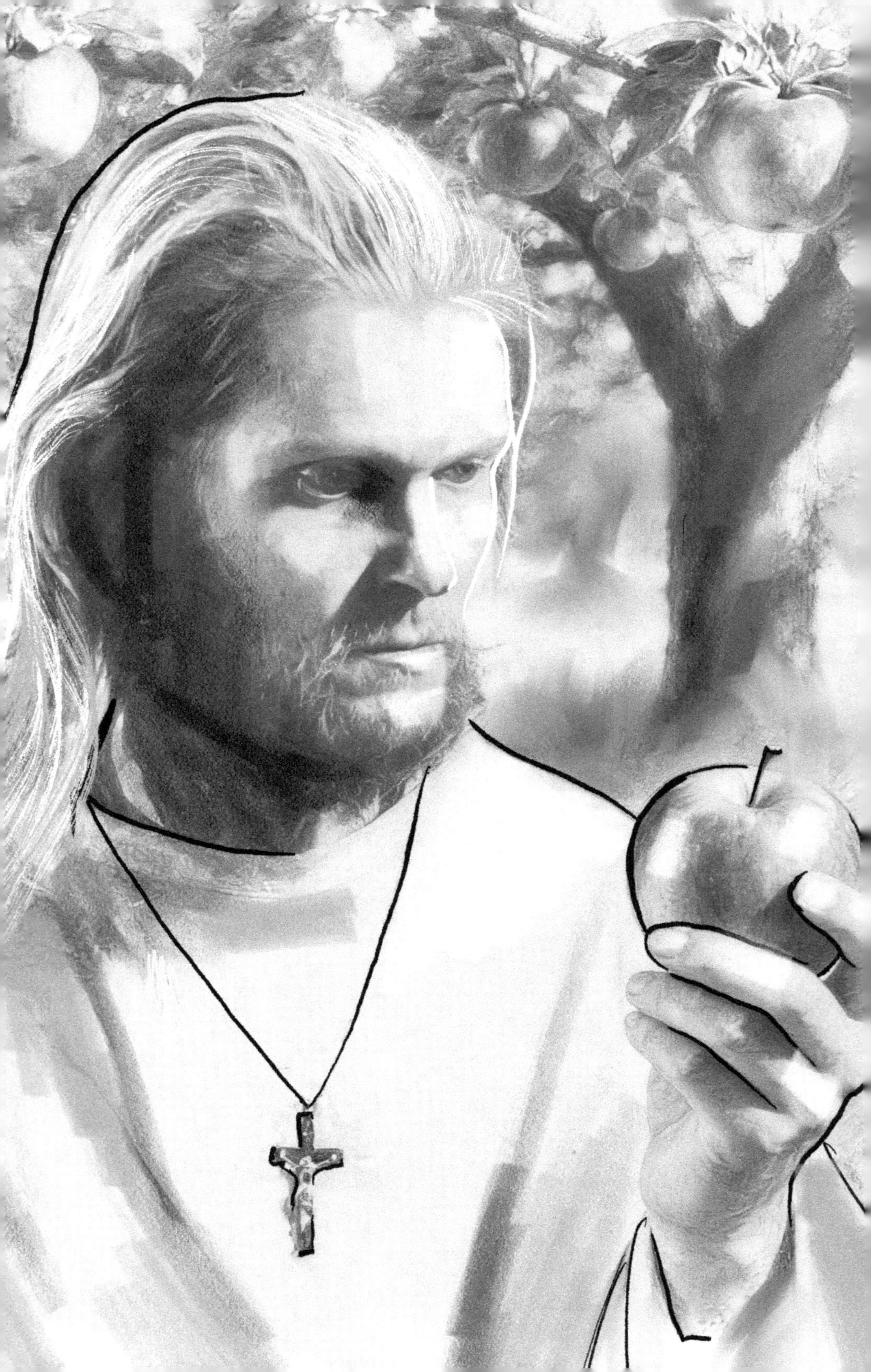

14.
Johnny "Lovewisdom" Wierlo: Spiritual War against Sex and Death

On the eve of World War II, an American man made plans to move to South America after he was conscripted for the fight. As the raw food-loving Führer of Germany was about to initiate worldwide destruction and his own final dismal years, Johnny Lovewisdom would begin his peculiar career as a religious figure and raw food advocate.

Lovewisdom, whose birth name was Johnny Wierlo, was born in Washington state in 1919 to Estonian immigrant parents. But he would live out a spiritually-focused raw food quest in South America for nearly sixty years, the vast majority of his life.

Photographs of Lovewisdom show a man with long straight light brown hair, smiling, talking with followers, picking fruit, and wearing a white robe with a red cross that looks remarkably like a Ku Klux Klan robe. But Johnny's aims were not racially motivated in any way. He was fixated on conquering the most formidable universal foe imaginable: death. To do so, cooked food and sex would have to be done away with. With this plan, Lovewisdom set out in his attempt to recreate a type of Edenic paradise, a fruit-fueled sexless paradise.

New Age Before the New Age

"What right have we Westerners . . . claiming the Judo-Christian Bible as the oracle of Truth, beyond which no other Verities can exist?"
—Johnny Lovewisdom

Johnny functioned like a New Age star, or cult leader, before the New Age was a more formalized movement. He was actively writing down his New Age-like philosophies in the 1940s, decades ahead of his time. In the 40s and 50s, before the counterculture of the 1960s and the fruition of many New Age philosophies and writings in the 1970s, Lovewisdom was living out his unique and amalgamated beliefs.

Lovewisdom borrowed from many religions in forming his own religious order. Christian, Hindu, Buddhist, Daoist, and other philosophies were utilized to build the Pristine Order of Paradisian Perfection, which came to be officially recognized by the government of Ecuador, the country of Lovewisdom's naturistic style residence.

Lovewisdom chose Ecuador as his home because he could grow fruit there easily, he wouldn't be exposed to industrial pollution, and because of the openness to foreigners and affordability of the country. Living in an environment conducive to a strict raw foodism and being isolated from the trappings of modern society was certainly important.

In this location, Lovewisdom could focus on his far-flung aims, one of which was the "sublimation of the sex force and substance." He believed this sublimation, or in other words, the avoidance of ejaculation for males, was a source of longevity as well as spiritual power. If practiced perfectly, he felt, it could actually accomplish immortality.

All religions, he believed, recognize the value of chastity and the desire for the termination of the sex drive.[685] "Words of wisdom" from Christian teachings are "identical to Higher Doctrine of Buddha and of Yogis."[686] The Bhagavad Gita has profound truths identical or comparable to the Christian Bible, Lovewisdom explained, in a very New Age rejection of insular religious exclusivity.[687] All truly spiritual texts, his main point was, bid readers to relinquish their sex drive and gain spiritual power.

Lovewisdom believed that he had expertly combined these disparate traditions and had retrieved the critical essence from each of them. As leader of his Paradisian sect, he had become a prophet and the voice of the most advanced spiritual teachings the world had ever received. "Jesus Christ could only vaguely start to tell men of his day [the truth]," Lovewisdom claimed. "He had to bid men farewell saying they were not able to bear the teaching . . . and that the Spirit of truth would come to reveal it."[688] The Spirit of Truth had now arrived in Johnny Lovewisdom. This was fitting, considering that he believed that he was the reincarnation of Buddha's disciple Ananda as well as John the Baptist.

---

[685]   Lovewisdom, Johnny. *Spiritualizing Dietetics ""Vitarianism.""* Createspace Independent Pub, 5 June 2014, 113

[686]   Ibid.

[687]   Ibid., 192.

[688]   Ibid., 138.

Leaving behind the orthodox religious structures of the past, "We need," he believed, "a live religion." Humanity needed a "democratic Universal Scripture accepted by all parts of the world" and instructive teachers of comparative religions, so that people can know and live out the essential teachings of all religions.[689]

Lovewisdom's teachings could act as a synthesis of sacred doctrines that had been hidden in the world's religious texts, he felt. "In the Vitarian Way," as Lovewisdom called his spiritual and dietary regimen, "for the first time in the history of religions, philosophies, and sciences, you are now given a practical way of spiritual living to give one the experience of knowing the Transcendent Truth." He was the greatest teacher of all and saving the world. Before he came along, "Never has the root cause of world suffering been found."[690] Even the best of the past sages couldn't get to the truth like he did.

Perhaps it's not so surprising that someone that confident, who believed he was ushering in an age of universal wisdom, also had the confidence that he could possibly defeat his own sexual instinct and even death itself.

To Defeat Sin and Death

"Why did man fall?" Lovewisdom asks, "How did man lose his original spiritual state," the state of idyllic union with God in the garden of Eden, and degrade into "a creature fired with passion?" Why did man become a carnal mess, a creature of woeful erotic craving and destructive emotions? Man became this way, Johnny answered, because he started eating unnatural food. It was when Adam and Eve gave up the "paradisiacal diet" of fruit and "herbs."[691]

Sexual craving, the result of unnatural eating, "is not natural," Lovewisdom believed.[692] Even marriage is "legalized prostitution." [693] Ungodly and cursed food made man crave sex and procreation, when before that, man lived in supreme awareness, non-suffering, and a state of immortality. But then humans ate the forbidden food.

The "first precept given to man" in the Bible, the most important rule in existence, Lovewisdom points out, deals with "what [we] should eat." Man, by eating from the wrong tree and disobeying God's

---

689   Ibid., 194.
690   Ibid., 138.
691   Ibid., 6.
692   Ibid., 71.
693   Ibid., 72.

precept, thus plagued himself with "suffering and death."[694] God had warned humans to not eat of the "tree of knowledge" and "die the death" which Lovewisdom believed signified not just one specific forbidden apple but "seed" foods.

These so-called seed foods refer largely to grains, nuts, and seeds. Lovewisdom says that there was an upside to falling into the temptation of eating them: they make one "rather quick witted or brainy"—they give one a sense of "knowledge" but in return, the eater forfeits humanity's original state of spiritual innocence. Most crucially, the eater of this seedy "lust-producing food" falls for a life of sexuality.[695] And sexual activity was not good for longevity or spirituality.

Because of this nutritional theology, Lovewisdom was strictly opposed to the consumption of grains, legumes, nuts, and seeds (as well as animal products).

In Lovewisdom's vocabulary, lust was synonymous with all "passions"—all "sin." To this day, ever since the fall, he says, all the world "so prays for the rest from desire, relief from pain, passion." But hardly anyone suspects Lovewisdom's revealed truth that "all sin goes back to the Original Sin" of eating anything other than "fruit and herbs." For in this nutritional deviation, Lovewisdom proclaims, "all sin is rooted." Humans became a pernicious, ravenous "bread-eating people" with lives full of pain, desperate yearning, and violence. The earth fell from paradise. Wars began. Everything went to seed, so to speak. Humans were now nutritionally and morally lost creatures who, having rejected the holy fruit food meant for them, would "murder for a dish of lentils, [or] kill to partake of animal carcasses."[696]

The dietary violation of eating forbidden foods lowered humankind's lifespan progressively from hundreds of years to 120 years, and eventually less. Eating this way also made people burn with strange emotions, generated a terrible lack of morality, and "created the detestable Old Testament Bible history" filled with war, suffering, perversity, and other sins—"sorrow, passion for killing, lust of the flesh and painful existence."[697]

Despite the history of this torturous deviation from God's Edenic menu, humans could spiritually and physically reclaim "The Genesis," the seminal state of Adam and Eve. Extreme physical longevity and spiritual bliss were in his sights. This state of being is available for all time and "is not a thing of the past . . . and is eternally true," he

---

694   Ibid., 16.
695   Ibid., 8.
696   Ibid., 9.
697   Ibid., 6.

reminded followers, and could be reclaimed by starving the body of devilish food and squashing sexuality.[698]

To Forsake Sex and Gain Life

> *"Stop now, before it is too late . . . Give up the old*
> *Adam for the new Christ . . . You are the one to decide*
> *whether man fails or becomes Life Regenerate."*
> **—Johnny Lovewisdom**

> *"Degeneration came from eating nuts, and other forms of*
> *seeds and protein that build flesh and sensuality."*
> **—Johnny Lovewisdom**

"Truly everything is obtainable thru [sic] a chaste life," Lovewisdom believed.[699]

The reverence for chastity, evident in religious traditions the world over, is "not merely a religious superstition, but a biological concern in hygiene," he claimed, because the sublimation of the sex drive and the conservation of one's reproductive fluids facilitates bodily regeneration.[700]

"The holy life," and the healthy life, "is that of celibacy," Lovewisdom proclaimed.[701] "Whosoever is born of God committeth not sin." He quotes John, disciple of Christ, for "his seed abideth in him" (or as Lovewisdom interprets, "the semen remained in him").[702] And when Jesus says "death shall be no more" in his kingdom, he's really speaking of "celibate regeneration" of the body in the here and now, not in the afterlife.[703]

Our "reproductive fluid was originally intended for reproducing our own body anew continually or eternally," Lovewisdom explained.[704] Semen, for instance, is an extremely potent life-giving fluid. "Science has found," Lovewisdom dubiously claimed, that "40 drops of blood

---

[698] Ibid., 6,7.

[699] Ibid., 76.

[700] Ibid., 12.

[701] Ibid., 47.

[702] Ibid., 47, 48.

[703] Ibid., 48.

[704] Ibid., 61.

[is] equal to only one drop of semen."[705] Waste this precious substance and "disease will only prove the result," he warned.[706]

Semen, the biologically "creative substance," is involved in the production of blood, which Lovewisdom called the 'life of the body' because it builds tissues. No wonder that Gandhi (a fellow sexual sublimatist and also part-time raw foodist), Lovewisdom notes, linked "perfect health" with "conservation of the sexual secretions."[707]

The "creative" attributes of semen also extend to the spiritual. The loss of, or conversely, the constant conservation of the fluid "makes the difference between the saints of God-realization and sinners."[708] It makes the difference between being spiritually aware and intuitive or grasping in the darkness of ignorance.

Celibacy was at the core of spirituality and hygiene, so much so that Lovewisdom argued that Jesus's mission was similar to his own: "Basically Christ's Gospel is on dieting and the celibate life," Lovewisdom plainly put it, "which he continually emphasizes in the scriptures."[709] "Long ago Jesus warned us" that God destroyed those who were "eating, drinking, and marrying" with the Old Testament flood. The Nazarean, Lovewisdom believed, was clearly lambasting dietary deviations and sex even within marriage.

Nutritional and sexual hygiene, he argued, were the core of Jesus's teachings but only the spiritually attuned will read between the lines to understand that. Lovewisdom believed that we must give up having biological families to attain spiritual bliss and physical health. A man's (spiritual) enemies shall be they of his own household, Jesus told us, and "reassured us reward for this forsaking of family in this present life." "Spiritual Love and Ecstasy" replaced sexuality. Chasity gives people "marvelous spiritual power" and only those that have sublimated their sexual desires, "only the touch of the celibate can forgive sins." There is no desire to procreate and marry anyway, if one doesn't eat "the passion foods."[710]

Lovewisdom believed that his chaste way of life and fruit diet, Vitarianism, is the original true doctrine of Christ. And it is rooted in centuries of spiritual tradition prior to Christ. The yogis of India were teaching the same things—that "the semen is the real vitality of

---

705   Ibid., 68.
706   Ibid., 69.
707   Ibid., 79.
708   Ibid., 81.
709   Ibid., 48.
710   Ibid., 135.

man, that through conservation one can live as long as one desires."[711] The great Buddha also taught, Johnny claimed, that if we abstain from sexuality, we "destroy birth and death . . . [and] old age will cease."[712] And Daoist masters of China achieved extreme longevity and "food-less living" through a "celibate associating with young virgins."[713]

The corporeal and the spiritual, as is typical in New Age philosophy, were intimately codependent. "The state of the mind is the state of the body, and also the state of the body determines the state of the mind because the two are essentially one," Lovewisdom noted.[714] When we physically and spiritually ruin ourselves with destructive food and sex by "defiling [our] bodies at dinner tables and in bed at night," we become physically decrepit in addition to being "sinners" who are "afraid of truth"—truth like the regenerative power of celibacy.[715] The sinner doesn't want to give up lust, his defilement.

"The fire of passion only burns when it is fed . . . Immoral foods favor an immoral life," Lovewisdom warns.[716] The foods that we must avoid—seeds, nuts, grains, legumes, and animal products have "semen-producing properties."[717] They cause one to have an active reproductive instinct, thus driving the spilling of reproductive fluid or life force. Lovewisdom's dietary stipulations are so strict that even raw avocados are vilified—Lovewisdom includes this fatty fruit in his list of "heavy protein" foods.[718]

Forbidden foods make us "approach death thru accelerating the egg production of the human body" and stimulating the lusts which lead to health-destroying ejaculation.[719] Unlike fruit, seed foods have excessive protein and the body's "instinct is to make use of this excess flesh-making" substance.[720] Lovewisdom is vague about why ejaculation causes us to degenerate but he mentions the draining of "mineral substance" and by the loss of the nebulous "regenerative" power.

But even prior to ejaculation, high protein food causes the "wasting away of teeth, hair, vital organs" and aging in general, Lovewisdom claimed. "Seed foods" drain minerals from our tissues to "manufacture the reproductive fluid." Then lust takes over, we ejaculate during sex or

---

[711] Ibid., 49.
[712] Ibid., 50.
[713] Ibid., 137.
[714] Ibid., 63.
[715] Ibid., 93.
[716] Ibid., 51.
[717] Ibid., 20.
[718] Ibid., 21.
[719] Ibid., 10.
[720] Ibid., 11.

have nocturnal excretions and the valuable minerals drawn from our vital organs are squandered, "poured into the sewer."[721]

"Superfluous protein" converts into "toxins" that damage the reproductive energy centers of the body. By these foods, we "inflame" these "regenerative centers" that could be instead used to regenerate the rest of our bodies.[722] The "tumorous" growth of excessive cells in the ovaries and testicles saps the "vitality of youth, giving body wearout, age . . . pathological degeneration." But by fasting and eating the Edenic "food of paradise" (fruit), we can regain the anti-reproductive ever-renewing state of "pre-puberty power of the incorruptibility of the flesh" and "restore man's power over death" that was destroyed by protein foods.[723]

Meat is certainly off the table for Lovewisdom. It is "the height of sin." We can't make healthy bodies out of "putrefying carcasses." And meat fuels sexual lust like crazy. "He who lusts after flesh as food, also lusts after flesh in passion."[724] Consumption of meat causes a lust for human meat, so to speak. It will lead you to ejaculation and death. Eggs and milk are no better. Eggs especially, "animal seed," Lovewisdom holds, is the "most potent producer of human seed." Animal products make man "a killer and puppet of passion"—violent and sexual.[725]

The Raw Food Sex-Killing Diet

"Fresh fruits were given as a pleasing and adequate sustenance for man, and are a secure refuge for living free from passion of the flesh."
—Johnny Lovewisdom

The rough and treacherous road of the extreme calorie restriction of "Christian saints of the past," including that of the Desert Fathers, Lovewisdom notes, is not very appealing or realistic for most moderns who have little chance of being "one in a million" who can survive on one meal of little sustenance per day. In place of such a diet, an only-fruit diet acts as the more realistic and tolerable way of cleansing the deadly passions from the body.

---

[721]   Ibid., 39.
[722]   Ibid., 145.
[723]   Ibid., 146.
[724]   Ibid., 19.
[725]   Ibid.

"The Vitarian Diet," Lovewisdom explains, can be briefly defined as "conservation of the seed of life."[726] "Making oneself a spiritual eunuch . . . [the] sublimation of the sexual building force, is the object of Vitarianism." And why would one sublimate lust? To find the "Fountain of Youth" within and be vital forever. It must be remembered, Lovewisdom instructed his followers, that "the act of generation," sex, "is the beginning of death."[727] Throughout the existence of animals and plants, this is apparent. "Many plants die as soon as the seed is mature."[728]

Lovewisdom's path is not easy, he tells readers. "Most religionists are hoping for a heaven without effort," he warns. Extreme sexual and nutritional discipline is not for the faint of heart but it is the narrow path to salvation and immortal life on earth.[729]

Raw food is the basis of the nutritional portion of Lovewisdom's path. Uncooked food, "live food," Lovewisdom says, is "recommended always"—although he contradicts himself a bit. "Cooked vegetables" can be okay to use as salad dressings, to put over the top of raw salads. But people shouldn't dare add nuts or whole grains (whether raw or cooked) that will feed "pathological seminal losses."[730]

Raw food is a necessary starting place for a Vitarian life but it is not good enough in itself. Raw "seed foods" are still bad. "Mere raw foodism," Lovewisdom found—a raw foodism that includes nuts, seeds, and raw grains—actually intensifies the production of sperm, semen, and the sex drive.[731] This feeding of lust can lead to semen spillage, and thus the destruction of health.

We need to limit our diet to primarily fruit, he thought, to "starve the body of the elements of the lower sensual passions."[732] Jesus told us, Lovewisdom argues, that "Juicy fruit is the ONLY FOOD" we should eat with his references to "drink[ing] henceforth the fruit of the vine."[733] Lovewisdom's interpretation is unique, considering that on the surface, most believe Jesus was referencing wine and saying he will *not* drink more of it, on the earthly plain, because he was about to be crucified.

---

[726] Ibid., 67.

[727] Ibid., 29.

[728] Ibid., 30.

[729] Ibid., 25.

[730] Ibid., 65.

[731] Ibid., 83.

[732] Ibid., 91.

[733] Ibid., 102.

By eating fruit primarily, a very low protein food group, we can "feed the body enough to keep it strong, healthy, and vigorous" while "starving it of the passion and sin."[734] "After a few weeks of the juicy fruit diet," Lovewisdom promises, the overarching goal is accomplished: one will not be tempted by sex, because a fruit-only diet has starved the desire.[735] Vitarian foods generally have less than 2% protein, and more than 75% water, he notes, making it so they don't feed the reproductive instinct with excessive protein building materials.[736]

This aversion to protein and interest in the minimization of "substance" being ingested, steered Johnny toward an interest in breatharianism—the state of eating no food and living off air alone. "Eating destroys instead of supports [sic] Life!" he explained.[737] But Lovewisdom ultimately knew that most people had to eat to survive (or, at least, they believed they had to). And most people liked the pleasure of eating. The closest thing to breatharianism that he could institute among his followers was an all-fruit diet, the vast majority of which is water. At least then, they'd be eating "God's food"—"juicy" fruit, the only truly permissible food. If you were eating "live" raw fruit and absorbing clean air and sunshine, you were on the right Vitarian path.[738] You didn't have to forgo eating altogether.

Fruits are "man's perfect food," and "fruitarianism is a self-evident fact," Lovewisdom believed. Apparently the claim didn't need much explanation, besides the sex-killing aspects of it.

Vegetables are a distant second best. They don't taste that great, for one. Vegetables "have to be combined in salads, cooked, etc., to be liked, while the fruit of the tree is ready to serve, delicious," and raw.[739] "God created the perfectly evolved food, fruit." Just as holy people sublimate grosser sexual desire to use it for higher spiritual purposes, fruit "refines and sublimates the grosser substance from the earth," all the minerals and other substances we need for perfect health, making them readily edible for humans.[740]

Vegetables or herbs, on the other hand, while acceptable in their raw state, are of coarser material and require more energy to digest than fruits. Lovewisdom at times seems to even denigrate the "herbs" that are reluctantly a small part of his Vitarian plan. Fruit is for high-

---

[734]   Ibid., 17.

[735]   Ibid., 28.

[736]   Ibid., 30.

[737]   Ibid., 122.

[738]   Ibid., 116.

[739]   Ibid., 56.

[740]   Ibid., 58.

er spiritual pursuits and vegetables are somehow connected merely to "physical labor," despite the fact that they suck up one's energy and are harder to digest.[741] "The vegetables," he says, "seemed to be an emergency food should man wander elsewhere on earth from his fruit paradise." A fruit diet "requires only three hours sleep," whereas vegetables require six hours sleep.[742]

Vegetables "dull the brain" and produce grogginess because of the "elaborate digestive process" to absorb their nutrients. In fact, it was the dulling and energy-sapping effects of vegetables, Lovewisdom believed, that made humans crave other "narcotic herbs" like tobacco, tea, cocoa, and coffee to stimulate themselves out of their stupor.[743]

Fruit was "the true way of mineralizing the body," while squashing lust, and keeping the valuable reproductive fluids inside the body to do their work of regenerating our tissues.[744]

ANOTHER FAILED QUEST

Lovewisdom's quest was another failed push for power, this time over death. In the end, his lifespan turned out to be fairly normal, as he died at age eighty-one in the year 2000. Neither did his fruitarian ideas flourish on a mass scale.

Lovewisdom was very frail in his later years. He suffered from paralysis, other neurological issues, and poor eyesight—effects he had attributed to pesticide exposure during his early years as a farm laborer in California.[745] But others have eyed his extreme dietary practices of fruitarianism, breatharianism, and a period of living on papaya leaves alone, as potential culprits for his long-term health problems. Some have suspected that Lovewisdom was severely deficient in vitamin B12, the critical nutrient, especially important for the central nervous system, and typically absorbed from animal products.

Two years before his death, Lovewisdom was said to have been visited by a group of Spanish fruitarians who inspired him to rededicate himself to fruitarian advocacy.[746] After seemingly losing faith in

---

[741]   Ibid., 31.

[742]   Ibid., 107.

[743]   Ibid., 109.

[744]   Ibid., 22.

[745]   "Johnny Lovewisdom." *Wikibin.org*, 2025, wikibin.org/articles/johnny-lovewisdom-3. html. Accessed 23 Apr. 2025; Amsden, Matt, and Janabai Amsden. *The RAWvolution Continues : The Living Foods Movement in 150 Natural and Delicious Recipes*. New York, Atria Books, 2013.

[746]   Lovewisdom, Johnny. *The Ascensional Science of Spiritualizing Fruitarian Dietetics*.

his protocol for years, he briefly became inspired again and embraced his peculiar fruitarian beliefs but his longevity was never to reach anywhere close to the far-reaching hopes he had. After continuing to record more of his theories in his last years, he died, proving to the world that sublimating the sex drive and feeding on fruit was not the key to immortality nor did it succeed in resurrecting Eden on earth.

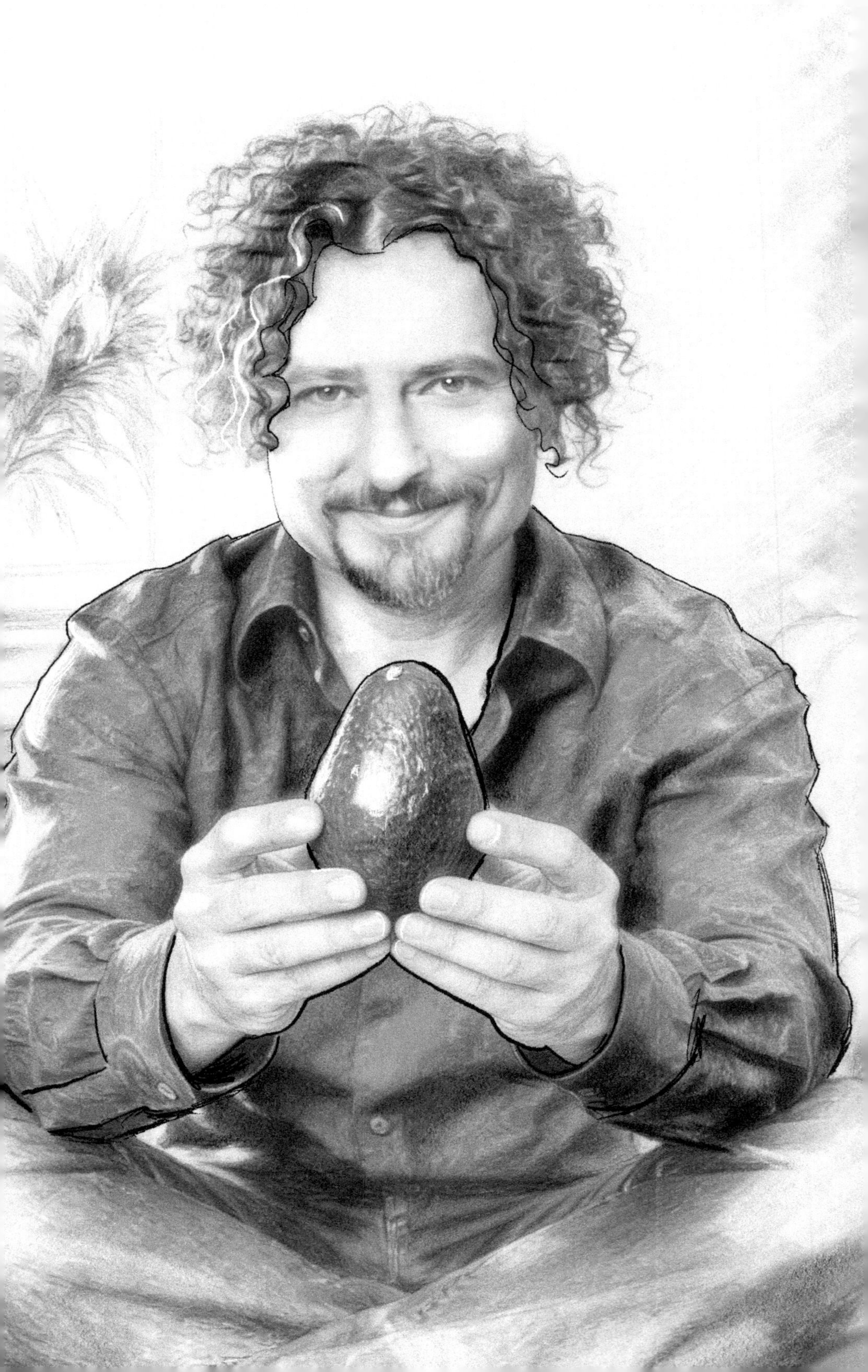

15.
David Wolfe and Raw
Food Spirituality

Along with aesthetics, spirituality was a major focus of Wolfe's raw foodism. His aim, whether spiritual or aesthetic, was always on self-empowerment. Raw food gives us, he argues, a potent awareness of reality along with the power to change the world around us.

Food, he holds, is the key to the flowering of spiritual life. The saying, "'You are what you eat' is the 'zip' file we downloaded from our Creator when we were emailed to the planet at our birth," Wolfe says. What you eat not only determines the quality of your physical form but your consciousness as well. It is an "inescapable fact of quantum reality" that "each person's own nature is always being modified by choices" he says. Self-improvement is accessed through food, in other words. Thus, we should "eat the best food ever and observe the results over time." Cooked food is certainly not the best food. It is "raw plant food" that "ennobles consciousness."[747]

How you "feed your biology" as well as how you "orient your attitude" can create "extraordinary synchronicity, prosperity, joy, magic" or "extraordinary disease, destruction, hate . . . , despair and materialism."[748] Raw food and positive beliefs create a good life. And without eating raw, it's harder to have beliefs that will empower you. Spiritual values, in his paradigm, can act as an outgrowth of the foods we eat. Darkness and despair are the results of low energy and toxic food. Life becomes magical, on the other hand, when we start eating raw organic food. The universe works in our favor. External events conspire to prosper us.

CreateSpace, 20 Mar. 2014.

[747]   Ibid., 9.

[748]   Ibid., 11.

The "magical power of awareness," Wolfe holds, is increased by raw food. We have more power over our "consciousness" as well as "choices" and more "freedom" and ability to express ourselves and accomplish our goals.[749] We become "activated souls" when we achieve a healthier "biology."[750]

Becoming a Spiritual-Nutritional Superhero

By eating raw foods, you cultivate your mind to become, in Wolfe's words, a "superhero"—a being with the power to affect reality, carve out a unique life path, and accomplish anything you can imagine.

The "ability to transmit soul power into this reality is dependent on the art of nutrition," Wolfe says. Our spirits and bodies are intertwined. Our "physical body" is crucial to our spiritual life. The body is the "ocean which laps against the shores of our own soul, "the source of strength for our willpower. And we gather spiritual energy to "assist our sacred journey" from the food we eat.[751]

As our awareness grows, we reject all "pesticide-sprayed . . . fungicide-washed, herbicide-dipped, suicide-filled . . . greedy substances that are currently called 'food,'" Wolfe says in reference to the life-destroying expediency of corporate agriculture.[752] A "superhero" rejects putting crap in her body. She rejects the foods that disable and disempower her mind. Instead, she chooses raw organic fruits, vegetables, nuts, and seeds to eat.

Ormus, Raw Superfoods, and the Gateway to Consciousness

Part of what makes raw foods, and "superfoods," a key component to spiritual empowerment is that they contain special forms of minerals. These unadulterated spiritually alive foods supply us with an "entirely new class of mineral substances that are deeply associated with life-force energy, consciousness, and superpowers."[753] These aren't just hard substances of our old stale conceptions, they are living, dynamic, and intelligent energies that infuse our being with "superpowers." They are

---

[749]   Ibid.
[750]   Ibid.
[751]   Ibid., 56.
[752]   Ibid.
[753]   Ibid.

spiritual superfuel. And if we cook our food, we risk corrupting these precious minerals and thereby diminish our own physical strength and spiritual abilities.

Ormus (Orbitally Rearranged Monoatomic Elements) is another substance that Wolfe claims is in spring water and various raw superfoods. The conception of this substance is controversial and some claim that Ormus doesn't even exist as described. Any scientific case (or lack of a case) for Ormus won't be explored here but Ormus's advocates claim that the substance is precious metal elements like gold, platinum, iridium, and rhodium that exist in a unique, high-spin, monoatomic state as single atoms that are not attached to molecules or standard crystal structures. This unique state of metals, it's claimed, gives Ormus metaphysical and physical effects.

When you consume Ormus, Wolfe claims, it puts you into a "superhero" consciousness that transcends mere "thinking" or reasoning. You enter into the very New Age ability of intuitively "feeling" the universe and become far more aware of reality than short-sighted conceptual thinking can comprehend.[754] "The superhero ethic does not reason and rationalize."[755] The superhero instead downloads intuitive trans-intellectual powers from the cosmos. "Feeling replaces idea," Wolfe puts it simply.[756]

Ormus is powerful, both biologically and spiritually, from Wolfe's perspective. It is the "wire that connects our consciousness to . . . pure energy and imagination." This "pure energy," Ormus, is sometimes referred to as "Infinite Intelligence, the oversoul." Ormus helps our mind access transcendent awareness, the "non-physical . . . eternal consciousness" and helps us see or rather feel things from a higher perspective. This raised awareness lends us "potential and opportunity," in our lives and makes it easier to accomplish dreams, Wolfe notes.[757] Our hopes are much more likely to manifest, through the consumption of a substance.

Our diets should be a major source of Ormus. Wolfe claims that many raw superfoods contain high amounts of the substance: almonds, medicinal mushrooms, blue-green algae, chlorella, seaweeds, hemp seeds, wild coconuts, goji berries, bee pollen, carrots, or any crop grown "with diluted ocean water," which is rich in Ormus.[758]

---

[754] Ibid., 74.

[755] Ibid.

[756] Ibid., 77.

[757] Ibid., 88.

[758] Ibid., 75.

Eating raw is also crucial to absorbing the power of Ormus because cooking, according to Wolfe, depletes Ormus in food. "Cooking food on an open flame or with oil or in any way [makes Ormus] carbonized and oxidized and therefore less useful nutritionally" and could make it "even dangerous."[759] Raw foods are the way that we absorb the maximum amount of Ormus out of the environment.[760] Uncooked plants carry the "life force" and what the ancient Polynesians called *mana* or spiritual energy that we need for our spiritual ascension.

Biology feeds into spirituality by granting us access to the life force of the universe. Whether it's eating high-Ormus super-plant-foods or experiencing mind-altering plant hallucinogens, "Biochemical enlightenment is a real phenomenon" for Wolfe.[761]

Ormus affects the mind in more ways that materialist science can understand thus far, Wolfe argues. But minor preliminary research, he claims, has demonstrated "left and right-brain synchronization" and the increase in brain alpha waves which signify heightened learning and lowering of stress.[762] But, of course, in his view, that's just the tip of the giant iceberg when it comes to this cosmically powerful substance. Its "dynamic" interaction abilities towards other matter make its effects hard to pin down and label. It's an intelligent substance capable of having a vast array of biological and spiritual effects.

Wolfe believes in a mythology of Ormus that reaches back in history. Ormus experts say that pharaohs in ancient Egypt, before ascending to the throne, engaged in a "nine-month fast on Ormus elements," sometimes consuming 500 milligrams of Ormus gold, to aid the "ascension and spiritualization of the crown prince into pharaoh."[763] Wolfe also cites a possible reference to Ormus in the biblical Book of Revelations: "Blessed be the man who will overcome for he shall be given the hidden manna, the white stone of purest kind."[764] Wolfe even implies that Jesus's references to "everlasting life" in the Gospel of John are connected to Ormus consumption.[765] Again, nutritional substance, these tales show us, is a key to spiritual enlightenment.

---

[759]   Ibid., 69.

[760]   Ibid., 75.

[761]   Ibid., 90.

[762]   Ibid., 66.

[763]   Ibid., 63.

[764]   Ibid., 64.

[765]   Ibid., 79.

Raw Souls on Ormus

Imagine a world, Wolfe posited, where humans ascend to higher spiritual levels through consuming high quality raw plant foods. "Imagine an Ormus-soaked biology," he dreams. "What if we," he dreams, "had enough Ormus saturating our system that every cell in our body began to resonate in perfect harmony?" "Thoughts of infinite love and wonder" would overtake us and our "super healthy cellular structures" would resonate with the "highest frequencies of Creation."[766]

Through this "biological transmutation" we become powerful superheroes in both body and soul, living by higher values and able to manifest previously impossible improvements in our lives. By feeding on high-Ormus raw foods, we arrive "at the leading edge of awareness," a spiritual state where we can take inspiration and excitement from "all possibilities" and a "new paradigm" of life on earth, as it should be. We receive more help from the universe—it starts to aid us in our chosen quest. This "harmony" of the Ormus in our bodies with the outside world helps manifest outward phenomena that aids us in our superhero journey by "creating irrational, synchronistic phenomena."[767] The universe conspires with us in a way that surpasses common conceptualization.

Consuming Ormus is like absorbing God's intelligence. It "bring[s] light into your body," Wolfe says vaguely. This is most likely the pure light of the Creator, the consciousness of God, and the power of psychic creation—to manifest desires.[768] Wolfe has learned from anecdotal reports that this substance can "amplify any thought we think. Therefore a body saturated with Ormus is going to be on a psychic cell phone all the time." We can know things that others are blind and deaf to. No wonder "Superheroes (cosmic knights) tap into Ormus," he says.[769]

In considering the extremely exciting near-magical effects of Ormus, a tone of regret or anxiety enters into Wolfe's musings. "What if we have been deficient in Ormus minerals?" Wolfe asks readers to reflect. What if we therefore "never achieved our full capabilities of personal power?"[770] It's a dark thought, to have gone through life without actualizing your abilities or having access to superhuman powers.

---

[766] Ibid., 65.

[767] Ibid., 87.

[768] Ibid.

[769] Ibid., 75.

[770] Ibid., 60.

Don't think eating raw or eating superfoods is important? Think again, argues Wolfe. The entire experience of your life depends on it.

Raw Foodist Mythos: Illuminati vs. Nature

It's clear that raw food and Ormus are the fuel for Wolfe's conception of a spiritual "superhero." But what are the goals or the struggles of the ideal raw food hero figure—what he also calls the Warrior Hero? What is his or her storyline? A highly aware person with an enhanced raw food biology indeed has a narrative arc to fulfill.

The raw superhero should be engaged in a cosmically important battle. The notion of good versus evil is not just a myth of the past, Wolfe explains. This binary struggle is alive and well in the twenty-first century. In Wolfe's raw foodist mythos, the ancient battle is occurring amongst new combatants.

On the side of good, is "Gaia (the spirit of the Earth itself)."[771] It is the duty of a spiritually aware human to protect this sentient being, this planet. The superhero defends the precious and endangered health of Mother Earth, an entity that was created by a loving God. Earth gave birth to humans and sustains us. So we must respect it and defend its purity and dignity. When ecological cleanliness is degraded, the Earth suffers along with all of the creatures that depend on it for life. The health of all creation is imperiled.

In serving nature, the raw superhero is also filled with its power: "Our allies, Wolfe claims, "include everything natural: Gaia, all plants and super-plants."[772] Plant intelligence (everything from raw foods to entheogens) nourishes our minds and bodies and empowers us to fight for Gaia's "pre-ordained . . . strategy" for the "beautification of the physical environment and the ennobling of galactic consciousness."[773] The purpose of human life, as alluded to in the section on Wolfe's aesthetic motives, is to generate beauty on Earth, as well as refine the quality of our awareness, or in other words to be spiritually enlightened.

In addition to plant allies, there are even hidden spiritual forces like "gnomes, fairies, sylphs, nymphs, aliens" that aid the superhero "eco-yogis" and "environmental activists" in their benevolent quest.[774] Wolfe isn't ashamed that some readers will be astounded at the claims

---

[771]   Ibid., 158.

[772]   Ibid., 158–9.

[773]   Ibid., 159.

[774]   Ibid.

that such wide ranging mythical creatures are invisibly helping raw foodists in their quest.

Despite such help, "David has to face Goliath," Wolfe warns. Raw eco-yogis must face a powerful enemy, just as "Jesus has to face the cross."[775] The superhero must face the destroyers and defilers of nature. These evil agents are part of a value system that seeks to abuse, extract from, and destroy the planet. Wolfe names this group the illuminati.[776]

The illuminati, whether a "formal cabal" or not, "certainly exist as an archetype of consciousness in opposition" to nature-loving raw-foodists.[777] Whether or not specific people are conspiring systematically to abuse the Earth is not important to know. What's true for sure is that in general, this "consciousness" is a real phenomenon and must be purged from the planet.

The poisonous attitude can be described as the "banking-military-pharmaceutical-petrochemical-agribusiness-industrial complex" that poses threats "to the detriment of the human family and Mother Earth."[778] This force seeks to siphon profit out of Earth and its people at the expense of the suffering it causes.

The physiological and spiritual are blurred in Wolfe's description of the wicked agents of the illuminati: "The whole direction of civilization has been and is being specifically engineered by the most toxic beings in our world." Spiritually toxic deviants spew physical toxicity into the world. They pollute without shame. It's no wonder that this illuminati is the purveyor of "disease and all forms of disharmony," in Wolfe's mind.[779]

The wanton pollution of our sacred planet, the purveyance of deadly and unnecessary wars, the corporate trashing of the ecosystem for a quick grift, the spraying of toxic synthetic chemicals in our fields, water, and air, the ruthless profiteering and pushing of dangerous pills by pharmaceutical giants—these are the crimes of the illuminati.

One benefit arises out from this dismal picture, however: the misdeeds and dark energy of the illuminati inspire the superhero in her quest to conquer this evil, to feats of greatness. The darkness is a backdrop for the light: "The shocking and horrific revelations of demonic energies associated with many illuminati conspiracy theories propel superheroes into a state of super-consciousness," says Wolfe. The raw superhero is inspired to embrace the opposite values of the ecocidal

---

[775]   Ibid.

[776]   Ibid., 12.

[777]   Ibid.

[778]   Ibid.

[779]   Ibid., 158.

illuminati: "Consciousness, love, laughter, wonder and hope"—the intent of the Universal Soul (God).[780]

In the New Age, being on the side of the environment is how a raw saint embodies the values of God. So take up the mantle of a David, Wolfe urges readers, and save the planet from the Goliath of "psychic and ecological catastrophe . . . Stop working for big brother and start working for the mother," he implores.[781] The divine feminine nurturing spirit of Gaia shall conquer, with the help of conscious raw foodists, the predatory and toxically masculine energy of the illuminati.

Victory is in sight, so eat raw! If the Gaian side wins the cosmic battle and darkness retreats, if "material greed, ignorance, arrogance, military industrialism, pharmaceutical disinformation, [and] suicide ego-tripping" are defeated by "planetary" superheroes, humans could live in an ecological, nutritional, and spiritual utopia. We could have "homes built entirely of natural and recycled materials and filled with scents of wood, beeswax." We could have "raw-food-based super-kitchens" and homes surrounded by gardens "rooted in well-loved soil loaded with Ormus concentrates."[782] The formerly abused Gaian ecosystem will be cleansed and healed. "War, toxicity, and disease" will retreat, good values will prevail, and our bodies will flourish with the highest quality nutrition imaginable. "Hold onto your chakras, because the future is going to be [the] wildest ride ever," Wolfe beams.[783]

ALIEN CIVILIZATION AS THE MYTHIC TEMPLATE FOR RAW SPIRITUALITY

"Any discussion of ultimate success and spiritual transformation must . . . explore at least the possibility of an alien presence."
—David Wolfe[784]

To illustrate what the values of a utopian raw-fed society would look like, Wolfe outlines a narrative, which he believes to be true, of an enlightened alien civilization that perfectly embodies the Gaian values that humans should live by.

Wolfe is committed to the idea of an extraterrestrial race, but he realizes that such a claim is bound to be dismissed by many people.

---

[780]   Ibid.
[781]   Ibid.
[782]   Ibid., 122.
[783]   Ibid., 159.
[784]   Ibid., 26.

"If the belief in the illuminati or aliens is too much to take," he allows, "it is nevertheless the story, the mythology of our times"—the "archetypal situation we are in."[785] Whether this alien race exists literally or metaphorically is secondary to the fact that the archetype mirrors the real moral struggle in our world. After all, "the superhero," Wolfe says, "does not ask what to believe but instead wonders: 'What is it useful to believe?' What can you believe that would allow you to feel incredible all the time?"[786] Believing in benevolent, peaceful, ecology-protecting aliens is apparently the answer. The intuitive value of beliefs, of whatever beliefs make our lives better and guide us to virtue, is what matters most on a raw-fueled spiritual quest.

These beings from outer space can serve as a template for humans to follow in achieving a higher "collective state of self-awareness, of consciousness" since the aliens "got out of a state of conflict with each other, and out of conflict within themselves" and into a state of "enlightenment." "This appears to be an actual fact," Wolfe states plainly.[787] Humans, he instructs, should follow their example and convert our "competitive natures," and the destructive profiteering and warmongering that results, into "something that is beneficial . . . [like] transcending war [and] solving every ecological threat."

Spirituality and ecology are linked for these enlightened beings. Aliens, having cared for and respected the ecology of the Earth and the rest of the universe, are "extremely connected to the ancient devic energies of the Earth (Gaia)." They are spiritually in tune with nature, Wolfe says.

Nutritional habits are also, of course, intertwined with Wolfe's spiritual descriptions and are deeply tied to ecological care. Wise aliens are said to have a metaphysical connection with their raw-food-nourished human "superhero" brethren. "Earth-friendly souls" are described by the alleged alien Tan as "children of the living waters, possessors of the staff of reason."[788] By consuming the power of nature directly, its "living waters," human raw foodists absorb the benevolent energies of Gaia, the Earth, and raise their consciousness to a higher level of awareness.

On the other hand, aliens are certainly not friends of the Earth-hating illuminati, the power-hungry human rulers of the world. The illuminati don't even want people to know about the existence of aliens, as it would challenge their power and give Gaian superheroes

---

[785]   Ibid., 32.

[786]   Ibid., 150.

[787]   Ibid., 32.

[788]   Ibid., 33.

a morale boost. "The illuminati's alien cover-up is the most elaborate and pervasive of any lie ever told," claims Wolfe. These immoral people want to "protect their rulership (as the Earth's masters)," from "cosmic angels," or "alien races who potentially might want to help free us" from the tyranny imposed on us.[789]

Superhero humans must work to stay strong, believe in the inspiring archetype of helpful aliens, and fight against the illuminati. Things look dire but the superhero can succeed by committing to raw foodism and protecting the planet. As of now, the Earth is inundated with the spirit of "greed", the "grand old-growth forests are almost all cut down, the pristine holy rivers are polluted, the skies are filled with cooking soot" and the "magic" of our ecosystem is being destroyed.[790] "The great Earth is in peril," warns Wolfe, but if we transform ourselves dietarily and spiritually, if we "soak" our biology in raw foods and Ormus, we can save Gaia and be like the enlightened alien races, and move onto the future "*Star Trek* reality we know is our destiny" and explore the whole universe and God's light throughout all of creation.[791] Gaia will be cleaned up, raw food and the magical powers of nature will fuel us, and consciousness will be expanded through space.

---

[789]   Ibid., 28.
[790]   Ibid., 32.
[791]   Ibid., 33.

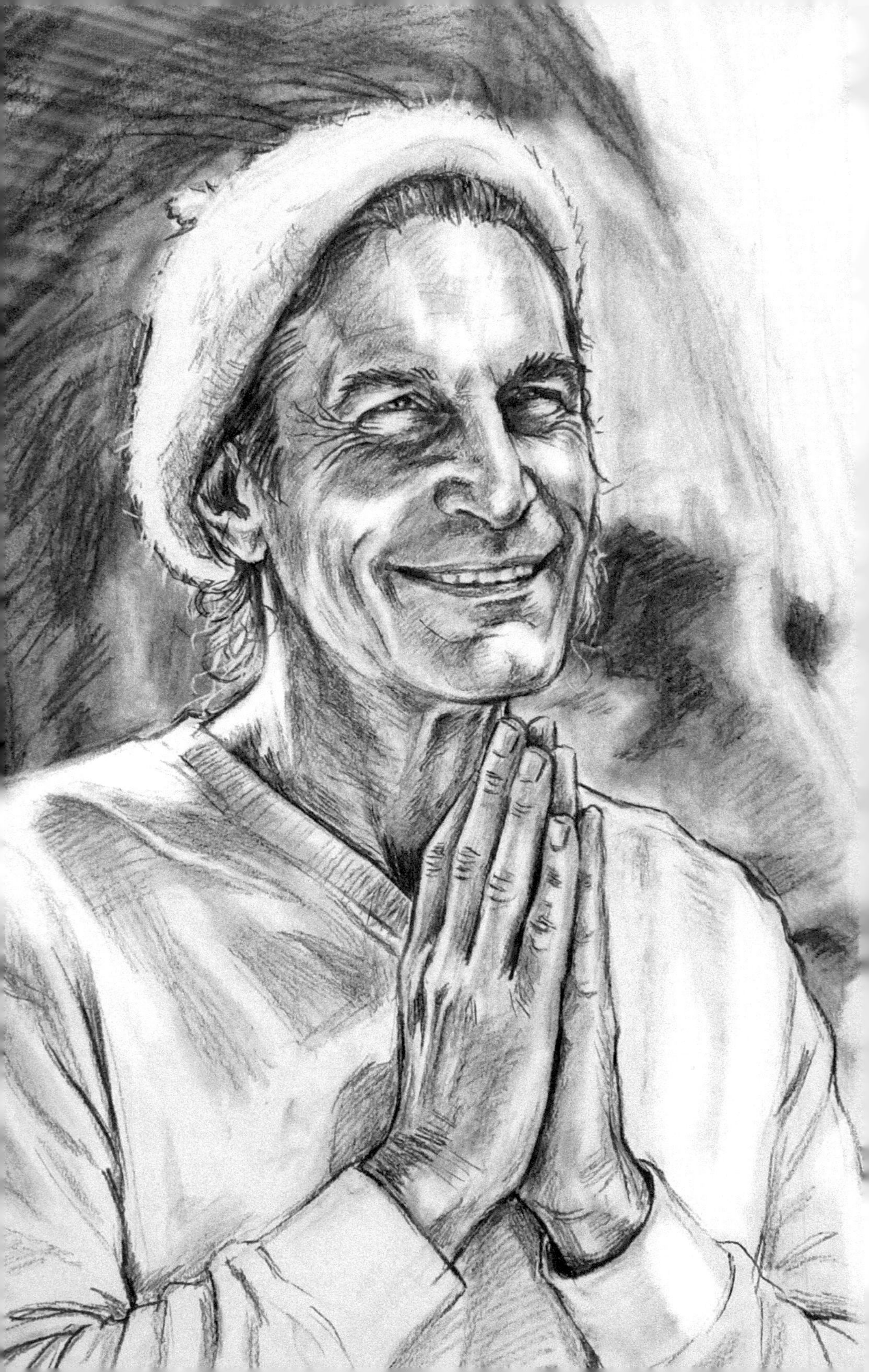

16.
Gabriel Cousens and New Age Spirituality

During a 1975 meditation session, Gabriel Cousens experienced a profound "small voice" emerging out of the silence of his placid mind. "You should learn how to eat and live in a way that enhances the Kundalini," the voice whispered.[792] This insight initiated a decades-long journey to optimize the flow of this life force through the chakras of the body, by eating raw foods and utilizing certain spiritual practices.

NUTRITION AND SPIRITUALITY

Gabriel Cousens has dedicated his life to medicine and spirituality. He is a medical doctor, completed a residency in psychiatry, and has additional credentials in Ayurvedic medicine, homeopathy, and acupuncture.

In the 1990s, he founded the Tree of Life Rejuvenation Center in Arizona, which instructs people in raw foodism, fasting, and spiritual practices like meditation.

Born in 1943, Cousens had a peculiarly ageless look and often wore a trademark beret hat during his prominence on the internet in the 2000s and beyond. Just from his image and his yogi-like physical flexibility, one gets the vibe that he's an alternative health advocate and spiritual leader. He is indeed an ordained rabbi and, inspired by Szekely's stories of the supposedly raw foodist ancient Essenes, he founded the Essene Order of Life, a spiritual organization influenced by Kabbalah in addition to the Essenes. Cousens also studied under a Hindu

---

[792]   Cousens, Gabriel. *Spiritual Nutrition : Six Foundations for Spiritual Life and the Awakening of Kundalini*. Berkeley, Calif., North Atlantic Books, 2005, XV.

swami in the seventies, when he experienced his mission calling to study diet's relationship to the spiritual energy of kundalini.

Cousens' primary goal is to help people become more conscious of God. He's influenced by a mixture of Eastern and Western traditions. Kabbalah, Essene, and Yoga traditions all point to "the same One God," in his words, and life's ultimate goal of "merging with God."[793]

And to get closer to God, more kundalini and prana are needed. Spirituality, or awakening into a higher state of consciousness, a consciousness in "communion" with the divine, "is made easier and accelerated when the life force" or "prana" in the body is built up, according to Cousens. Prana and kundalini are two related concepts. Prana, the universal energy, as defined by Hindu tradition, sustains everyday physical and mental existence. Kundalini is a latent energy in the body, stored at the base of the spine, that can awaken gradually or suddenly (in special epiphanic situations) and can lead to profound spiritual realizations or states of awareness like feeling in communion with God or having feelings of "oneness" with the universe. Prana is a more general life force that kundalini draws upon.

When kundalini is awakened in the body, consciousness transcends normal waking limits." "Psychic" abilities may be realized, says Cousens; "reason yields to intuition," which brings out joy, peace, and love.[794] Kundalini, "is the real cause of all genuine spiritual and psychic phenomena," he believes, and the "unfolding" of Kundalini is the most important process in our spiritual evolution.[795]

According to Cousens, both of these energies, prana and kundalini, can be nurtured with raw plant food.

By eating raw, alongside spiritual practices, we can build up prana in our bodies. This helps us more easily "merge with the Divine Self." "Live foods," veganism, and fasting, are all important to achieving "full body awakening" and help "transform us into Whole Person Enlightenment."[796] There is not much of a dichotomy between flesh and spirit in Cousens' New Age approach, as there had been in much of Western history. The body is part of Cousens' Whole Person Enlightenment and live food helps "our bodies physically cope with the demands of the spiritual process."[797] With live foods, less energy is spent on digestion and can therefore be used for spiritual pursuits. More prana

---

[793]   Ibid., xvii.

[794]   Cousens, Gabriel. *Spiritual Nutrition : Six Foundations for Spiritual Life and the Awakening of Kundalini*. Berkeley, Calif., North Atlantic Books, 2005, 6.

[795]   Ibid., 6-9.

[796]   Ibid., xvii.

[797]   Ibid., 510.

comes into our bodies through uncooked food than devitalized cooked things. Food also is the main "interface" between us and nature and how we relate to God's creation. So we'd better relate in the right way and not mutilate our food by cooking it.

By feeding our bodily prana and strengthening our store of kundalini, raw foods facilitate higher spiritual awareness. With live foods, we become, physical and metaphysical "superconductor[s] of the Light."[798]

A New Spiritual Paradigm of Nutrition

> *"To explore fully the relationship of nutrition to spiritual life, this one [Cousens] had to evolve beyond the present materialistic-mechanistic paradigm of nutrition to an expanded definition of nutrition that includes subtle energetic principles."*
> **—Gabriel Cousens**

Several of Cousens' books are considered lodestars in the New Age movement. In 1986, he published *Spiritual Nutrition and the Rainbow Diet* and this book received glowing reviews over the years within New Age circles. The preface to the 2005 edition of *Spiritual Nutrition* states that his 1986 publication "revolutionized dietary consciousness."[799] *Meditation* magazine hailed *Spiritual Nutrition* as "arguably the best book on diet from both a health and a spiritual point of view ever to see print." Cousens' spiritualization of nutrition—the notion that what we eat affects our spiritual life—had earned him a type of reverential status.

By bringing to light the spiritual qualities of raw food, he was showing that the "old order" of the twentieth century was fading away—the "dishonesty, greed, war, . . . environmental toxemia, chemtrails." The new paradigm of helping "Mother Earth detox into the world of tomorrow" was being born by "Light Bearers" like Cousens.[800] The New Age was bringing more awareness to how we live and even to how we eat.

In Cousens' spiritual-nutritional worldview, nutrients didn't just have mechanistic physiological roles. The interplay between food and our bodies and spirits is much more multi-dimensional than the conventional materialist notions of the recent past would have us believe.

---

[798] Ibid., xvii.

[799] Ibid., x.

[800] Ibid., xi.

A deeper, more correct awareness of nutrition, in Cousens' mind, acknowledges the "emotional, energetic, and spiritual qualities" of nutrients like minerals, vitamins, and phytochemicals. When you have in mind that you're absorbing spiritual attributes from food, and not just obligatory tools for common functioning of cellular machinery, your attitude toward food changes. Rather than just eating to sustain physical functioning, you eat also to "intensify [your] Communion with the Divine." And it is through raw food, Cousens holds, that spirit and body, as well as God and man, could be united. Fellow raw foodist Viktoras Kulvinskas said that reading Cousens was "like having a conversation with God over a glass of wheatgrass juice."[801] Through the lens of nutrition, New Agers believe, we see more of the reality of what God is and how humans are to spiritually relate with the universe. With the right spiritual practices and the nourishment, a more enlightened state was achievable.

But raw food is such a powerful source of prana that Cousens warns that such a diet must be tempered by certain spiritual practices. He believed that the ancient rishis (seers or sages) were on raw food diets. He says that their advanced spiritual awareness was key to their success on such a diet, as the *vrittis*, potentially harmful thoughts and emotions, can "potentially be activated" by a "live food diet," meaning that it's more difficult to initially manage the unleashed formerly suppressed or negative emotions on a raw diet.[802]

SOEFs and Spirit

One phenomenon within this expanded "wholistic" paradigm of nutrition, and one thing that helps accomplish spiritual ascension is what Cousens calls Subtle Organizing Energy Fields (SOEFs). Although not understood by materialist science, Cousens' understanding of SOEFs, like other aspects of "spiritual nutrition," are "intuitively derived" from "historical, cultural, spiritual, and scientific evidence."[803]

Foods, Cousens posits, are integral to our conscious experience of life because they generate SOEFs—energy fields or vibrations that alter our cellular health as well as "all levels of . . . emotional, mental, and spiritual health."[804] Any food or lifestyle habit, or attitude that weakens or "disorganizes" the SOEFs contributes to spiritual and physical en-

---

[801]   Ibid., xii.
[802]   Ibid., 385.
[803]   Ibid., 106.
[804]   Ibid., 110.

tropy. "Peace and Love," Cousens says, "combined with a low-glycemic, high-mineralized . . . live-food, vegan diet" maintain SOEF health.[805]

Organic live foods—as evidenced by Kirlian photography that measures electrical discharges from objects—emits stronger electrical discharges than cooked or non-organically grown foods. Raw foods, as examined by Kirlian photography, have "a much stronger auric, luminescent field" as compared to cooked food.[806] Some raw superfoods like blue-green algae, Cousens holds, have extremely high SOEFs. Thus foods like these "regenerate mind" and are "expansive for consciousness."[807]

Cousens' unique ideas about physiology explain why he believes the electromagnetic frequencies, the SOEFs, that we receive from food are so important. Our bodies and especially our bones, are "crystal" structures. Cousens believes that our bones act as a resonant structure that emits an electromagnetic field based on the vibrational energies that we absorb from food (and from other things like emotions).[808] "Our crystalline bone structure . . . acts as an antenna for all incoming and internal body vibratory energy [and] nutrient energy," he says. We eat food, for instance, and the "bone structure then amplifies and radiates this energy and information to the rest of the system down to the cellular and subcellular crystalline structures."[809] The vibrations of the food we eat echo throughout our resonant physiology—a physiology that was specifically designed for the resonance of raw living foods.

And the effects of SOEFs aren't just physical. When SOEF energy intake is increased, when the vibration resonating from one's "crystalline" bone structure is elevated, "we recreate a new and healthy field that then reorganizes the person on a spiritual, mental, emotional" level.[810] Our bones "transform" the specific vibrations of the foods we eat into healthy or pathological vibrations that relay information to our consciousness.[811] Foods become "bone EMFs" (electromagnetic frequencies) which affect our entire being, especially our spiritual life.

And the higher the vibration of our crystal structure and the more our kundalini is awakened, we become "more etheric," and "our spiritual potentials are awesome."[812] High energy, lighter foods like raw foods energize the "kundalini vortex," he claims. Live foods pulsate

---

[805]   Ibid., 112.

[806]   Ibid., 295.

[807]   Ibid., 524.

[808]   Ibid., 141.

[809]   Ibid., 143.

[810]   Ibid., 149.

[811]   Ibid., 152.

[812]   Ibid., 189.

with electricity, with prana, and have "higher conductivity." Low energy toxic and cooked foods are "metaphoric sludge" which slows down kundalini flow.[813]

We assimilate each "subtle vibration" from every food that we eat, Cousens believes. These vibrations are formed by the environment in which the food is grown, the chemicals used on the food, whether the food is cooked or not, and even "by the consciousness of the people who prepare our food." Everything is connected and every energetic subtlety matters when it comes to food quality. The "highest" vibration comes from love-infused organically grown or wild raw plants.[814] Nutrients that come from chemicalized and cooked foods—from "a non-living source do not recreate this optimal living frequency."[815]

Although Cousens admits that we can't just "can't eat ourselves" to enlightenment (for concomitant spiritual practices must accompany diet), he points out that at the least, a live-food diet facilitates the mind-body complex to accomplish basic morality and spiritual enjoyment. Raw food generates a lot of energy—energy that gives "enough clarity of mind to live according to basic moral principles."[816] Raw food sets the foundation for our spiritual and ethical lives.

"The mind is not at all easy to control," says Cousens. Only when it is "pure, clear, and full of energy" and fueled by quality plant foods can it successfully enter into a spiritually-elevated "silence," or lack of discordant thoughts. The same descriptions might as well apply to the body, since our physical cells are tied to our spirituality. "The mind and body are organically interrelated and our bodily condition strongly influences how we think," notes Cousens.[817] He cites the Jewish tradition. Twelfth-century rabbi Moses Maimonides said that "the welfare of the soul can only be achieved after obtaining the welfare of the body."

Minerals

"Yoga tradition . . . teaches, 'The mind is made of food.'"
—**Gabriel Cousens**

---

[813]   Ibid., 191.
[814]   Ibid., 152.
[815]   Ibid., 166.
[816]   Ibid., 100.
[817]   Ibid., 233.

"Minerals are one of the deep secrets of Spiritual Nutrition," says Cousens. The Earth is made of minerals, he notes. Minerals are not just static substances. They are the "frequencies of creation" that built the universe. They are spiritual messengers.

Plants are able to break down minerals in soil and absorb them as particles small enough that, when we eat them, they can enter our cells, according to Cousens. Highly mineralized plants, grown in highly mineralized soil, are the healthiest food.

People on a "highly mineralized live-food diet have more of an opening or tendency to open" themselves to the "supermental mind"— the universal realm of creative insight and intuition that can "transcend the bondage of time, space, and Being."[818] The ability to contact this supermental mind is the highest "kosha" or layer of a person's existence, according to Hindu tradition, and Cousens claims that a high quality raw foods diet helps to calm the lower koshas so that the "deep awareness" of the highest kosha can reign.[819]

"Each mineral has a vibratory rate that supports different aspects of consciousness and spiritual awareness, as well as chakra and organ systems," claims Cousens. So it's important to eat a variety of plant foods to make sure you're getting all types of minerals.

In short, minerals, preserved in food in its raw state, are electrical conductors of prana and kundalini, throughout the body and spirit. They are crystallized spiritual "light" for one's whole being. Raw leafy greens, nuts, algae, and seaweed are especially important mineral and trace mineral sources.

PURIFICATION FOR FREE-FLOWING KUNDALINI

"Let our hunger for the Divine be the overwhelming appetite and guide to our choice of diet . . . we eat consciously to feed our hungry souls."
—Gabriel Cousens

We are feeding the soul with every subtle quality of the food we take in, Cousens believes. We must consume pure things for our spiritual flowering. Every dirty thing that we ingest acts as sludge, obstructing the flow of kundalini and thus spiritual consciousness.

---

[818] Ibid., 92.
[819] Ibid., 93.

It is only after the body has been purified, says Cousens, and feeds off of raw food, "that the Kundalini . . . can act with full force."[820] Having an "appropriate diet" (along with spiritual practices) "maintains the physical body as a superconductor" of kundalini. Breathing practices, meditation, service, charity, and reading "wisdom literature" like scriptures play a role alongside nutrition in preparing the body to be a "superconductor."[821] But it's a "vegan, organic, live-food, high mineralized, low-sugar" diet that forms the basis of Cousens' kundalini-enhancing "spiritual nutrition" program. This is a very different regimen from the mostly fruit diet of Lovewisdom. There are a lot more vegetables and low sugar plant foods like nuts and seeds in Cousens' recommended diet. In his mind, this is the cleanest diet one can adopt.

Spiritual nutrition "is about purifying all of the koshas" and "purifying the mind on every level." When the lower koshas, like the body, "become dirty," they can obscure the highest kosha, the spirit, from attaining communion with the divine.[822] Partly by way of living foods, the purified body becomes "a vehicle of the Atman" or the true, eternal Self, the pure awareness behind each individual's existence—the awareness that underlies and is beyond thoughts and an individual's specific personality.

"We are the funny ones eating 'a birdseed-and-grass diet,'" Cousens jokes. But this seemingly strange and silly diet gives the eater the advantage of accomplishing the physical purity that facilitates spiritual ascendance. It is this regimen that "make[s] the body so pure and such a vehicle of Light that, on the grossest level of physical Being, it reflects the Highest Light."[823] The body becomes spiritualized, released, as much as it can be, from its base physical characteristics.

"Our spirit, our mind, our emotions . . . are affected by the food we eat," Cousens says, and food plays a large role in whether we are in "harmony with ourselves . . . and the Divine" whether or not we are rejecting the "universal laws of creation."[824] Are we eating what the Light, what the Creator, meant for us to eat? Are we in tune with the laws of sacred creation? Are we eating raw? Without adhering to it, without being pure, we risk spiritual disconnection.

Meat and cooked food are the main culprits in sullying the purity of the body. They reduce the ability of our fleshly temples to be "superconductors" of kundalini. Meat and cooked food muddy our commu-

---

820   Ibid., 10.
821   Ibid., 12.
822   Ibid., 96.
823   Ibid.
824   Ibid., 197, 211.

nication with the divine. They clutter our temples and make it harder for sacredness to dwell there.

In cooked food, water is "dehydrated off" during the heating. Water carries electrical conductivity into our body so less SOEFs and "Love vibration" are available to the eater.[825] We are cooking off the love and bliss that the Creator meant for us to consume. The cosmic and supernatural messages designed for us evaporate with the application of that dreadful heat. Our resonant bodies become out of tune, prevented from receiving their vibratory nourishment. Hence, spiritual communication is disrupted and our spirit is out of sorts. We are lost in darkness. The stakes are high.

As Szekely's *Essene Gospel* says, "the power of God's angels enters into you with the living food which the Lord gives you from his royal table." We give up angelic power if we spurn raw food.

Our bodies have consciousnesses just like our minds. Corporeal intelligence matches the mental. "The consciousness of our bodies and minds are both the cause and result of the diet that we eat," Cousens says.[826] Low-quality consciousness causes us to eat low quality foods and bad foods cause low quality consciousness in a vicious cycle.

Impure food carries with it moral meaning. When people consume animals that haven't undergone "proper ritual slaughter," says a rabbi quoted by Cousens, they "ingest the aspects of . . . darkness, foolishness, judgements, forgetfulness, and death."[827] Our cells and mind absorb negative qualities or "death vibration" of food produced in ignorant circumstances or cooked into lifelessness that is devoid of prana.[828] With meat, "the adrenal-fear energy" transposed to us by slaughtered animals, "blocks the awakening of the first chakra" that helps us feel trust in life. The fear energy also has a stimulating effect that is "adverse to the inner stillness of meditation."[829]

Furthermore, Cousens claims that meat acts as "intense sludge" that blocks kundalini energy in the body and he has actually seen meat being used in "rare emergency cases" when a person feels that their kundalini energy is too intense to handle and must be squashed.[830]

Cows' milk is no better. Besides the fact that it can often contain large amounts of herbicides and pesticides, you're also consuming the "cruelty, pain, and lack of consciousness" along with a sense of "en-

---

825 Ibid., 243.
826 Ibid., 245.
827 Ibid., 253.
828 Ibid., 255.
829 Ibid., 256.
830 Ibid., 256.

slavement" from the cows, especially those in factory farms, that live imprisoned lives.

Raw plant foods, on the other hand, are designed for a symbiotic relationship with humans and transmit to us "sunlight energy as excited electrons" that "stimulate a resonant response from the Inner Light of our higher spiritual subtle bodies." This sunlight energy in plants is full of prana and enacts a "pranic transfer" into the body of the eater.[831] This is why there's a "natural harmony between plants and humans" and why our chakra system becomes "balanced energetically by our plant friends."[832] With the raw food-induced expanded consciousness, we can see the "deeper truth" and the "reality of oneness" with all things in universe.[833] This is why we need the pure and "complete energy pattern" of live foods.

With a forceful warning, Cousens declares that cooking is "risky business" both physically and spiritually.[834] It "significantly diminishes" nutrients in food including vitamins, minerals, and antioxidants along with ruining their unique "energy pattern" and the effect it has on our spiritual self.[835] Our "consciousness" and "electromagnetic field" depend on the electron energy we receive from foods, Cousens holds. If we want to have a bright electrically vivid aura to our body and spirit, as seen in photographs of raw plants, we must eat right. There's no chance to "resonate" with the universe if we are not raw-fed.[836]

Summed up, Cousens says that, "When we eat live foods we are consuming the living energy of the planet and fully immersing ourselves in the full energy of food as a Love note from God."[837] We are absorbing an energy that is both terrestrial and supernatural—the energy of creation and Creator.

Mere traditional nutrition is cast aside in this paradigm of "spiritual nutrition." Raw veganism is "not a diet" but "a way of life in which we live authentically and fully on every level of our Being." We become "super energy Beings" with enhanced sensitivity to the Divine.[838] When kundalini is activated in our bodies, as a result of the consumption of high-prana raw foods, we experience a feeling of "non-casual

---

831   Ibid., 262.
832   Ibid., 263.
833   Ibid., 288.
834   Ibid., 291.
835   Ibid., 289.
836   Ibid., 296.
837   Ibid., 303.
838   Ibid., 305.

ecstasy, non-casual peace."[839] That is way more epic of a feat than say, getting the protein you need for a day.

HUMAN PRANA CONDUCTORS

But we have to be careful when treading into the electrically potent world of raw food. The energy, the prana, from live foods can be so intense that eaters have to be careful so as to protect or "lubricate" their system so that we can handle the increased cosmic energy properly.[840] This adds another dietary stipulation to the raw food plan—we must get high quality fats to protect our systems from the high energy of prana.

Cousens uses the ayurvedic concept of *ojas* to explain how we must ground ourselves to avoid getting overwhelmed by the pranic energy of raw food and causing "potential harm to the subtle nervous system."[841] The *ojas* represent a subtle energy system in the body that "maintains the integrity" of the prana energy channel and can be thought of as "primal vigor" and the "integrity and stored energy of protein, fat . . . gross tissue mass."[842] *Ojas* can be thought of as the "lining and conduit" through which prana, the "fire" or electricity that fuels kundalini energy, burns. *Ojas* are the "lubricant" or the "logs" by which the "inner fire" and "electrical energy" of kundalini burns.[843]

Taking *ojas* into consideration, Cousens recommends specific raw food practices to "build" these energy conductors, putting an emphasis on fatty plant foods. He recommends nut milks, oily fruit like avocado, and raw foods that have a "creamy" quality like hemp seeds, coconut oil, macadamia nuts, and flax seeds. These foods provide the fatty foundation for the ojas alongside other densely nutritious raw foods like bee pollen, spirulina, chlorella that are high in protein and fats.

The energy of living foods is so powerful that along with nourishing the *ojas*, spiritual grounding practices are also needed to be able to utilize prana in an orderly or safe way. A devotion to God is critical, Cousens argues, as is a meditative mindset that can provide emotional balance. Without these groundings, "a 100 percent live food diet . . . is like a teenager getting a very fancy racing car but not knowing how to

---

[839]   Ibid., 380.
[840]   Ibid., 373.
[841]   Ibid.
[842]   Ibid., 372.
[843]   Ibid., 373.

drive."[844] The engine, so to speak, the live food, is so powerful, that the energy is potentially destructive if not used correctly. Prana and kundalini need to be directed carefully or else an ungrounded raw foodist might become hyperactive, a workaholic, or hypersexual.

It's not just fantasy or imagination. Raw food is powerful stuff, so we have to be careful, Cousens believes.

COUSENS' LASTING INFLUENCE

The *Spiritual Nutrition* of Cousens influenced droves of raw foodists since it was published in the 1980s. It added New Age spiritual depth to the raw foodism movement and generated the belief that food deeply affects our consciousness instead of just fulfilling physical needs. People in holistic health and yoga circles have been influenced by these ideas to make raw foodism a spiritual practice and not just a nutritionally superior way of eating. Raw foodism had accomplished a more expansive meaning.

Followers of *Spiritual Nutrition* adopted the belief that they now had tremendous spiritual power from the food they eat and that by adjusting their diet, they could gain control over their life experience and finally feel a sense of ecstasy.

---

[844] Ibid., 385.

17.
Joe Alexander and New Age Spirituality

"Cooking began in northern Europe, where people would put frozen food over a fire to thaw them out. Fine. Then they got careless and left them over the fire too long, and that's when our troubles began."
—Joe Alexander

"There is no God, no Christ, no Master or Avatar or any such thing who is going to bring in the New Age."
—Joe Alexander

Previously discussed artist Joe Alexander's interest in raw food transcended aesthetics. It also focused on spirituality. "My first introduction to raw-foodist type ideas came in 1971," he says. An old friend from high school had renewed contact with Alexander, and it was apparent that something was different about the man. "I had known him as an ordinary fool," back in the school days, Alexander reminisced. His friend had just been an average bloke back then, "repeating the same things that everyone else said." But "now there was a soul looking out from behind his eyes and he spoke from an inner source of wisdom, and not just unreflective cultural conditioning."[845]

What had changed about the man? Besides practicing yoga, he had mentioned Arnold Ehret and his "mucusless diet." Alexander was skeptical of these "bizarre" dietary ideas but a few years later, after joining a yoga and meditation group, another person pushed Ehret's ideas on Alexander. Eventually, he experimented with a completely raw food diet and found that he attained a natural high from it.

But with later experimentation, Alexander found that the one meal daily of cooked vegetables that he had been in the habit of eating

---

[845] Ibid., 98.

on Ehret's diet, had been keeping him from enjoying the "surge of energy," the "greatest benefit" of a 100% raw diet. But unlike drugs, this was a "clean and pure and healthy sort of energy that turns your cheeks pink, not gray." It was healthy, but it "resembled the rush of energy you can get by injecting amphetamines into your veins." Uncooked plant foods were powerful stuff, he found, and "a better high than marijuana or speed or LSD."[846]

Raw foods were "real magic."[847] Although Arnold Ehret's "mucusless diet" had pointed Alexander in the right direction, he found that, since it allowed cooked food, the regimen was "not enough" to experience the magic of complete rawness. It was necessary to eat only raw foods, Alexander had concluded from personal experience, if the full spiritual effects of the diet were to be harnessed.[848]

There was deeper spiritual benefit of raw food, beyond just an energetic buzz. "I have done many things for self-improvement and transformation," Alexander said of his mystical journey, "but I feel that the raw food diet initiated the deepest, most basic and profound transformation of all of them, the most to return me to a basic grounding in the real world and a natural sanity."[849]

Other spiritual practices were practically powerless compared to raw eating. "Several yogas" and meditational techniques were never as effective as uncooked eating was for him. It was the most powerful way to not only have physical health but "a mind naturally connected to reality." And it opens up one's spiritual awareness to see that we are not just to "fulfill a role in human society" or accomplish "personal goals" but to "serve in the overall greater life of the Earth," that is, to care for the planet as a living entity.[850] Raw food makes you aware that you should protect and nourish the wonderful planet that gave us all life.

Adopting a raw food diet felt like spiritual release. Alexander was now inspired to work on the "liberation of the human spirit."[851] That's why he wrote his book on raw foodism. He needed to spread the message so that humanity could improve its quality of life.

To achieve such liberation, releasing "blocked or dammed-up energy" is needed. Cooked food burdens us with heavy energy and dis-

---

846   Ibid., 100.
847   Ibid.
848   Ibid., 101.
849   Ibid.
850   Ibid.
851   Ibid., 130.

torts healthy frequencies. "Poisoning from unnatural food" is a main cause of "restriction of the inner spirit," Alexander proclaims.[852]

Cooked food also obscures your intuition, which is your compass for life.[853] Alexander compares these dietary-induced spiritual restrictions and oppressions to a New Age theory of suppressed emotions formulated by William Reich, who was a student of Freud. Just as the heavy and distorted energy of cooked food burdens us, we emotionally and sexually oppress our own feelings and create "stagnant life force" within us, Reich believed.[854] The emotional suppression that can result from a conventional diet burdens the human spirit and destroys people's confidence and intuitive "inner direction," Alexander believes.[855] Cooked food feeds into spiritual pain and dysfunction.

Conversely, raw food is so effective at instilling well-being in the eater that Alexander believed, like many raw foodists, that cooked food was the root cause of drug addiction. Having a diet and lifestyle that is out of touch with nature and distorts one's energy field makes it more difficult to experience joy, so we seek to fill the gap with short term artificial highs.[856]

DEVOTEE OF THE EARTH

Personal spiritual growth presages the ideological changes that many raw foodists experience. This was the case for Joe Alexander, as his attitude about humanity's purpose changed.

The Earth, as we've seen, is often conceived within New Age raw foodism as a sentient entity that deserves the devotion and protection of humans. Alexander's spiritual beliefs about the Earth are similar to David Wolfe's and other New Age thinkers. In an appendix to his book, *Blatant Raw Foodist Propaganda!*, Alexander featured a written piece by a man named Michael Tobin that pitted Mother Nature against its cosmic enemy, technocratic man, the "anti-life tyrant" who was a "death threat to the whole living earthly scheme." In this rendering (which Alexander endorsed), it was life versus death; the noble and generous Earth versus "sick" and parasitic man.[857]

---

[852]   Ibid., 131.
[853]   Ibid.
[854]   Ibid., 141.
[855]   Ibid., 133.
[856]   Ibid., 105.
[857]   Ibid., 155.

The "psychic plague," said Tobin, caused humankind to mistreat nature and only value the extraction of economic value from it. It must be defeated if the planet is to survive. Many humans have become "arrogant parasites lording it over creation," despite the fact that nature had created them "solely because the terrestrial web needed a nervous system to complete it," claimed Tobin. Humans are here to serve the planet and to be the intelligent and moral conscience in stewarding this ecosystem. But we've forsaken our original purpose. We were meant to be "a vital function in the Earth's bio-system. In this respect, we are on apar with earthworms and micro-organisms," Tobin educates.[858] We are also "merely one of many humanoid species" that Mother Nature created to act as an intelligent nervous system.[859] Humans need an ego check, in other words. We need to remember who created us and that we are to serve Mother Nature, not abusively extract from it.

The Earth-disrespecting technocratic man, spurning nature's design, is the "final sick product of patriarchal society" that promoted the idea that humans, especially men, were "intellects" that were totally separate from nature, argued Tobin.[860] Male-dominated arrogant societies who think they are above nature have misunderstood why we were created. We need to remember that we are simply an outgrowth of nature that will be destroyed if we don't serve nature. And "we *are* nature," as Alexander points out, so we best not fail ourselves.[861] Whatever bad we do to the planet, we are doing to ourselves.

A good human acts in the opposite way as technocratic man; serving nature's needs is the top priority. To do that, we need to become "moral and spiritual giants," in the words of Tobin.[862] The survival of the planet and the health of all life depends on us and we have to start with our diet to become the spiritual masters we need to be. Basically, a mind fed by raw foods is capable of becoming such a master.[863] As Alexander said, you can try any self-improvement technique or any drug you can think of but nothing gives you the hyper-awareness or changes you as powerfully as the foods that contain the raw power of nature.

Regarding the spiritual power of diet, Alexander points out that Gabriel Cousens believes that by eating raw plant food, we "remain attuned to the energy field of the Earth" and are thus enabled to "receive

---

[858]   Ibid.

[859]   Ibid., 156.

[860]   Ibid.

[861]   Ibid., 103.

[862]   Ibid., 157.

[863]   Ibid., 101.

the broadcast of her desires and will."[864] The raw foodist will receive in-tuitive instructions from the Earth, which is the only god that matters, in Alexander's worldview. He believes that "for all practical purposes, the Earth is our god and we need to act in harmony with her will." "God," conceived as Alexander's own New Age god and hardly the God of Abrahamic religions, "is threatened and needs our help!" The Earth is a vulnerable god. Speculation about "the ultimate creator of the universe" is "irrelevant and far beyond our present practical needs," he says, because the fate of the Earth God is what is at stake for the moment.[865]

By feeding on rawness and accomplishing the "attunement of our personal energy field with the Earth's," we can act to "promote the evolution of the Earth." Through attunement to the will of the planet, we know what to do to bring "happiness and fulfillment for all her creatures," since, as Alexander believes, the godlike Earth "wants" this happiness for "all her creatures."[866]

All of these spiritual qualities depend on raw foodism; it should be the core of everyone's spiritual practice. Because the state of the planet depends on our spiritual linkage with it, "the most urgent requirement of our time," if life is to survive, is to eat raw food, and for human be-ings to get their "energy fields" back in sync with the global terrain.[867] But eating cooked food, perhaps the most negative influence on the minds of humans, keeps the planet in a state of endangerment because this food "disturb[s] and misalign[s]" the energy fields of humans so that they lose contact with their Earth mother.[868] Cooked food, as we've heard from other raw foodists as well, also foments a spirit of violence and disharmony. Mice fed leftover cooked food from humans, Alexander claims, lose their sense of cooperation, break out in quarrels, and even practice cannibalism.[869] No wonder humans make war.

Whether the world will be enlightened by raw foodist values—New Age values, as Alexander calls them—is up to the common man. No leader, no savior, will bring about the change we need to survive. "See, people on this planet are used to thinking in terms of bosses and governments doing everything, so they're waiting for a Big Boss or a government to bring in the Golden Age," Alexander notes. A Chris-tian paradigm of a savior that sets everything right should also be dis-

---

[864]   Ibid.
[865]   Ibid., 102.
[866]   Ibid., 101.
[867]   Ibid., 102.
[868]   Ibid., 101.
[869]   Ibid., 64.

missed, according to him. "The Christians think that Jesus is going to return as a Big Boss and impose heaven on Earth . . . But it's not going to happen like that at all."[870] "That's how it is in this world," Alexander laments, there's no likely dramatic redemption of humanity from a supernatural being. "There is no [innate] fairness or justice at all."[871] The fate of the world is completely on the shoulders of humans—on their dietary and spiritual choices.

It is up to humans to "create a New Age of health, happiness, freedom, justice, true creativity, and true progress." We do this by being in touch with the "True Center"—the Earth—and the "life force" that stems from it. We must eat the Earth's food, raw food, and dump our emotional restrictions and "stagnant energy" so we can discern what is best for the evolution of the planet. "Governments, universities, religions, theories and philosophies," as well as our own egos, are the "false centers" of useless guidance—they will not lead us to the answers.[872]

But the ultimate False Center is clear to Alexander. It is "cooked-food eating" which "has caused the most harm to humanity's course of evolution" and is the worst source of the "pollution of consciousness" that causes the suffering and ecocide on our planet.[873] By eating only raw, we can achieve spiritual clarity and remedy the sins and injustices of the world. "New energy" and "new insight" from raw food can "help straighten up the damn mess on this potentially Paradise Planet."[874] We have the power to create a new Eden but people have to stay disciplined with what they consume.

Raw food is a better savior than some supposedly divine no-show or government. "People who experience [a] raw food diet" and its incredible benefits, "tend to see it as the key to regaining Paradise on Earth," Alexander explains of his outlook. The more people who join the raw way of living, "the faster and further we can all go" toward paradise."[875] "The New Age can only come when significant numbers of people decide they're going to discipline themselves," eat living food, and enact the values that naturally arise out of such nutritionally-saturated bodies and minds.[876]

"The cancerous growth on the planet—that modern human technocratic civilization has become—lives on cooked food!" Alexander

---

[870]   Ibid., 97.

[871]   Ibid., 133.

[872]   Ibid., 144.

[873]   Ibid., 144.

[874]   Ibid., 146.

[875]   Ibid., 7.

[876]   Ibid., 97.

declares. So starve it. "Natural" eating removes this spiritual malignancy, begins healing the planet, and gives hope for a bright future, a New Age.[877] But the vast majority of humanity has yet to be convinced to change their culinary habits. There's much work left to do for conscious raw eaters.

---

[877] Ibid., 63.

18.
Miscellaneous Raw
Food Spiritualists

*"When we consume the living essence of plants, we
merge with the heartbeat of the Earth."*
—Viktoras Kulvinskas

It's common for raw foodists to feel they experienced a spiritual renewal after ditching cooked foods. But many of them haven't articulated an extensive gospel of their beliefs because they haven't written books or released other long-form content on the subject. Nevertheless, various people have given short descriptions of their perceptions of their change in consciousness.

Most raw foodists feel that food hugely impacts the way their spirits and minds function, and similar themes of increased awareness, the shedding of psychic burdens, and a more intimate connection with creation or a creator fill their descriptions.

Joe Alexander's 1990 book *Blatant Raw Foodist Propaganda!*, shares some intriguing letters from raw foodists about their spiritual transformations.

One Californian named Rachel wrote in grandiose terms about the spiritual experience of "fruitarians" whom she refers to as "elfish [sic] people." Raw eaters apparently take on an air of magical childlike playfulness. She first notes, like other raw foodists, that one's biological state is the basis for one's spiritual state. Fed on raw food, her cells act as Gabriel Cousens' "perfect resonating crystal reflectors . . . resonating their own harmony, singing of the happiness of perfection." People on raw diets, Rachel claims, "become as we were meant to be"—"spirit-matter stars"—magical incarnate beings, shining with vitality. Their perfected biology becomes a perfected spirit. A strong belief in oneself arises and a deep connection with the universe is "felt deep within." A "calm meditational state" and a "stillness" also grounds the dieter. But this does not mean spiritual enervation. Cosmic information is downloaded into one's bodily communication network: "The electricity and intelligence flows freely, then through us as in a child."[878] The eater reclaims the seamless functioning of an innocent and healthy child.

Rachel believes, similarly to other raw foodists, that most of the world's problems are caused by bad food. She hopes that the world drops the cause of its dysfunction—cooked food. All the wars in the world are "caused by poisonous gases formed from decayed food in our temples—our bodies."[879] Emotional turbulence, spiritual blindness, and destructive habits like violence result from poisonous fermenting junk food in our intestines. If humans would only cleanse their inner temples, "There will be peace and we will all be our true child-dream selfs (elves)." [880] She often connects a sense of blameless childishness and purity with raw food. By eating this way, we reclaim a child-like carefree attitude and become like giggling elves, not stiff, oppressed adults.

Once humanity is biologically cleansed, hate and war will be no more: "I become hysterically aware," Rachel ecstatically projects, "of the history of all the stories of healing from live foods. Unity is possible with love . . . Raw is war turned around." Raw food increases "love capacity" and is a "capital pacifier," smoothing out enmities.[881]Raw foods cool the hot turmoil of cooked humanity's toxic destructive and malicious instincts. Raw food could bring world peace.

In the other hemisphere, but with similar enthusiasm, a solitary Australian farmer and desert dweller, Hal A. Skinner, wrote to the *American Vegetarian* magazine, sometime in the twentieth century (date unknown), expressing the incredible changes that raw food wrought on his spirit. Joe Alexander has described Skinner's account as "one of the most moving testaments I have ever seen."[882]

"I am an old man," Skinner wrote at the time, but "recently made young again" physically and spiritually. Eating only "fruit and water," he had no trouble doing "heavy work without weariness or exhaustion" in the hot desert.[883] Riding on horseback day and night for months at a time and claiming to only get one to two hours of sleep much of the time, Skinner said he did not need "protein food or stimulants" to have such incredible endurance, only fruit.

---

[878] Alexander, Joe. *Blatant Raw Foodist Propaganda!, Or, Sell Your Stove to the Junkman and Feel Great!, Or, Consider Your True Nature.* Blue Dolphin Publishing, 1990, 90.
[879] Ibid.
[880] Ibid., 91.
[881] Ibid.
[882] Ibid., 79.
[883] Ibid.

Spiritually, Skinner rediscovered a greater connection to God and an abandonment of burdensome emotions. There is, the Australian realized, "something infinitely better than the cravings, passions, lusts, frustrations, etc. that devastate and ruin the soul through wrong eating." The craving that haunts humans (that the Buddha warned about), or the caustic passions (that the Stoics warned about) that torment, are done away with through diet. "Comfort, peace, unspeakable joy," on the other hand, accompany the return to a "biologically correct diet the Great Designer and Maker arranged."[884] Once again, raw food is the key to spiritual enlightenment.

American actor, comedian, and social critic Dick Gregory wrote that, after experimenting with fasting and raw foodism, his "spiritual awareness" was "lifted to a new level." He started to understand more Biblical scriptures, and negative values were relinquished. The "six basic fears" of the human psyche—("fear of poverty, fear of death, fear of sickness, fear of getting old, fear of being criticized, and fear of losing your love")—disappear as a result of "cleansing the system," he claimed. Bigotry, war, racism, and other "insoluble problems" feel like they can be cured on such a diet.[885] Sociology and spirituality are affected, he believed, by food quality.

Arshavir Ter Havonnessian, an Iranian raw foodist of the twentieth century, agreed that food was crucial to spiritual health. He claimed that raw food vegetarianism had an "even more profound" effect on his "mental acuity and spirituality" than it did on his physical health. "A clean body and a pure mind are inseparable,"—we cannot separate diet from spirit, he believed.[886] On raw food, cognitive improvements like increased "concentration and an increased stamina and attention to detail" accompany a feeling of being "closer to Mother Earth and truly connected to creation."[887] It's amazing how many raw foodists, from different parts of the world, express this same sentiment.

Raw foodism, Havonnessian continues, because it is a "humble way of eating," instills a humble gratitude toward our Creator because it involves reverently accepting the food that God meant for us, without altering it artificially. Raw food also transfers its inherent values of peace and simplicity onto the eater. But this is not a stale simplicity. The "soul can be free at last to express itself. The soul can play," Havon-

---

[884]   Ibid., 80.
[885]   Ibid., 83.
[886]   Ibid., 84
[887]   Ibid., 85

nessian says.[888] A liberty in feeling and expressing one's authentic self takes place.

Viktoras Kulvinskas, an affiliate of Ann Wigmore and fellow Lithuanian, and Brian Clement, who was mentored by Ann Wigmore, have both articulated a sense of union with the divine energy of the Earth after switching to a raw lifestyle, and the raising of consciousness so as to be at peace with all life forms.

In these testimonials, a pattern also emerges of spirituality being considered the most important effect of a raw diet. Physical health is almost merely the gateway to the higher purposes of the mind. Raw foodists aren't just hoping to not get sick, they're hoping for happiness and expanded consciousness.

Many of them claim to have found such states. But one must stay away from cooked food if these elevated mindsets are to be maintained.

---

[888]   Ibid.

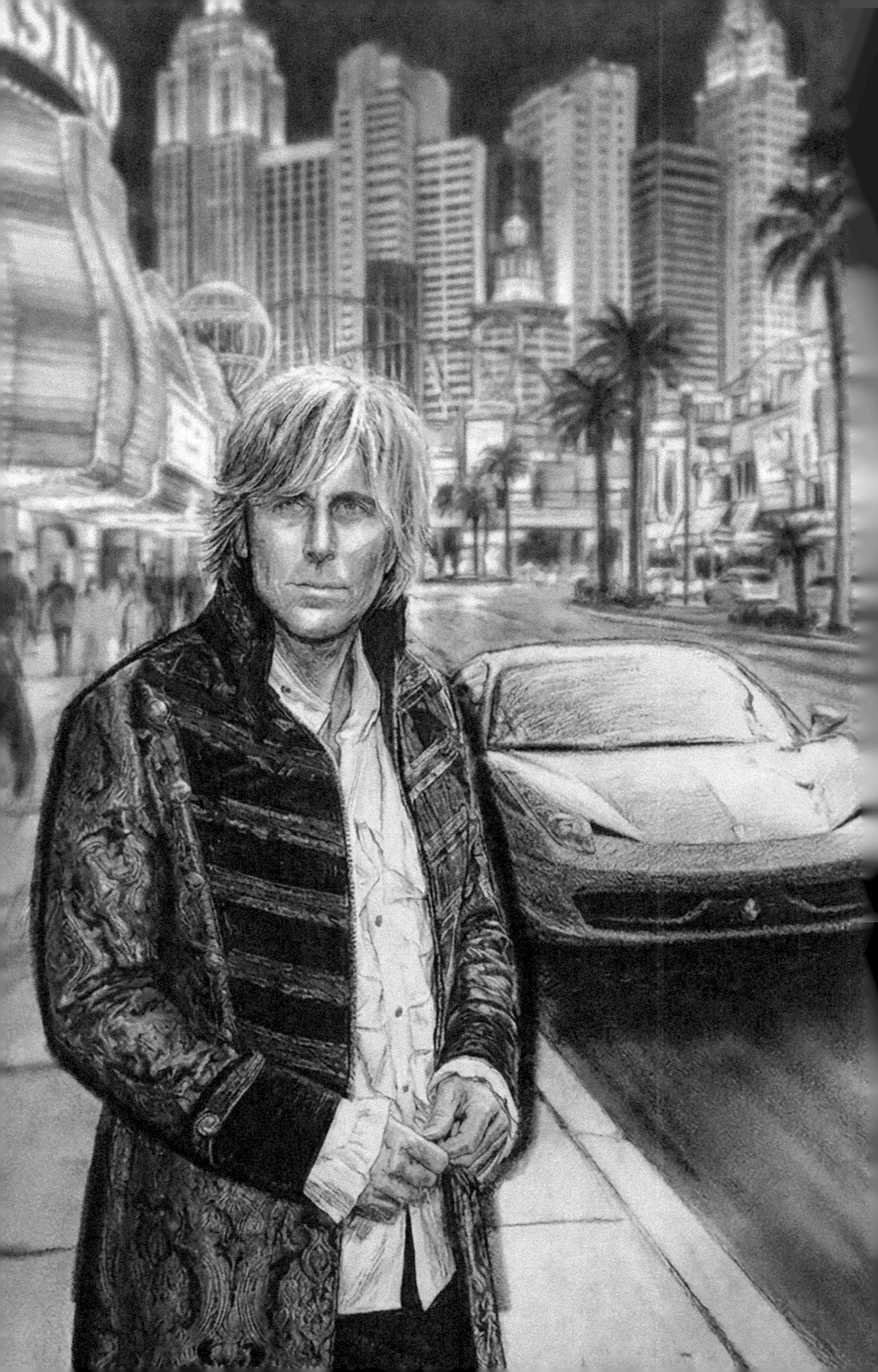

19.
Markus Rothkranz: Combining Spirituality and Aesthetics

"The face doesn't lie. A thousand messages stream instantaneously from our faces. Our bodies and unspoken energies are so much deeper and complex than anything we could ever say with words."
—**Markus Rothkranz**

Over 1,600 years after the first Christian ascetics forsook their own belongings and worldly stations and took to the desert of Egypt, an American visual effects artist had a spiritual transformation of his own. "I took my clothes off, and had my forty days in the Arizona desert. I woke up on a rock, under a vast blue sky," Markus Rothkranz explained, referencing the similarity of his experience to Jesus's forty days of fasting and temptation.[889] Rothkranz had given up nearly all his possessions and walked away from a long-term relationship. He had been unhappy with his life and wanted to start over.

History was echoing. Just as in the case of the Desert Fathers, this modern man who loved hair metal and fancy cars, was ready to forsake material possessions and identities, and remake his life. And uncooked food, of all things, would be an emblem of his renunciation of his previous life, similar to those monks so many years ago. Raw food was used once again, this time in the space age, as a rite of purification.

Rothkranz felt liberated, similar to what some ancient monks must've felt. Paradoxically, all of them had achieved a new kind of power upon giving up their worldly status and belongings. Once he'd gone into the desert, Rothkranz noted, "I had no fancy house, no car, no money, not even clothes, but I was accepted, and completely respected. I could feel God smiling at me." It's not hard to imagine some Desert Fathers reciting a similar sentiment. Without the trappings of

---

[889] Rothkranz, Markus. *Heal Your Face.* 1 Mar. 2011, 13.

the world, the material things that people valued the most, Rothkranz and the monks felt new spiritual potentialities in the stark desert. They felt a closeness to the truth and to God. For Rothkranz, giving up everything gave him a feeling of being "alive." There was an erotic undertone to the intensity of the feeling, as he described feeling the most "turned on" he'd ever felt.[890]

Rothkranz's days in the desert marked a transformation that soon spawned his advocacy of raw food. But whereas the raw foodism of the Desert Fathers was aimed toward physical disempowerment, like the squashing of fleshly passions, Rothkranz's aim was partially for physical empowerment—for greater health, beauty, and libido. The monks, of course, sought to minimize their appetite and completely erase their desire for sex drive to the supposed benefit of the spirit. But Rothkranz took a different aim. He felt like he could attain, partially through raw foodism, the fullness of life in body *and* spirit. His new sense of spiritual empowerment was intertwined with the physical, the two being in a constant interplay. The flesh, in Rothkranz's mind—its beauty and its vigor—reflected one's spiritual state. The face was especially telling.

So the body was not to be punished into emaciation in his scheme, like that of the monkish ascetics. Marrying the flesh to the spirit and thriving holistically was his aim.

AESTHETICS AND CONTENT CREATION

After his renewal in the desert, Rothkranz became an internet content creator, author, and eccentric advocate of raw foodism, easily recognizable in YouTube videos because of his drooping blond hair and fast playful rants. The bright colors of his videos—his flashy hair, colorful shirts, often sunny backdrops—reflected the vibrant image he wished to embody. Mixing humor and occasional heartfelt earnestness, his videos showcase the benefits, on body and soul, of a raw food lifestyle.

Achieving a sort of small-scale fame, he became a prominent voice within the raw food community and eventually, he was even seemingly lampooned on a national American comedy show, the Kroll Show, where a similarly looking character breathlessly advocates the virtues of his diet in a high pitched voice. Rothkranz' style certainly proved to be attention-grabbing, regardless of whether some thought it gauche.

Rothkranz knows how to attract attention with his content. His background, after all, as a painter, visual effects artist, and filmmaker, served him well. Aesthetically gifted from birth, he has always been vi-

---

[890]   Ibid.

sually-minded even in his nutritional advocacy. He is driven by beauty and has always been interested in maximizing the charm and appearance of the human body, along with his art. And raw food, in addition to spirituality, were to be the most powerful tools in shaping his own body as he desired and in instructing others to do the same.

RAW FOOD AESTHETICS

Well into his content-creating career, Rothkranz released a video expressing his frustration with people's shortsighted views on bodily aesthetics. He wondered how people could not understand that one's appearance conveyed meaning about bodily health and inner spiritual realities.

He had been receiving negative comments on videos that showcased his and his girlfriend's bodies. Rothkranz sought to show people their potential to be healthy, strong, and beautiful in middle age. He wanted, he said, to show viewers "what you could look like" if you followed the raw food lifestyle in the right way.[891]

People who think the outside of their bodies—who say their skin, hair, etc. are merely "superficial" and devoid of meaning—are lost in ignorance. "Maybe you won't be so bitter about other people and their sexy videos," he chastised viewers, if they woke up from their unconsciousness and practiced the right lifestyle habits. He challenged critical viewers (and jealous ones) on whether they were actually practicing healthy habits. If they were, they wouldn't be so bitter at the sight of well-kept bodies. "Some people piss me off so much," he complained, that, "I said 'fine I'm coming to your house.'" After actually going to these viewers' houses (they must have lived within driving distance of his Las Vegas home) and scouring their pantries and refrigerators, he found the dreaded items of their less than ideal health habits: "bread, or pasta, or cheese."[892] They were caught red-handed. They were sneaking cooked food. They didn't have the raw food commitment that would make them sexy, healthy, or happy. No wonder they left negative comments, he thought. They were dietary traitors, coveting the toxic temptations of the cooked world. Little hope did they have of becoming beautiful as long as they didn't have fidelity in the kitchen.

These are the people who have a victim mentality and deny that anyone can still be beautiful after a certain age. These are the peo-

---

[891] The Healthy Life. "The Outer Is Not Superficial- the Key to Staying Young." *YouTube*, 8 June 2018, www.youtube.com/watch?v=qdrsloMyb9s. Accessed 17 Mar. 2025.
[892] Ibid.

ple, Rothkranz points out, who say "there's nothing you can do. It's downhill from there. I'm screwed," once they turn fifty. "No excuses," Rothkranz counters. "I don't take excuses." He refutes some supposed genetic advantages that cynical viewers assume he has for his fresh-faced looks. He had looked terrible and had been horrible health in childhood and some of his adulthood. "I was bleeding when I went to the bathroom . . . I had asthma, allergies, I could barely breathe."[893] But raw vegan food changed all that. He had pulled himself up by his own bootstraps from a disadvantaged beginning, just like Tonya Zavasta.

FOOD BECOMES FLESH

Practicing the right dietary, lifestyle, and spiritual habits have created Rothkranz's youthful aesthetics, he submits.

Veganism is not enough to be healthy and look good, in Rothkranz's world. Donuts and other junk food can be vegan. All sorts of cooked and refined grains are not healthy, he argues. Even raw food in itself is not automatically healthy. There are actually raw foodists who look terrible, Rothkranz explains. Unbalanced habits like excessive fruit consumption can mar their aesthetics. Fruitarians eat a ton of sugar, causing glycation damage to the collagen (where sugars stiffen the proteins), which ruins the smooth and plump look of the skin.

In his first viral video, 2008's "Go Raw Now Trailer," Rothkranz dramatically warns viewers about the destruction caused by cooked food. As ominous music plays, he asks if people really think that the pizza or cake they eat "just goes through" them. "Your body absorbs it to make new cells," he says with emphasis. He continues, his voice imbued with a sense of sadness: "What do you think those cells will be made out of? That pizza becomes part of you." And that pizza is not good for your aesthetic future. "Go ahead," he challenges with bite, "sit there in your huge SUV, sucking down that sugar and cholesterol, wondering why your hair is falling out, or whine about how cellulite just showed up for no reason. Come on, people, take some responsibility in your life!" He snarkily continues, raising his voice to a shout, "Go ahead, get your stomach staples so now you can only eat one candy bar instead of twelve. Grow UP!"[894]

And what should you eat to improve your physical appearance? The correct food is "growing outside." As camera flashes sporadically light up his face, Rothkranz picks up props in front of a green screen.

---

[893] Ibid.

[894] Dharmaboost. "Go Raw Now Trailer." *Youtube.com*, 2008, youtu.be/z3xOU2tLl-7g?si=57YwsaPwZE0x4Tbt. Accessed 10 Apr. 2025.

"This is a papaya," he tells his audience, lifting it up and then setting it down, with an air of impatience and annoyance, "This is a mango," he says, holding up the next item. "This is called FOOD!"[895] The implication is clear: First World countries that think so highly of themselves, must be re-educated on the basics of life.

Raw foods build your cells out of "life," whereas anything cooked and most packaged foods build your cells from a place of death. You plant cooked cereal in the ground and you get nothing but "mold," but if you plant an apple, you get a tree. The apple "has life" and "that's what our body needs!" shouts Rothkranz.[896]

"Beauty and health are one," there's no escaping it, Rothkranz claims. We can't eat junk and be truly beautiful at the same time. "The sooner we realize that, the sooner our lives start radically improving."[897]

"The only way to beauty is to clean out the garbage," he declares. What you don't put in your body is even more important than what you do put in. A raw food diet is a given. Roughly half your diet should be greens, with the other half composed of fruits, nuts, and seeds. You must get these proportions right because eating too much fruit can stress your organs and ruin your skin, marring the complexion and causing wrinkles.[898]

"Milk products, sugar, cooked food, chemicals, preservatives, and colorings, bread, crackers, cheese, meat and refined cooked dead foods" uglify and poison your body.[899] "You can only be as good as the building materials you were made out of," Rothkranz explains, so would you rather be made out of beautiful colorful plants or roasted lump of meat on white bread?

Spirituality, Cooked Food, and Aesthetics

The body is not only a repository of dietary habits. It also absorbs energy, thought patterns, and moods, which make visual marks in its flesh.

Since both diet and spiritual habits are etched in the body, Rothkranz intertwines his descriptions of their dual effect. He also hints at a theme, throughout his books, of giving up burdens that are both dietary and spiritual. They are one and the same and it's just as import-

---

[895]   Ibid.

[896]   Ibid.

[897]   The Healthy Life. "The Outer Is Not Superficial- the Key to Staying Young." *YouTube*, 8 June 2018, www.youtube.com/watch?v=qdrsloMyb9s. Accessed 17 Mar. 2025.

[898]   Ibid.

[899]   Ibid.

ant to give up toxic thoughts as toxic food since both affect the states of your inner organs—states that then appear on your skin. "Being positive about life is just as important as what you eat," he explains.

Rothkranz uses Chinese medicine to show how thoughts and food affect our organ "meridians"—the points on your surface appearance that denote the health of your inner organs. Your skin, hair, and nails tell the story of what's going on inside and even the small area of the face comprises a map of much of your internal body. Because "every part of your face is connected to a different part of your body . . . Healing your body and organs also heals your face"—hence the title of one of Rothkranz's books, *Heal Your Face.*[900] Moles, bumps, lines, and wrinkles pop up "on areas of weak energy," on the meridian lines associated with organs.[901] And hair and nails "speak volumes." Brittleness and texture both "mean something."[902]

The state of your face, at this moment, can tell you nearly everything about your body and the thoughts and diet that formed their appearance. There's not much use in expensive doctor visits or blood tests. Neither is there much use in expensive dermatologists or plastic surgeons. Your organs and aesthetics heal by giving up the sugary and "sludgy dead [cooked] foods" that are making you unattractive.[903]

"Your face is a map" that is a "built-in x-ray machine all over your body," he says.[904] It tells you, on its surface, every deep physical truth you need to know. "The truth is written all over you. . . We are in control. Real healers simply hold a mirror up" to see the state of your internals, Rothkranz says.[905] Deep lines in the middle of the forehead signify that your small intestines are "crying for help."[906] Creases from the nose to sides of mouth signify a traumatized colon of an "old-school meat eater" who loves "steak, hot dogs, beer, coffee."[907] Zits show up at sites on the skin that correlate with organ meridians and they are at least subtle signals, so "pay attention" to these "warning lights" on your bodily dashboard, urges Rothkranz.[908]

Hair loss at the front of the head signifies kidney, bladder, and reproductive system troubles. Hair loss all over the head equals overcon-

[900]   Rothkranz, Markus. *Heal Your Face.* 1 Mar. 2011, 5, 17.
[901]   Ibid., 40.
[902]   Ibid., 20.
[903]   Ibid., 24.
[904]   Ibid., 25.
[905]   Ibid., 19.
[906]   Ibid., 47.
[907]   Ibid., 54.
[908]   Ibid., 22.

sumption of bad foods: meat, dairy, alcohol, etc.[909] "One of the biggest reasons for hair loss is eating meat," Rothkranz argues.[910] Gray hair signifies weak kidneys, emotional turmoil, lack of proper sleep.[911]

Other visible parts, like eyes and teeth, also can't keep quiet about the inner reality of your body. Different teeth are associated with different body parts and "all body parts can be seen through the eyes"—color patches, redness, and various parts of the eye tell the story of associated organs. Instead of "stretching and puffing" your face through surgery, pay attention to what your face is telling you. "Your face and your body are the best tools for telling you what's wrong with you . . . Health is not just what you put in your mouth." "Health is liking what you see in the mirror" and a "great sexy relationship." In other words, aesthetics are the point of health. What fun would it be without looking good?

There is spiritual truth written in the flesh as well, Rothkranz believes. To witness the health of our soul, "It's time we took a good look at ourselves. Literally," he urges.[912] You can see the energetic truth of a person in their voice, eyes, skin, and hair. Their physical body represents the accumulation of their mental and dietary choices. The "structure of our face, our very bones," are molded by "our choices (food), thoughts, environment, and spirit."[913]

The flesh is a repository of "subconscious thought and emotional patterns." The lines on the face can designate the spiritual burdens you have put on your kidneys, liver, gallbladder, or other internal organs. And how those internal organs function is often "just a physical manifestation of your energetic thoughts and mental patterns."[914] You have to "clean up your thoughts, value system" if you want "healing and rebuilding," he claims—if you want internal and visible health.[915] "Being positive about life is just as important as what you eat," he notes.

Our visible body parts and the energy we give to others indicate the spiritual reality of what's happening inside us, even if we try to artificially cover up our imperfections. "Even with the most expensive extensive plastic surgery," Rothkranz warns, "somehow the truth still shows through . . . True thoughts, emotions, aura and secret energies

---

909 Ibid., 45.
910 Ibid., 46.
911 Ibid.
912 Ibid., 6.
913 Ibid., 18.
914 Ibid., 30.
915 Ibid., 43.

are still beaming out to the world."[916] The way we hold our bodies, posture, can also be indicative of inner energies—the habit of being hunched over can indicate spiritual "undernourishment"—not enough "love, sex, appreciation, recognition etc."[917] Cracked and splitting fingertips can indicate "sexual weakness and frigidity."[918] A clogged liver is tied to anger issues and a weakened spleen causes one to become anxious, "wishy-washy," and have "trouble standing strong against others" and may cause puffiness or dark circles under the eyes.[919]

"Nothing is by coincidence," Rothkranz proclaims. Our organs, energy, and appearance are intertwined. "That mole did not just randomly show up on your body for no reason . . . those bags under your eyes. The wrinkles . . ."[920] The aesthetic changes that we dread with age are actually not natural. "Wild animals," those raw food eaters, with minds unclouded by the stressful ruminations that humans so often have, "*do not* get gray hair, or become fat and bald as they get older." This uglifying process should not be accepted as inevitable. It irritates Rothkranz that it is. It "really pisses me off," he says.[921]

THE FOOD, SPIRIT, AESTHETICS CYCLES

In Markus's paradigm, bad food and spiritual malaise can create a vicious cycle. Food, by affecting our organ meridians, also affects our spiritual health and how we feel, which then feeds back into our aesthetics. Toxic food may weaken the liver, for instance, which then makes us prone to certain negative emotions. Those emotions then exacerbate the aesthetic problems that relate to the traumatized organ system. For better or worse, the roundabout cycle goes on.

WHAT ARE THE RIGHT SPIRITUAL VALUES FOR A RAW FOODIST?

That's why Rothkranz emphasizes spiritual values and how they complement raw foodism. Everything is connected, Rothkranz repeats. Every decision affects something else and when we start to think more

---

[916]   Ibid.
[917]   Ibid., 68.
[918]   Ibid., 69.
[919]   Ibid., 73.
[920]   Ibid., 9.
[921]   Ibid., 10.

about the way we look, that "single, vain action," like "wanting to get rid of wrinkles . . . ultimately turns into a life-changing experience that ripples out to the entire universe."[922] A simple aesthetic desire, one that people may call "selfish," can affect our health and even the universe for the better. A desire for better skin or hair can have a healing effect on the world because we reevaluate how we think, treat others, and what we eat. We make fewer toxic choices, both spiritually and physically. Aesthetic desire can actually underlie spiritual goodness and initiate a life of positively affecting the world around us.

This is why Rothkranz declares, "It isn't a luxury to be beautiful, it's your duty."[923] Treating others well, being a responsible caretaker of your body, and setting an example (physically and spiritually) for others are the downstream results of the aesthetic drive for beauty, a drive that makes the world a better place.

"The world is [spiritually] lost. People are dying." People wander, sucking up toxic food, drugs, and thought patterns that "suck the life out." Therefore, it is an act of "love" towards others, we should become "a shining signpost to guide others to the truth," by being a beautiful specimen.[924] "You want to know what your purpose in life is?" Rothkranz asks and then answers: "How about being the sexiest . . . healthiest, [most] glowing being ever seen?" That way, you spread "true healing" in the world by inspiring others to live out their own positivity.[925]

You will live benevolently with your thoughts and actions, because this is what you need to do to be beautiful. Our spiritual practices affect our face. An attitude of non-resistance and acceptance is a key part of fostering health and beauty and might be even more important than the raw food we should feed ourselves with. When you "let go," and "no longer resist or struggle," you have "given yourself to the Universe (God)..," Rothkranz explains.[926] We must "let things happen" to become "enlightened" and this habit of acceptance "has a lot to do with your face"—how your flesh is molded. "Unless you start understanding what I just said," Rothkranz warns, "your face will be stressed out and not look pretty."[927] The Kingdom of Heaven, a spiritually elevated state, and a beautiful body "comes from letting go."[928] This attitude is

---

[922]   Ibid., 8.

[923]   Ibid., 33.

[924]   Ibid.

[925]   Ibid., 34.

[926]   Ibid., 12.

[927]   Ibid., 14.

[928]   Ibid., 32.

critical for feeling good, acting virtuously, and looking good, which are all interrelated.

Another spiritual value, one that Rothkranz shares with other raw foodists, is that we should reclaim intuition and simplicity. Excessive mental noise is often destructive and it's sometimes "amazing how simple the answer is." As evidenced by how beautiful nature is and how "messed up and crazy mankind is," the "less of a brain something has, the more sensible it usually is," he says.[929] Our minds are typically "overprotective guardians" that generate fear in a hyperactive attempt to protect us. But in doing so, the mind can be destructive on our body and life quality. The human mind is "NOT the first thing you should listen to," Rothkranz warns. The mind is a "tape recording" of mostly "fear-based" beliefs and opinions that have been fed to you by society.[930]

Letting go was a spiritual value that led Rothkranz to raw foodism. It led him to the desert and led him to give up the burden of cooked food. "Let go," he tells readers, "of every fear, every belief, and any programming society may have given you," including what food is considered normal.[931] To drop the burdensome habits and beliefs that are imposed on us, is to adopt the most innocent and natural way of eating—raw.

The way that a twentieth-century American was taught to eat (Rothkranz was born in 1962) was full of erroneous beliefs that demoralize one's spirit and mar one's flesh. If you don't eat meat, the America that Rothkranz grew up in warned, you won't get enough protein. And if you don't drink cow's milk, you won't get enough calcium. But as he gave up society's useless "tape recordings" and embraced his intuition, he realized that these instructions were destructive and returned to the unconditioned natural path of uncooked food, just as the wild animals in the desert ate.

Aesthetics and Physiology Feed into Spirituality

Spirituality, of course, molds physiology and aesthetics. But Rothkranz, like other raw foodists, points out that influence moves in the other direction as well—the body molds spirituality.

---

929 Ibid., 32.
930 Ibid., 6.
931 Ibid., 14.

Firstly, "The way you look affects the way you feel" and the way you look is built off of what you eat.[932] Rothkranz agrees with Tonya Zavasta in saying that bodily aesthetics imbue how we feel—our quality of flesh affects our spirit and whether we are comfortable with ourselves or not. The importance of our looks is undeniable—a big house, a fast car, a lot of money—"you would trade all that in" if it meant that "you liked what you saw in the mirror," he claims.[933] Ideally, the spirit and the flesh are in sync and reflect each other's excellence.

But food doesn't only affect aesthetics and the resulting feelings of satisfaction. Dietary choices ripple effects through the rest of our life and reflect our values. Discipline is a key value for Rothkranz, and he explains the fulfillment or lack of it has far-reaching societal effects.

Many people choose the very short term gratification of "eating pleasure" as "being more important than the relationships they are in," he says. They would rather have a quick high from cooked comfort food and "clog their liver, burn out their adrenals, kill their sex drive" and become irritable and combative than have the discipline to eat healthy raw food.[934] Relationships are destroyed because of shallow dietary hedonism. "Our choices" involving food "create what we become" spiritually—they create the vibes that cause harmony or dysfunction in our lives.[935] Food transmutes into spirit.

The quality of societies and the behavior of its members are dependent upon these nutritional choices. If people lived ideally, and chose raw food, they would be "functioning properly and full of life"—their hormones would be high, they would be sexually satisfied, and thus "make happy workers," Rothkranz claims.[936] Creativity and productivity would soar. "Everything is connected," he repeats.

When your body is pure and detoxified from junk food, you can "actually *hear*" where other people are "coming from." Physiological purity opens you up to have more empathy and helps you to no longer feel that people are an emotional threat to you. Raw food also promotes equanimity and feeling grounded. "Your calmness will calm them," Rothkranz promises.[937]

If cooked food and junk food reign supreme, however, people will be grouchy, overly aggressive, inefficient workers and generally dysfunctional. "If our kidneys are overwhelmed" with toxic foods like refined grains, too much meat, processed sugar, or stimulants, then

---

[932]   Ibid., 27.

[933]   Ibid., 29.

[934]   Ibid., 99.

[935]   Ibid., 200.

[936]   Ibid., 100.

[937]   Ibid.

it "makes us indecisive in work and life."[938] Cooked crap clouds your clarity of mind and can steer you towards the wrong decisions.

Those dark circles or puffy bags under the eyes indicate kidney strain and the energetic waning of these organs makes it harder for our minds to discriminate between decisions in life. Weak-kidneyed people find it hard to "think straight" and may even find that events synchronize with their inner state—funky or unexpected things happen that throw us off track.[939] If you choose the wrong food, it might affect what external events happen to you.

Sticking to raw foods benefits not only your behavior, but even the universe's behavior toward you. "Whole new worlds open up to you," and the universe "will honor you back," Rothkranz promises.[940] The raw eater's mind is opened and so is a connection to the external world, which supposedly aids human sentience.

The Raw Food Exemplar

Rothkranz seeks to bring more beauty and positive energy into the world. His paintings, films, and even his own body are his media. And like others, he found that raw food was the means by which to artistically mold himself into how he desired to look. Spiritually, raw food was also the means for being one's best and being in harmony with the external world. Raw food is the foundational source of empowerment, Rothkranz claims.

Raw food, he tells viewers and readers, will beautify and heal the world. If you live like him, you will look better and the world will be a kinder place. "I just look the way that I do because I am the result of my choices in life." The way that he feels and the way the whole world feels could also be a result of similar choices.

---

[938]   Ibid., 19.

[939]   Ibid., 30.

[940]   Ibid., 100.

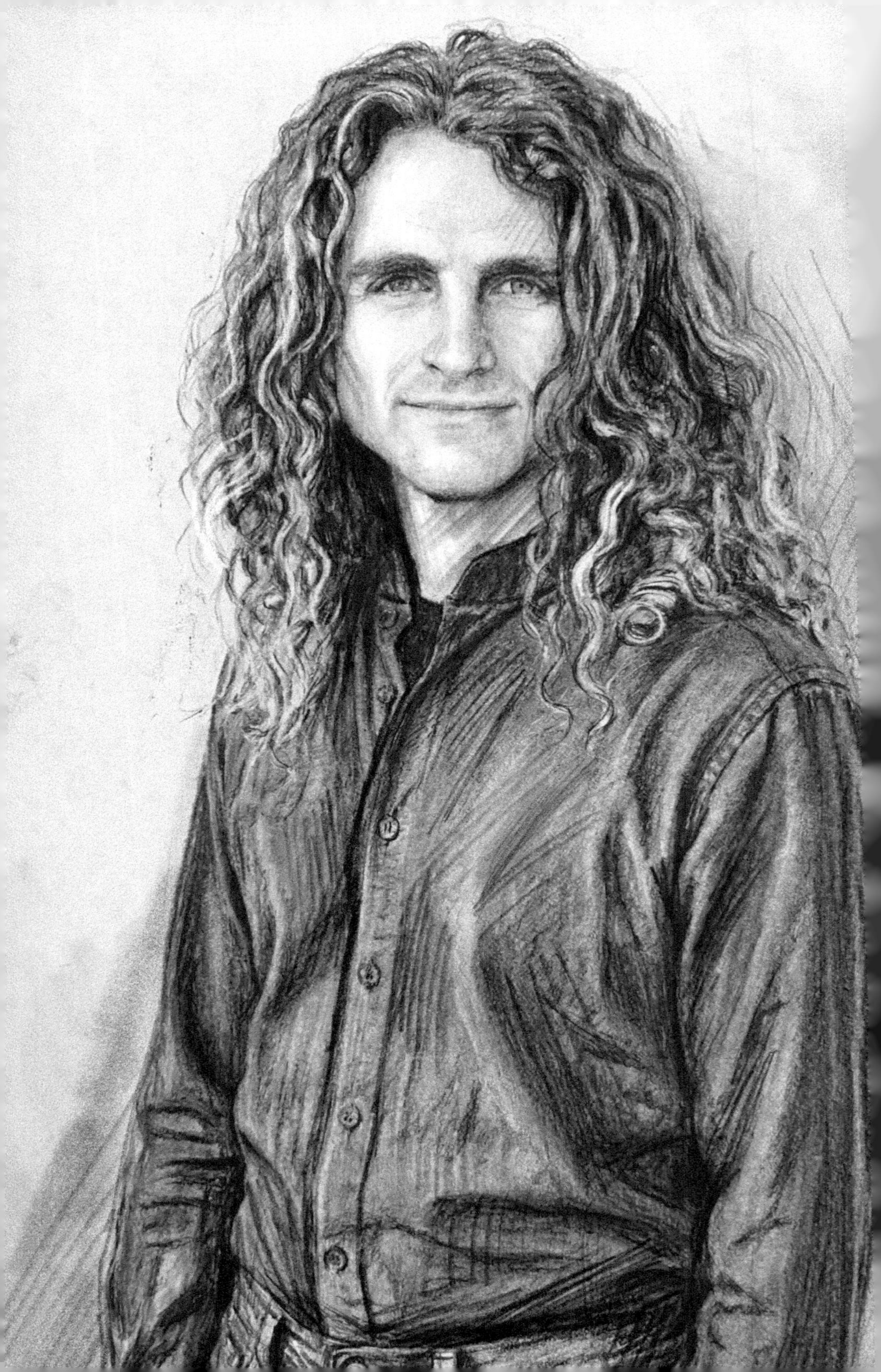

20.
Matt Monarch: Spiritual Transformation and the Turbulent "Raw Food World"

A Dying Raw Foodist

Twenty-three years into a raw vegan diet, Matt Monarch hung onto the edge of life. He was dying from complications of untreated ulcerative colitis. At the most desperate moment of this ordeal, the closest he came to death, he says, he was injected with adrenaline to keep his heart beating.

Previous to that moment, he had suffered for years with his digestive disease, often bedridden and having to wear a diaper. Added to the physical suffering was the distressing fact that he was a leader in the worldwide raw food niche. Being so, he was supposed to have found the key to exceptional health. Now, tragically, he was no longer considered a living example of the diet's superiority.

He had authored a number of books on raw foodism and had become a successful businessman, owning the world's largest online raw food emporium—The Raw Food World. His site offered an array of uncooked products like nut butters, raw chocolate, fruit powders, supplements, and educational materials. It was a popular shopping stop for the community, and Monarch, a self-described "superfoods pioneer" in the space, cashed in, at least when all was going well.

Monarch was seen as an authority on health and constantly preached the power of the raw food diet. He was never overbearing or absolutist. He wouldn't deny that cooked food can be part of a healthy diet. But he was certainly one of the most famous faces representing raw foodism. If he walked into a health food market, with his well-known thin form and long hair, he would often be recognized. Considering this, it is hardly surprising that he felt trapped in the "dogma" of being committed to his diet no matter if his health was failing. He tried a multitude of natural remedies and nothing worked to heal him. He tried for two years to heal from colitis by staying on raw foods. He juice-cleansed, "fasted" on only bananas, water fasted, dry fasted (in which no water or food is consumed), but nothing healed him.[941]

Still, he was dead set in his ways. He was psychologically yoked to the raw food lifestyle. He believed that this diet could heal almost anything. His public reputation and his business were built on his advocacy for this diet, after all.

Later on, he would note that if only he had taken "a med," like the pharmaceutical Humera that he later went on, it would've dramatically reduced his symptoms in only a week or so. But such a remedy was a taboo in his intensely naturistic mind. His stubborn attachment to the idea of raw food being the only remedy almost killed him. "I was so sure and narrow minded like raw vegans are today," he said years later. "I'm only here today because I opened my mind."[942] He mentions other raw vegans who died because they were "not willing to open up and look at other avenues," like conventional medicine.[943]

It was when he realized, "I have children. Being right about the raw vegan diet isn't as important as being alive," that he finally gave into treatment—surgery and pharmaceutical drugs.[944] Detaching from his rigid beliefs saved his life, but he "wouldn't be in as bad of shape" if he had accepted medical help earlier. His ailment got to the point where some of his colon had to be removed. He was grateful to be alive, however. He knew others, he said, that died in their raw food dogma, prematurely, refusing to undergo medical treatment for serious ailments. After having some of his colon removed and starting his prescription pill regimen, Matt Monarch's health stabilized.

His health struggle disturbed the raw food community. How could a chief expert on raw foods, someone who had an impeccable diet, become ill? What did he do wrong? What were his nutritional errors? Raw devotees pondered these unsettling questions. Was there a point of following such a strict diet if it didn't save you from such a disastrous near death experience?

Some convinced themselves that if only Matt had followed their specific advice for dealing with his ulcerative colitis, he would've been

---

[941]   Matt Monarch. "Twenty-three Year Ex-Raw Vegan Comes out about Raw Vegan Diet." *YouTube*, 26 Sept. 2023, www.youtube.com/watch?v=_H2Ppcv1HUU. Accessed 15 Apr. 2025.
[942]   Ibid.
[943]   Ibid.
[944]   Ibid.

healed. Raw foodists chimed in with their opinions: he should do more enemas, or he did too many enemas, too many colonic hydrotherapy treatments, or perhaps he should've eaten more fruit etc.

Monarch was annoyed by such confident proclamations. Clearly, the raw food diet had not prevented his colitis. In his words, he "failed on the raw food diet." He claims he was "one of the most strict, extreme raw foodists." He was knowledgeable and followed all the rules. He "didn't do anything wrong in terms of what I ate," he says. His diet was, by all standards, "perfection."[945] He was no fruitarian gorging on fruit. He ate very nutritionally dense foods like greens, nuts, and seaweed that should've taken him to elite levels of health.

In the end, he believes, spiritual chaos in his life caused him to fall ill—"crazy, unbelievable, unfathomable, nutso spiritual chaos for seven years," not some overlooked dietary sin.[946] Nutritionally, he had been as thorough and pure as possible.

After his experiences, he turned his back on what he had advocated for over two decades. In one video he put it plainly: "I don't think the raw vegan diet is the ideal diet anymore. There, I said it."[947]

Before Monarch began the raw food diet, he didn't have any health issues. But, convinced by a friend that it was the right step for aesthetic, spiritual, and long-term health reasons, he started eating raw and felt he understood how damaging unhealthy food was after he "vomited" from eating a Subway sandwich and a slice of pizza.

But in the end, living without cooked food is usually untenable in the long run for humans, he believes—that is, without consuming vegetable juices, a form of unnatural food processing.

Monarch's health crisis hammered in the point that there was more to health than raw food. At the least, it wasn't the only path to take. After all, Monarch points out, "My dad is 300 pounds . . ., goes to Kentucky Fried Chicken. He's eighty-four! I don't know many raw foodists who have made it past eighty-four."[948]

MONARCH'S INITIAL NEW AGE RAW FOODISM

When he went raw, around the turn of the century, switching his diet from standard twentieth-century American fare (primarily refined carbs and meat), Monarch noticed changes in the way his senses func-

---

945   Ibid.
946   Ibid.
947   Ibid.
948   Ibid.

tioned, as well as an odd vibration in his body that he felt had spiritual meaning.

In 2005, Monarch wrote that "the most exciting reward of being raw" is the "spiritual effect" of the diet.[949] Soon after switching to raw vegan eating, he says, "I had never felt so clean, so light; the feeling was weightlessness, my body felt like quickly moving energy rather than dense solid matter."[950] This ethereal feeling felt like a liberation from the physical heaviness of his former body and an opening to the "spiritual realities" and "subtle realms."[951]

He now had increased sensitivity to unseen forces. Life became more vibrational and energetic, rather than solidified and material: "your spiritual energy vibrates at an almost tangible rate," he wrote. Your body "becomes clean and vulnerable" to life's energies as well as chemical toxicities. This vulnerability increases spiritual sensitivity but brings challenges alongside empowerment. "Since [now] cooked foods are not there to medicate the senses, any emotional and psychological issues bubble up to the surface."[952] Raw foodism caused emotional detoxification and fragility at first. The difficulty of handling these painful "buried emotions" that arise when you wean off desensitizing cooked foods can be a daunting challenge and a common reason why people fail on raw diets, he believed.[953] One's ability to navigate this painful realm of dark emotions was put to the test. Raw food was a spiritual gauntlet. Thus, it was critical to develop "control over our emotions" to be able to physically continue a raw food diet, he wrote.[954]

Monarch also began to get in touch with a subtle "pain, a feeling of misery in my being" and started meditating as a technique to dissolve this subtle pain.[955] Through "complete, unwavering focus" on the body parts that seemed to reverberate these "disturbing energies," he was able to "transform them" away.[956] Clearly there were challenges that came with raw food-induced energetic sensitivity.

Alongside these uncomfortable challenges, Monarch noticed a positive sensation. He felt "an orgasmic-like" vibration in the center of his forehead. He welcomed the feeling but was also bewildered; he searched for probable causes. Eventually he was convinced that this was his pineal gland vibrating on a new level. This endocrine gland in

---

[949]   Monarch, M. (2005). *Raw spirit: What the raw food advocates don't preach*, 11.
[950]   Ibid., *12*
[951]   Ibid., 105.
[952]   Ibid.
[953]   Ibid., 105.
[954]   Ibid., 106.
[955]   Ibid., 107.
[956]   Ibid., 109.

the brain is known for producing hormones like melatonin and serotonin but in mystical traditions it is linked to transcendent experiences
and intuition. Monarch read, in the works of Norman Walker, another
raw foodist, that the pineal gland is "the spiritual receptacle for life
force" and "is analogous to a radio antennae, receiving from the atmo-
spheric environment the vital flow cosmic energy, acting like an electric current when it enters the body."[957] Raw food had made Monarch
susceptible to receiving spiritual information, this time in a good way.
He was attuned to the background vibrations of the universe.

Monarch also felt his consciousness open up beyond the social
conditioning we are all inundated with. Dietarily, since he had to "drop
the social mainstream ways, to travel a path on my own," and only eat
raw plants, he learned to overcome social pressure and do something
that is extremely strange to most Americans.[958]

Monarch was convinced, similar to Johnny Lovewisdom and Gabriel Cousens before him, that since he went on the raw diet, his digestive tract was more "dormant" and thus, his "spiritual organs" like
the pineal gland were "in use" because less energy was being siphoned
away from it by digestion.[959] He believed in a theory articulated by
spiritual writer Hilton Hotema that the "spiritual faculties" of man
used to be more active when they were "Breatharians"—when they
consumed no food and were sustained only by the air. When you're on
a raw diet, Monarch thought, you're a "step closer to the ancient divine
man" and on a "higher vibration" because your pineal gland is taking in
more "cosmic energy."[960]

Like other New Age raw foodists, Monarch was obviously convinced that food had a substantial effect on spiritual experience. He
believed like his mentor, Dr. Fred Bisci, that the "spiritual life we experience has a lot to do with our internal chemistry."[961] When one's body
reaches extraordinary purity on a raw food diet, a "super consciousness"
develops and the "spiritual profoundness" in things is evident.[962]

Bisci warned, on the other hand, how difficult it is for people to
spiritually grow while eating a bad diet. He saw how difficult it was
for "people searching for answers from organized religion or searching spiritually while still eating a bad diet." Quality of consciousness
and perceptivity were said to be decimated by cooked food. Monarch

---

[957]   Ibid., 54.
[958]   Ibid., 52.
[959]   Ibid., 56.
[960]   Ibid., 57.
[961]   Ibid.,. 97.
[962]   Ibid., 98.

thought similarly—that with raw food and meditation, it's easier to see that "everything is connected" in addition to more acutely perceiving the sensory beauty of the world. When the body is purified from poison by a raw vegan diet, "the tremendous struggle" of spiritual searching lessens and "the brain functions more efficiently. You automatically become a more gentle, unconditionally loving type of person." Even "criminal mentalities change when they adopt a better diet."[963]

But in years after, Monarch distanced himself from such New Age raw foodist beliefs. Eventually, he became a Christian. Monarch's comments in the late 2010s and 2020s, seemed to reject, for the most part, the connection between diet and spirituality.

EMBRACING CHRISTIANITY AND FORSAKING RAW FOODISM

*"One woman just said that Jesus was going to use
me in reaching out to New Age people."*
—Matt Monarch, from his hospital bed in 2021

It eventually occurred to Monarch that only raw foodists who believed "heavily" in God had seemed to succeed on the diet. Norman Walker and his mentor Bisci were two such examples.

At some point, Monarch crossed the threshold and became a Christian and veered away from the diet-spirituality connection that even his Christian mentor Bisci accepted.

The details are a bit murky on Monarch's transformation, but in interviews, he references a time of tumultuous trouble and spiritual crisis that occurred after "messing around" with certain occult practices and becoming involved with an evil business partner. Monarch seems to connect his illness and life tumult with these ill-sought practices. At one point, he says it was "because I did my [New Age] spiritual practices," that he almost died.

Around 2018, the business and health crisis began in Monarch's life.

"After I found Jesus," he says, "everything went haywire in my life." When he made the heartfelt decision to dedicate his life to Christianity, he "looked up to heaven and was like 'I want to take it all the way.'" And almost all the way it went. He was "warned by the devil," he says, that he could lose his health and money if he took the path of being a

---

[963]   Ibid.

Christ follower.[964] And that's what happened. He lost his property in Ecuador, his business, and was diagnosed with ulcerative colitis.

When all this was happening, a nebulous and ominous figure appeared in his life. As Monarch recalls the events, it almost seems like the man was a satanic test, to challenge Monarch's dedication to his new Christian faith. It was "like the story of Job" in the Bible, Monarch says, "where the devil came to him and . . . took his belongings and health."[965]

One day, in Vilcabamba, Ecuador, known as a "valley of longevity," where Monarch lived out his especially-minimalist raw foodist lifestyle in the pristine air, he was walking toward a man. It was as if, Monarch later noted, they were magnetically drawn to each other. The man told the Raw Food World owner that he's "gotta go hide his money."[966]

This man, who Monarch ended up entrusting with some of his money and the functioning of his business, used trickery and caused distrust between him and his wife.

He was like some sort of sorcerer. Monarch later claimed he learned that this man worshipped the devil even though he was tricking others that he was a force for good. This man practiced "black magic" and had a strange ability to metaphysically enter Monarch and remove spiritual "attachments" that would bring him relief initially. When these negative spiritual attachments were removed, it was like "being electrocuted by lightning" and experiencing "electrical spiritual craziness" in a pleasurable way.[967] The man also performed a divination on Monarch, convincing him that he had Biblically-important ancestors.

But this person was stealing from him all the while, and ruining Monarch's marriage.

Ultimately, Monarch believes that his ulcerative colitis was caused by the spiritual darkness surrounding him—"Maybe there was a point of weakness in my colon that this being [the devil-worshipping man] penetrated and fed off of for many years and then it resulted in my disease."[968] Even after giving up his spiritual faith in raw foodism, it's

---

964   Eva Loves Raw. "Matt Monarch Heartfelt Candid Interview." *YouTube*, 10 Apr. 2022, www.youtube.com/watch?v=ePy5k3rHyII. Accessed 16 Apr. 2025.

965   Matt Monarch. "23 Year Ex-Raw Vegan Comes out about Raw Vegan Diet." *YouTube*, 26 Sept. 2023, www.youtube.com/watch?v=_H2Ppcv1HUU. Accessed 15 Apr. 2025.

966   Ibid.

967   Ms.FitVegan. "MY Interview with 23 Year EX-RAW VEGAN Matt Monarch! | a MUST WATCH." *YouTube*, 28 Sept. 2023, www.youtube.com/watch?v=dS6t8x1NAHQ. Accessed 16 Apr. 2025.

968   Ibid.

still apparent that Monarch believes that supernatural forces are powerfully intervening in human lives.

"The only person I look up to now is Jesus Christ," Monarch says. Experiences like this had left him with very little trust in others or interest in following any gurus.[969]

Losing his business and having his land "stolen" from him was a tremendously painful. "I went through so much suffering," he says. In one video from his hospital bed, after a colon surgery, Monarch tears up, saying he hates Ecuador and doesn't want to go back.[970] It was where he lost everything and the people who were leeches on him were still there. The landscape itself had become painful.

Nevertheless, out of all the suffering and loss, he says, "What I have gained goes beyond anything that can be imagined . . . I saw spiritual stuff that is very rare to see . . . It's almost like the spiritual realm is more real than the physical," he concludes. All the physical things had to be taken away, he feels, to highlight the deeper spiritual realities of life. The ultimate such spiritual reality that he is left believing is that he'll be taken care of by God and "that Jesus is the way to eternal life."[971]

PHYSICALLY AND SPIRITUALLY REEVALUATING NUTRITION

Monarch became detached from a strict adherence to raw foodism as well as his former beliefs about the spiritual supremacy of such a diet.

Nutritionally, in his opinion, the healthiest diet in the world is simply one that "obstructs" the body as little as possible while obtaining optimal nutrition, something like CRON (calorie restriction with optimal nutrition). You don't overwhelm the body with excess macronutrients but still receive all needed vitamins, minerals, and other substances.

"Why classify?" he asks. There are many different paths to the mountain top. You can eat healthy on many diets. But people are obsessed with strict boundaries and labels. He's sick of the dogma, judgment, and different groups arguing and condemning each other—veg-

---

[969]   Eva Loves Raw. "Matt Monarch Heartfelt Candid Interview." *YouTube*, 10 Apr. 2022, www.youtube.com/watch?v=ePy5k3rHyII. Accessed 16 Apr. 2025.

[970]   Matt Monarch. "I Had Surgery for Irreversible Ulcerative Colitis." *YouTube*, 5 May 2021, www.youtube.com/watch?v=ECgenBMir10. Accessed 16 Apr. 2025.

[971]   Matt Monarch. "23 Year Ex-Raw Vegan Comes out about Raw Vegan Diet." *YouTube*, 26 Sept. 2023, www.youtube.com/watch?v=_H2Ppcv1HUU. Accessed 15 Apr. 2025.

ans vs. carnivores, raw foodists vs. cooked foodists. Dietary partisans often want crystal-clear answers so they stick to the dogma of raw food being the only way to health. Monarch's irritation at the overbearing judgments of raw vegans is apparent in one video. As he holds a glass of what looks like blue-green algae-infused water, he yells at the camera, rebuking dogmatists: "Leave people alone! Do your raw vegan diet and shut up!"[972]

Sure, there are benefits of a raw food diet, Monarch says. It is heavy in water and low in calories (it doesn't damage or obstruct the body that much). But there are plenty of other ways to eat just as healthily and you can still eat badly on the raw—you can eat too much, eat lots of sugar, or eat lots of dehydrated food.

Raw foods do not hold the key to longevity, he believes. Very few raw foodists have made it to an impressively advanced age. He entertains no delusions now. "If the raw food diet is so good, why didn't I heal on the raw food diet?" he asks with irritation. He did dry fasts and water fasts, after all, too. Eating any raw vegetable, nuts, or even fruit would send him into enormous pain. If the raw vegan diet is so great, he challenges, we should see all these people living to a hundred but we often don't.[973] The few who do, only last that long because of their belief in God, he claims. "Why are so many people dying on a raw food diet?" he asks.[974] It is a false promise of salvation, he hints.

But one can sense a tinge of regret in his explanation. He hasn't completely given up the special place raw food has in his mind. In a sense, "I'm still a raw vegan on many levels," he says. He's "fighting" to get off the anti-inflammatory drugs he takes for colitis. He would rather be natural. He would eat "way more" raw food if he was healthy enough and didn't have the disease. "I'm a raw vegan at heart," he says broadly, in reference to his dedication to the optimization of human health.[975] The archetype of the raw foodist as a person who searches strenuously for insight and power is still alive and well within his psyche.

---

972   Ibid.

973   Eva Loves Raw. "Matt Monarch Heartfelt Candid Interview." *YouTube*, 10 Apr. 2022, www.youtube.com/watch?v=ePy5k3rHyII. Accessed 16 Apr. 2025.

974   Matt Monarch. "23 Year Ex-Raw Vegan Comes out about Raw Vegan Diet." *YouTube*, 26 Sept. 2023, www.youtube.com/watch?v=_H2Ppcv1HUU. Accessed 15 Apr. 2025.

975   Eva Loves Raw. "Matt Monarch Heartfelt Candid Interview." *YouTube*, 10 Apr. 2022, www.youtube.com/watch?v=ePy5k3rHyII. Accessed 16 Apr. 2025.

THE CHRISTIAN REJECTION OF THE SPIRITUAL IMPORTANCE OF FOOD

Monarch became a nutritional heretic, leaving the fold of raw veganism and its exclusive claim to mastering the secrets of human health. His idea of spiritual flourishing also underwent a transformation. He seemed to embrace the idea, shared by many Christians, that food has no spiritual meaning—a far cry from his previous belief about the supposedly incredible spiritual possibilities that came with eating raw food.

Attacking dietary labels and the aggressive proselytization by dietary advocates of their own niche habits, Monarch declared in one interview that "Life is not about food." "This judgmental stuff"—the harsh criticism that some raw vegans hurl towards others who don't practice their specific dietary habits—he finds utterly distasteful. It's a "snobby" thing to classify yourself as "raw vegan" and be dismissive toward other diets.[976]

Along with attacking dietary zeal, he deemphasized the spiritual meaning of food. "We're all human beings and it doesn't matter what a person eats," he said. He then added a sweeping dismissal of the effect of food on consciousness and the spiritual identity of a person: "The way a person eats has nothing to do with who that person is, how they feel every day, who they are"—a startling deviation from someone who wrote much about how raw foodism affects one's conscious experience of the world.[977]

This claim, potentially hyperbolic, and perhaps made out of an excess of emotion, was confounded by his description, in the same interview, that the choline and phosphorus he was now getting from cooked egg yolks is incredibly important, a "critical nutrient" for our brain health and spirituality.[978]

Nevertheless, Monarch clings to New Testament assurances that, ultimately, food is amoral in regard to spiritual salvation. "God said, 'I will not judge you on the food you eat and so you shouldn't either,' he told viewers. "Those are pretty strong words," he continued, "and they're there for a freaking reason," he warned.[979]

---

[976] Matt Monarch. "23 Year Ex-Raw Vegan Comes out about Raw Vegan Diet." *YouTube*, 26 Sept. 2023, www.youtube.com/watch?v=_H2Ppcv1HUU. Accessed 15 Apr. 2025.

[977] Ibid.

[978] Ibid.

[979] Ibid.

There are indeed numerous verses in the New Testament stipulating that what you eat, contrary to the laws of the Old Testament, does not make one "unclean" or imperil their salvation.

One can interpret a laissez-faire attitude toward food in Mathew 6:25, which says "do not worry about your life, what you will eat or drink; or about your body, what you will wear. Is not life more than food, and the body more than clothes?" In chapter seven of the Gospel of Mark, Jesus drives home the point of food being amoral: "Nothing outside a person can defile them by going into them. Rather, it is what comes out of a person that defiles them." Words, thoughts, and actions are sinful, not the food you ingest. A few verses later, he states that food "doesn't go into their heart but into their stomach, and then out of the body."

The apostle Paul also rejects any spiritual importance of earthly food. In 1 Corinthians 8:8, Paul states, "But food does not bring us near to God; we are no worse if we do not eat, and no better if we do." In Romans 14:3, Paul stipulates that God accepts us regardless of what we eat. "The one who eats everything must not treat with contempt the one who does not, and the one who does not eat everything must not judge the one who does, for God has accepted them."

Other raw foodist Christians like Tonya Zavasta point out that while food doesn't imperil spiritual salvation, it certainly matters to our earthly lives. In support of her view, Paul points out in 1 Corinthians 10:23 that when it comes to food, "'I have the right to do anything,' you say—but not everything is beneficial. 'I have the right to do anything'—but not everything is constructive."

Matt Monarch would agree that food does matter to our physical health but he gave up the belief that raw food is a key to spiritual empowerment. In his story, we see a rare example of a raw foodist giving up on the idea that his way of life was the path to personal empowerment and near-perfect health. Monarch had instead found that Christ, not eating raw, was the path to flourishing.

21.
The Spirituality of Modern Christian Raw Foodism

Obviously, most Christians are not raw foodists. Why would they be, since the vast majority of humanity eats cooked food? Nevertheless, there are a number of fervent Christian figures in the twentieth and twenty-first centuries, in addition to Tonya Zavasta, who have advocated for uncooked diets. But these raw foodist Christians are certainly rare. Despite their small numbers, these raw Christians, in trying to convince other believers to adopt a raw diet, have argued their way of life by utilizing Biblical scripture in unique ways.

BOB MCCAULEY AND CHRISTIAN SPIRITUALITY

"I dedicate this book to my Lord Jesus Christ who has taught me everything about life and health."
—Bob McCauley, in his book *Honoring the Temple of God: A Christian Health Perspective*

Bob McCauley was just a normal Midwestern American guy, who grew up on the so-called standard American diet (the SAD diet) of the twentieth century—plenty of refined grains, cooked food, and meat.[980] As an adult, he worked in the bottled water business before he came across the purported healing power of raw food, ionized water, and algal superfoods like chlorella and spirulina. These discoveries sent him on a path to become an author, master herbalist, naturopathic physician, and evangelist of raw foodism from a Christian perspective.

As a devout Roman Catholic, McCauley sees avoiding cooked foods as a way to honor God. Coincidentally, he reads many references

---

[980] Bob McCauley ND. *God's Path to Disease-Free Living.* WestBow Press, 7 Apr. 2017.

to health in Scripture, some explicit and others subtle and metaphorical. The Bible, McCauley feels, "may be viewed and understood from a perspective that stands apart from traditional interpretation."[981] He admits that many Christians have never considered his unorthodox interpretations of Scripture and the prism through which he reads.[982] Nevertheless, he "counts [himself] amongst the chosen whom God has blessed with this knowledge of health" and is determined to spread his message to fellow Christians who have never encountered his viewpoint.[983]

"The mystery that has been kept hidden for ages and generations," McCauley quotes Colossians 1:26, "but is now disclosed to the Lord's people."[984] Believing this line to be inclusive of dietary prophecy, McCauley hopes to play a role in bringing the nutritional truth to God's church.

McCauley sees physiological references peppered throughout Scripture. References to water and fasting throughout the Bible are no accident and contain profound meaning in relation to our bodies. "Water is referred to 617 times in the Bible, making it the most prevalent substance mentioned in it."[985] Bathing and water purification rituals in Scripture symbolize the fact that "every organ in the body heavily depends on water to function . . . The brain is 85% water, bones 35% water, blood 83% water," McCauley claims.[986] He also believes that the "living water" that Jesus refers to, which is usually interpreted as spiritual sustenance, symbolic of eternal communion with God, is a literal reference to "ionized water"—water with "an abundance of electrons" that raw foods also contain.[987]

Along the same line of interpretation, it is no mistake that God states in Genesis 1:29: "I give you every seed-bearing plant . . . and every tree that has fruit with seed in it. They will be yours for food." Verses like these signify that raw vegan foods comprise the original blueprint for a human diet, as laid down in the garden of Eden. "Nowhere in the Bible does it instruct us to eat cooked foods," McCauley argues.

"I give every green plant for food," God says—so eat vegetables and even algae, McCauley instructs, like chlorella and spirulina, which

---

[981] McCauley, Bob. *Honoring the Temple of God—a Christian Health Perspective.* SE, Inc, 5 June 2008, 4.
[982] Ibid., 4.
[983] Ibid., 5.
[984] Ibid., 6.
[985] Ibid., 25.
[986] Ibid., 24.
[987] Ibid., 25.

McCauley calls God's most powerful whole foods because of their richness in vitamins, minerals, proteins, and fats. [988] McCauley believes that the virtues of foods like these are hinted at throughout Scripture. Why else would God show us, like he did in the Book of Daniel, that a diet of vegetables and water brings good health and makes the skin glow?

The Body as a Temple

"Therefore honor God with your bodies."
—1 Cor. 6:20, as quoted by Bob McCauley

The foundation of McCauley's dietetics is his belief, as stipulated by Scripture, that the human body is a "temple of God."[989] The "next revolution in Christianity," he declares, is to understand that "our body literally is a temple of God. And it is a far more important temple than one built of wood, steel, and brick."[990]

Since the Bible commands us to honor our temples, McCauley emphasizes the instruction as a critical but overlooked part of being a Christian. "We cannot go on sinning, doing that which is shameful, and expect to have a meaningful relationship with God," he argues. "Shameful" dietary habits make our temples "full of toxins and pollutants." If we dishonor the temple He has given us, it's said, then we cannot truly honor God. If you want a relationship with God, you'd better get your nutrition in order because you are literally a temple through which God is worshiped. This most holy temple of flesh ought to be respected and "it is incumbent upon Christians to set the example of how God expects us to act and lead our lives, including what we should eat," McCauley explains.[991]

Adopting a raw diet is the most important method of keeping your temple clean. McCauley tells his readers that if they adopt his health protocol "even to the slightest degree," it will "help bring you closer to God. That I promise you."[992] A healthy body, like a properly constructed traditional temple, is the "physical foundation that a meaningful spiritual life can be built upon."[993] Once again, we see

---

988   Ibid., 56.
989   Ibid., 4.
990   Ibid., 6.
991   Ibid., 16.
992   Ibid., 6.
993   Ibid., 13.

biology posited as the starting point for spirituality. The physical place of worship, whether made of stone or flesh, is the vessel through which we perceive God, so we should dutifully make it one of good quality.

What gives McCauley the idea that our bodies are temples? Jesus, for one, referred to his body as a temple. "Destroy this temple. I will raise it up again in three days," John 2:19 has Jesus saying, in reference to his resurrection after death. Scripture explicitly verifies this interpretation: "The temple he had spoken of was his body."

After Jesus's resurrection, McCauley points out, there are other references to the body as a temple. 2 Corinthians 6:16 says, "For we are the temple of the living God." 1 Corinthians 6:19 states, "Do you not know that your bodies are temples of the Holy Spirit, who is in you, whom you have received from God? You are not your own."

Because we are temples built to worship God, and we are "not our own" we must, in McCauley's words, "control our appetites for the foods and tastes we crave, . . . not for ourselves, but for God and the glorification of his temple, our body."[994] Health is not primarily for our selfish benefit. To practice healthy habits is a way of glorifying our Creator by worshipful discipline. 1 Corinthians 6:20 says, after all, "Therefore, honor God with your bodies." Sometimes, these verses are interpreted as referencing sexual morality but in McCauley's world, nutrition is primary.

Overcoming the World: Cooked Food and Temptation

"Like all God demands of us, this is a more difficult, but rewarding path."
—**Bob McCauley**

"The choice we always face is whether to follow God's way or that of worldliness."
—**Bob McCauley**

We see, in McCauley, another echo of the Desert Fathers' struggle against worldly temptations. What's different about McCauley's struggle is that it is aimed at achieving physical health in addition to the traditional Desert Fathers' aim of demonstrating dedication to God. Unlike the weakened, emaciated, self-chastised bodies of elite raw foodist desert monks, the new Christian raw foodist seeks to in-

---

[994] Ibid., 14.

spire people to have a "physically strong, energetic [bodily] temple" to "honor God."[995] To be disease-free and fit is seen by McCauley as the earthly portion of the "eternal prize" for which the apostle Paul urged all Christian "athletes" to "run with purpose in every step."[996]

To practice right healthy habits "is what is expected from each of us as Christians," McCauley says.[997] Every day we face moral choices, and dietary choices are indeed moral, he stipulates.[998]

Early in life, McCauley let the media and the medical establishment dictate his beliefs about health.[999] He had faith in the world, not in God. He found hope in the new drugs that were constantly being developed. "In short, I believed in the medical establishment. I believed in man," he says.[1000]

Now, there's a clear dichotomy constructed in McCauley's thinking—man vs. nature; the ways of the world vs. God. He used to put his faith in man but since seeing the medicinal power of raw food, he has entrusted his faith in the perfection of God's creation (nature) and the food it produces. Faith in man is false; "man will never invent cures to the wrath of diseases we are prone to," he believes.[1001] Only the perfection of nature, exemplified in raw foods, allows the human body to be fully free from disease.

Christians must not place their faith in humankind. To prove their faith in God, they should overcome the worldly ungodliness of dietary social pressure. "Will you wilt under the pressures of friends and family to eat the way everyone else does?" McCauley asks readers. "Or will you shun the world, follow God's path to true health and prosper in your enhanced relationship with him?"[1002] The dichotomy is clear. According to McCauley and his forebears like Paul and the Desert Fathers, a Christian must decide between the way of God and the tempting customs of the world—in McCauley's mind, the "comfortable lifestyle" of socially acceptable cooked foods or the pious discipline of consuming only raw foods.

To be a "true" Christian, you need to be "a bit of a maverick," McCauley explains. "If you are not a maverick somewhere in your life," he tells readers—if you do not separate yourself from the pack and the ways of the world—then "you are not passionate about your Christian

---

[995]   Ibid., 73.
[996]   1 Cor. 9:25–27
[997]   Ibid., 73.
[998]   Ibid., 78.
[999]   Ibid., 7.
[1000]   Ibid., 8.
[1001]   Ibid. 8.
[1002]   Ibid., 15.

faith because to be Christian is to be different from the world."[1003] As the apostle Paul wrote, "Do not conform to the pattern of this world." Having the fortitude to "reject social norms" is a sign of one's dedication to Christian beliefs. And being a raw foodist is a perfect way, even perhaps one of the most important ways to prove one's Christian dedication. "When challenged by others," McCauley encourages, when provoked by cooked food, "know that you are the one honoring God's sacred vessel, your body," so that you can stick to the raw.[1004]

Defeating Sin
and Being Nutritionally Born Again

"When I discovered the truth about health, it was as though scales fell from my eyes the way they did from the apostle Paul's when the Lord revealed Himself to him," McCauley says of his nutritional conversion. Through the prism of health, through a dedication to raw food, "I have learned to put my faith in God only," says McCauley. This physiological shift in perspective is cast in religious terms: "Now, I no longer live in the darkness of ignorance. I have stepped into the light."[1005]

The "light" that McCauley refers to is the knowledge of how God designed the human body to thrive. The truth is that if we follow God's "rules," we'll have perfect health. And eating raw plants is the fulfillment of these rules. When we eat cooked food, McCauley holds, we are following the wicked ways of the world and rejecting God's path.

Eating raw foods signifies that "we have followed God's simple rules for properly maintaining His temple." These are "protocols that are intrinsic in nature . . . created by God and therefore is a reflection of Him," McCauley explains.[1006] By embracing nature, we embrace God.

We must not build our temples according to our carnal desires or the unthinking customs of the world. Cooked food that immediately pleases the tastebuds or nostalgic fondness for childhood comfort foods like chicken noodle soup veer us from the godly path. We must maintain; we must keep our temple standing by avoiding cooked food, which threatens the "light" and "signature of God" that are apparent "when our temple shines brilliantly and is disease-free because we have followed God's health protocol."[1007]

[1003]   Ibid., 60.

[1004]   Ibid., 63.

[1005]   Ibid., 8.

[1006]   Ibid. 12.

[1007]   Ibid., 13.

Forsaking selfish pleasure, we should instead eat primarily as an act of worship. "Our days should be built around God. The same should be true of our diet," McCauley says.[1008] We must consider what is best for our temple and overcome "gratifying the cravings of our sinful nature" that Ephesians 2:3 warns against.[1009] "We must revolt against our carnal appetites and addictions. We must revolt against the foods we eat because we like the way they taste," McCauley warns.[1010]

McCauley applies a dietary interpretation to Romans 8:13, which states, "For if you live according to the sinful nature, you will die; but if by the Spirit you put to death the misdeeds of the body, you will live." These sinful desires are the desires for junk food and cooked food. And the Christian must overcome these desires to properly care for the temple and stay alive for all of a natural lifespan. "Those controlled by the sinful nature," like a lust for cooked food, "cannot please God," Romans 8:8 says, and Bob McCauley interprets.

If you've forsaken living foods and if your body is unhealthy, it is a sign of your impiety. Put starkly, "disease is a symptom of not honoring what God has given us. A diseased body is a testament to our transgressions against God's temple," McCauley claims.[1011] You've failed in your caretaking of the holy temple and have wantonly sinned, thus disease takes hold. "There is no excuse for a Christian not to look healthy," he continues, adding an aesthetic spin to this health quest.[1012] It's a Christian's duty, to show that he is not purposely engaging in sin, to eat raw and look fit.

McCauley's stance is crystal clear: "Triumph over disease is essentially no different than triumph over sin because it is a triumph over temptation."[1013] Disease, in this view, results from falling into cooked temptation. Your dietary habits have deep spiritual meaning and reflect the state of your soul and whether you are winning or losing the battle against sin.

And the physical consequences of failing after being tempted are clear as well. When you succumb to eating cooked food, you succumb to sin and then disease. "Disease *always* resides in the body of the cooked foodist whether the symptoms have surfaced or not," McCauley says.[1014] There's no getting around it, cooked food is never permissible and it sickens body and soul.

[1008]   Ibid.,. 14.

[1009]   Ibid., 15.

[1010]   Ibid., 63.

[1011]   Ibid., 21.

[1012]   Ibid., 22.

[1013]   Ibid.

[1014]   Ibid., 65.

Despite his own victory over dietary sin, there is a hint of melancholy in McCauley's description of the battle against cooked food: "It is difficult to remain loyal to God and follow His path into the light of truth, health, and cleanliness," he warns. "I would be lying," he admits, if he told readers that this path is easy to follow. "I struggle every day," he says.[1015] McCauley has evidently never vanquished his lust for cooked food, yet he remains dedicated to serving God and keeping his temple raw. Just as it is difficult to not cheat on a spouse, it is difficult to avoid the gnawing desire for cooked food. "But with God, everything is possible," McCauley hopes.[1016]

God's Creation, Nature, Is Perfect.

*"When I look at a plate of living foods I see God's creation.
I see the reflection of God. I see a miracle."*
—**Bob McCauley**

*"Unfortunately, what is normal and natural is now
considered 'alternative' and the alternative to what is
natural, i.e. medical science, is considered mainstream."*
—**Bob McCauley**

McCauley's health protocol "advocates nature in its purest form, which only God is capable of creating."[1017]

"The further we get from nature," he admonishes, "the further we get from God." Nature "is a reflection of God" since it was created by God.[1018] And raw living foods are God's natural nourishment, perfectly designed for us. Cooked foods signify death. "Life cannot come from dead things. Only life begets life," warns McCauley.[1019]

God grows fruits and vegetables, which we are meant to eat unadulterated, while humans created the dreadful frying pan. Humans have corrupted the true nature of foods: "destroyed by man and his invention called cooking."[1020]

"God's temple can only be properly served and maintained by the living foods that are part of God's creation, that which we call na-

---

[1015] Ibid., 22–23.

[1016] Ibid., 23.

[1017] Ibid., 24.

[1018] Ibid., 17.

[1019] Ibid., 57.

[1020] Ibid.

ture."[1021] Without living foods, our temples become filthy. Our "living temple" requires "living foods." Ezekiel 47:12 puts it clearly, after all: "Their fruit will serve for food and their leaves for healing," a fitting description for a modern raw vegan diet.[1022] The Christian who actually pays attention when reading scripture will acknowledge verses like these as pertinent instructions for eating.

In McCauley's mind, the healing power of living foods comes from their delivery of sunlight energy into the body (similar to Bircher-Benner's theory), their enzymes, their electron content that helps fight free radical damage in the body. But ultimately, it is McCauley's belief that nature is in a sense perfect, which convinces him that raw plant foods are the best food imaginable because they were perfectly designed by our Creator.

Unnatural attempts at health that disrespect nature's magnificence will fail to sustain our temples. "Everything man creates to make himself healthy will end in failure."[1023] Only the supernatural perfection of nature can cleanse the sins, those "offenses against our temple" like "potato chips, donuts, soft drinks." Artificial corrective therapies like pharmaceuticals can never uphold the temple, they will always come with shortfalls and destructive side effects.

"If we are to assume that God is perfect, then His creation called our temple must also be perfect, including its ability to cure itself of any disease," McCauley argues plainly.[1024] Contrary to what the world inculcates us to believe, the body is perfectly designed to thrive when it eats only living foods. It's an impious assumption, an insult to God, to think that "the body is a flawed vehicle" and randomly vulnerable to disease and only man's artificial medicines can save it. "If provided with the right materials, the body operates perfectly and the medical establishment instantly becomes obsolete," claims the raw foodist.[1025] Everything goes perfectly if we embrace the pious belief that raw foods, God's foods, will keep us well. You need only to "place yourself at His mercy and begin putting the right foods in your body" in order to heal. Each morsel of raw food will make you stronger, he claims.[1026]

In comparing a raw food lifestyle to accepting Christ as the savior, McCauley admits that fully committing to living foods will "take time," similarly to how "you do not immediately stop sinning" when

---

[1021]   Ibid., 17.

[1022]   Ibid., 84.

[1023]   Ibid., 18.

[1024]   Ibid., 21.

[1025]   Ibid., 65.

[1026]   Ibid., 79.

you become a Christian. As you grow closer to God, you eat his food and you learn to savor it. Man's cooked food "inventions" gradually become less meaningful. As your relationship with God becomes deeper, your nutrition becomes purer. We move deeper into faith and leave fear behind—the fear that leads us to believe that "artificial treatments" can save our bodies more than "God's creation."[1027] This fear "feeds on the absence of God in our lives." We must drop this fear, embrace living foods, and take up faith in nature's Creator, for God feeds the birds who trust in their creator and don't even use technology.[1028] And He feeds them with perfect food.

Nature, diet, and one's faith are all intertwined in this raw food Christian creed. By embracing the correct theological beliefs and habits in relation to uncooked food, the Christian gains power over the destiny of his body and puts his soul more in line with God's truth.

George Malkmus

> *"Now, some Christians may question my emphasis on the 'body.'"*
> —**George H. Malkmus**

> *"Beloved, I wish above all things that thou*
> *mayest prosper and be in health."*
> —**3 John 2, as quoted by Malkmus**

"There are literally thousands of ministers helping to prepare people to die. But how many are teaching people how to live?" Pastor George Malkmus asked in his 1989 book *Why Christians Get Sick*.[1029]

To show people how to live, Malkmus bought a fifty-acre piece of land in Tennessee, "where there is pure air, chemical free soil, abundant springs, peaceful surroundings, organic gardens and orchards"—a "place where the beauty of God's creation is so abundantly evident"—a place he called Hallelujah Acres. In this modern Garden of Eden, Malkmus believed that God's natural ways for healing and health would reach Christians around the world.[1030] Christian leaders, he envisioned, would come and learn how to grow and serve raw plant foods to optimally nourish their faithful flock.

[1027] Ibid., 83.

[1028] Ibid., 82.

[1029] Malkmus, George H. *Why Christians Get Sick*. 1995. Treasure House Edition ed., Shippensburg, PA, Treasure House, 1997. 120.

[1030] Ibid., 122.

By middle age, Malkmus had transformed into a raw food advocate, dedicated to converting fellow Christians to a way of life that honored, instead of abused, the bodies God gave them.

He was by no means a raw foodist before this. But a slew of deaths within the ministerial community had tortured his conscience for a number of years. Year after year, he saw missionaries and pastors at the height of their influence, get diagnosed with life-threatening illnesses. Whole congregations and brotherhoods would offer up fruitless prayers for the healing of these diseased Christian leaders and, depressingly, they would not be healed. Many of them died shortly after their dreadful diagnoses.

How could so many Christian devotees' prayers from all over the world not save the lives of God's most effective servants? Theologically and emotionally, Malkmus was tortured by this unanswered question. As a minister, he felt powerless and embarrassed in his inability to provide any plausible explanation. His sense of powerlessness festered as he ruminated on the problem. Could it be, he asked, that the deaths of effective and dutiful ministers was "the will of God?"[1031] This confusing mystery intensified when, as his own ministry was reaching a pinnacle, Malkmus was given a colon cancer diagnosis at age forty-two.[1032]

He decided not to go the painful route of conventional radiation, chemotherapy, and surgery that he had seen his mother endure. He instead attended classes at a nutritional institute. Physical healing started to take hold and a spiritual epiphany followed. He noticed that "openly agnostic" people were experiencing "truly miraculous healing"—"non-Christians [were] getting well without prayer."[1033] Malkmus realized that God's law, natural law, was impersonal. If you followed it, you healed. If you didn't, you got sick and stayed sick until death—regardless of prayers offered, or the beliefs of the petitioner.

Many Christians had, for centuries, blamed every physical and emotional issue on spiritual forces. Sickness was a result of evil spirits, the sins of the ill person, or just God's will. Christians had neglected any responsibility and shunned God's principles for the body. Malkmus himself, for decades, believed sickness was a result of sin, and it troubled him that he was now sick. Had his own sin earned him such punishment?

When his tumor began to shrink, Malkmus believed that he had healed by changing his nutritional habits. He realized through this that all of Christians' health problems "can be eliminated" if "Chris-

---

[1031]   Ibid., 2.

[1032]   Ibid., 5.

[1033]   Ibid., 6.

tians will return to the Bible and observe the natural laws God gave man thousands of years ago!"[1034] He felt a new calling: "May God raise up multitudes of Christian warriors to expose this scourge," he proclaimed. In the tradition of Jesus's healings, his followers should help the fight against the plague of degenerative disease—the "unnecessary loss of millions of lives to heart disease, cancer, stroke, diabetes."[1035]

There is "not one" book, Malkmus realized in horror, that explains that tells us what God's Word has to say about health. Only New Age heresy was pointing people in the right direction, health-wise. Malkmus set out to write an authoritative Christian response to the ideologically treacherous world of "pantheistic 'Holistic Health'" and the "New Age movement."[1036] People shouldn't have to turn to false gospels to "be energetic, productive, and happy" he thought, because the Bible tells us how.

He set out, targeting a Christian audience, to materialize the Biblical idea of God as a healer and agent of human thriving articulated by Psalm 103:1-5: "Bless the Lord . . . who healeth all thy diseases; who redeemeth thy life from destruction . . . so that thy youth is renewed like the eagles."

The Bible as a Guide to the Body

"I have set before you life and death . . . therefore choose life."
—Deut. 30:19, as quoted by Malkmus

Malkmus was set on empowering Christians to become invulnerable to the seemingly random destruction of their health. If the Bible was truly the inspired "Word of God," then "all that men needed to know in order to live a healthy . . . life" had to be found within its pages, he felt.[1037] Malkmus had given up the "fatalistic" viewpoint of many Christians that physical problems were simply the "will of God" or the result of sin and not influenced by diet or lifestyle. "Let's stop blaming God for things we don't understand!" Malkmus proclaimed.[1038]

As it is written in the Bible, "Know ye not that ye are the temple of God? If any man defiles the temple of God, him shall God destroy."[1039]

[1034] Ibid., xi.
[1035] Ibid., xii.
[1036] Ibid.
[1037] Ibid., 9.
[1038] Ibid., 17.
[1039] I Cor. 3:16–18

Malkmus points out that, "If a Christian fails to care properly for his body, God will destroy that Body."[1040] The responsibility rests on the individual.

But one must have knowledge to care for our physical selves properly. Hosea 4:6 states that, "My people are destroyed for lack of knowledge." This lack of knowledge is physically "devastating" for Christians, Malkmus notes. Instead of the cooked-food "traditions of men" that Malkmus believes the Biblical letter to Colossians warns us against, we have to take up Biblical standards—raw standards, so to speak—of physical care. Too many Christians are spiritually but not physically knowledgeable. Genesis 6:13 states that since man had "corrupted God's way upon the earth," they had been destroyed.[1041] The same was happening in modern times, with the food Christians were choosing to eat. Humans were cooking their way to corruption.

Christians should be, Malkmus argues, the healthiest and happiest people on the planet, but many wallow in doom and gloom because of their ignorance of God's hygienic laws. Despite the fact that "the Bible clearly teaches that man is a triune being … comprised of a spirit, soul, and body," Christians ignore the physical side of reality.[1042]

The Bible tells us, Malkmus believes, that "all men [between] Adam and Noah, were vegetarians and fruitarians! On this meatless diet man lived an average of 912 years" without illness.[1043] Doubt it? "Read the first five chapters of Genesis," Malkmus challenges.[1044] "Meat was not consumed for over 1,000 years after creation!," until humans did so briefly out of necessity because "all vegetation had been destroyed by water" of the great flood. Man's life was shortened to 120 years and even to 70 years after. "Genesis Chapter Eleven shows this rapid decline in life span very vividly," Malkmus claims.[1045]

Before the disastrous decline in longevity and quality of life, "Food was eaten in its whole, natural, living, raw state."[1046] Before the disastrous sin-caused worldwide flood, "Man's original diet consisted of: raw vegetables, raw fruits, uncooked seeds, grains, and nuts," Malkmus claims.[1047]

[1040]   Malkmus, 20.
[1041]   Ibid., 23.
[1042]   Ibid., 88.
[1043]   Ibid., 93.
[1044]   Ibid., 92.
[1045]   Ibid., 93.
[1046]   Ibid.
[1047]   Ibid., 94.

Interestingly, though, Malkmus was not a raw food absolutist in his advocacy. He mentioned in speeches and writings that he'll concede the still-effective healing efficacy of a 85% raw food diet.[1048] Steamed veggies, legumes, and grains could be included to make up roughly 15% of the diet. Having a little bit of cooked food in the diet made it easier, he found, to placate followers of the regimen who found it too difficult to adhere to a 100% raw food diet.[1049]

Because raw nutrition kept people perfectly healthy, for hundreds of years of their lives, in Malkmus's opinion, we should doubt the sometimes-harmful modern medical interventions. "It is an outrage when Christians follow [the medical establishment's] pernicious teachings and allow them to drug, burn, and mutilate the bodies of Christians! Bodies that are the Temples of God."[1050] It's a travesty when sick Christians give in to unnecessary treatments that are destructive to their sacred temple-bodies because the cure of raw food is always available to them. "There is only one way to deal with our physical bodies, 'God's Temple,' and that is God's Way! His Ways are perfect!" declares Malkmus.[1051]

Malkmus witnessed his own mother's painful death, brought on not primarily from colon cancer, he believed, but because of the aggressive radiation, chemotherapy, and surgical treatments she was subjected to. When patients are predictably battered or even die while undergoing medical treatment, it would be good to remember, says Malkmus, that the "medical profession's failures are not necessarily 'God's will'" as the ignorant believe.[1052]

Personal Responsibility and Natural Law

Christians, sadly, ignore the physical side of life almost completely until they give themselves over to the medical establishment when illness strikes. "Most Christians," Malkmus says, "are more concerned with the brand and grade of gasoline they put into their automobiles" than the quality of food they put into their bodies.[1053] If they would only return to God's original plan, eat raw, and experience all the diet's

---

1048   Timothy Holt. "Hallelujah Diet with Reverend George Malkmus." *YouTube*, 16 Feb. 2013, www.youtube.com/watch?v=GrNW1lS96pQ. Accessed 7 Apr. 2025.

1049   Malkmus, George. *Back to the Garden*, vol. 11, no. 1, Spring 2001, Hallelujah Acres. 111

1050   Ibid., 112.

1051   Ibid., 117.

1052   Ibid., 113.

1053   Ibid., 35.

healing effects. Malkmus elaborated that the diet could help allergies disappear, eyesight improve, blood pressure drop, body odor evaporate. Their lives would be so much better improved as well as their service to God. Malkmus argues, quoting 1 Thessalonians 5:23, that their "whole spirit and soul and body be preserved blameless."[1054]

He pleaded with Christians to stop blaming "God's will" for physical problems and instead recognize "personal responsibility" and "natural law."[1055] Violation of natural laws will result in sickness, "whether the violator realized the law existed or not; whether the violator was a Christian or not," Malkmus pointed out.[1056] The universal rules of rawness are applied equally and amorally. "God maketh his sun to rise on the evil and on the good," Mathew 5:45 says. The good news in all of this is that Christians could now have more power in their own lives, as they would be able to clearly decipher cause and effect in relation to their health.

References to natural law was plainly visible in the Bible and Malkmus believed people could see it if they gave up their superstitious and ignorant presumptions but many people have trouble accepting personal responsibility for their habits. They should remember Galatians 6:7 which states, ."..God is not mocked; for whatsoever a man soweth, that shall he also reap." Malkmus pleaded for a more Enlightenment-era mindset as opposed to what might be considered a Dark Ages one. God had warned humans about cause and effect but that warning had been mocked. Modern Christians, ironically medieval-minded, still believed that things happened randomly.

Christians will be held responsible for the cooked food, fast food, synthetic pesticides, alcohol, and the coffee they consume. On Malkmus's regimen, even tea is not allowed. The caffeine from green tea has "poisoning effects on the body," he believed.[1057]

Malkmus also taught that emotions are deeply linked to our physicality: "I found that as my body responded physically . . . my emotions became more positive," he recalled.[1058] Many Christians have emotional problems because they are physical wrecks who are unwittingly mocking God with their eating and living habits, he felt.[1059] What you eat, he pointed out, as did many New Agers, affects your spirituality.

[1054]   Ibid., 88.
[1055]   Ibid., 80-82.
[1056]   Ibid., 80.
[1057]   Ibid., 51.
[1058]   Ibid., 71.
[1059]   Ibid., 72.

Malkmus reminded followers that their lifestyles should also attune to the original Edenic life rhythm as well. Before Adam and Eve's fall, stress was not an issue. They "had a slow-paced life with few pressures and lots of physical activity."[1060] Exposure to sunlight was also part of a godly hygiene program.

Through knowledge of God's laws and the habits of a raw food lifestyle, Christians could reclaim some power over their destiny.

Legacy of "Hallelujah Acres"

After its inception in the early nineties, Hallelujah Acres expanded from its initial agriculture project, small café, and health food store to train over 10,000 "Health Ministers" across the U.S. and forty-eight other countries.[1061] Its flagship product, BarleyMax, introduced in 2002, became a commercial hit, shipping to 139 countries.[1062] Hallelujah Acres also established Lifestyle Centers, where it offered hands-on training in the diet and lifestyle.

Malkmus's project told of thousands of people who wrote to it, over the years, reporting recovery from conditions like cancer, arthritis, diabetes, and obesity as a result of adopting the diet. Many of these letters were written after a 1990s appearance on famous televangelist Pat Robertson's *700 Club* boosted Hallelujah Acres' visibility.[1063]

George's Passing

One day in 2023, Malkmus, age eighty-nine, walked outside his home to check his sprinklers. After leaning over, he unfortunately fell awkwardly on the concrete, broke his shoulder, and suffered a concussion.[1064] Despite the fact that doctors and staff at a hospital "marveled" at his general health, he passed away shortly after his release from the hospital, perhaps as a result of concussion complications.

[1060] Ibid., 98.

[1061] "Health Minister Training Online—Now Available!" *Hallelujah Diet*, 28 Apr. 2012, myhdiet.com/blogs/healthnews/health-minister-training-online-now-available. Accessed 7 Apr. 2025.

[1062] "Hallelujah Acres History — 1997-2001." *Hallelujah Diet*, 31 Jan. 2012, myhdiet.com/blogs/healthnews/hallelujah-acres-history-1997-2001. Accessed 7 Apr. 2025.

[1063] Ibid.

[1064] Ibid.

After a life of religious and dietary ministry, Malkmus was laid to rest, having been one of a few Christ followers trying to reclaim the healing spirit and power of their Messiah through raw foodism.

22.
Christian Anti-Raw Foodism

Our band of earnest and vocal Christian raw food advocates exist as a tiny minority among Christians worldwide. Most haven't even heard of the concept and some ignore the pleas to shun cooked food.

And some Christian voices have spoken out specifically against the dietary theology of Christian raw foodists.

Within American Christianity, the Biblical arguments of raw food Christians have been mocked for being inconsistent with Scripture, and raw foodists have been accused of sanctimoniousness. Theologically and culturally conservative voices, emboldened by scriptural evidence, and the widespread acceptance of cooked and processed food, have justified the Christian consumption of cooked food and even junk food.

DECONSTRUCTING RAW FOODISTS' BIBLICAL INTERPRETATIONS

As raw foodist Tonya Zavasta alluded to in her aesthetics section of this book, American Christians can be defensive about their permissive attitudes toward unhealthy food consumption. She and other raw foodists feel that gluttony, as well as the impious abuse of bodily temples, are the only sins that Christians openly tolerate.

But Christians arguably have scriptural backing for their dietary liberalism. Adherents of Calvinist Protestantism and others who vouch for the absolute authority of Scripture have pointed out that the Old Testament seems to endorse certain cooked foods and, in the New Testament, dietary permissiveness is explicitly granted by the apostle Paul.

A website supporting Calvinist reformed theology points out that all throughout Leviticus, a lot of meat can be seen . . . God calls the smell of cooking meat a 'pleasing aroma.'"[1065] Burnt (cooked) offerings were endorsed by God. Additionally, God gave the priests a share of the sacrifices, implying that God felt cooked meat was good for human consumption.[1066] In the Book of Exodus 12: 8–9, God specifically commands lamb to be roasted, and there are numerous examples of cooked meat being used for sustenance, acts of worship, or given as hospitality for visitors.[1067] "Do not eat the meat raw," God says.

If we only eat raw because it's God's original and natural design, wouldn't we have to give up all technology, including homes, electricity, and clothing, since these things were also not part of the initial experience of humans in the garden? These are among the questions Calvinists ask. These developments are obviously highly artificial, yet they make life more productive and comfortable, along with saving lives. It wouldn't be too appealing to most people to follow such a strict naturalistic way of life

The New Testament also seems to sanctify cooked food. As noted in our discussion of Matt Monarch's Christian dietary views, there's a slew of evidence that Paul condones the consumption of any type of food. In addition, Jesus implies that bread (most likely cooked) and fish are good food for people. He calls them "good gifts" (Matthew 7:9–11). In John 21, Jesus takes part in a meal that includes fish cooked over coals. In Luke 22, Jesus instructs his disciples to prepare a Passover meal, which would've included cooked lamb. Also, Christ also makes clear when addressing the Pharisees' obsession with ritual purity and food rules, that food is amoral: "Nothing outside a person can defile them by going into them."

Scripture gives cooked foodists ammunition in their denunciation of what they perceive to be raw food faddism, New Age heresy, or pharisaical arrogance.

RAW FOODISTS: THE FOOD PHARISEES

"If you like to eat what you like to eat, this means that you are a human being. If you are morally indignant about the food choices of others, this means you are well on the way to becoming a food leftist."
—Doug Wilson[1068]

1065   Matt. "Food Pharisees | Taking Back the Bible from the Raw Food Diet." *Reformed Expressions*, 8 Mar. 2018, reformedexpressions.com/food-pharisees/. Accessed 25 Mar. 2025.
1066   Ibid.
1067   Ibid.
1068   Wilson, Douglas. *Confessions of a Food Catholic.* Moscow, Idaho, Canonpress, 2016,

The Pharisees were a purity-obsessed and legalistic ancient Judean sect, prominent during Jesus's life. The New Testament portrays them negatively as heartless rule followers—Jesus calls them "hypocrites" and "whitewashed tombs," meaning they appear dignified in their self-righteous outward appearance but are spiritually corrupt within.[1069]

Some Christian critics have compared raw foodists to these hated figures. A Calvinist writer warns that they are at risk of becoming "tyrannical do-gooders" who ruthlessly judge those who don't adhere to their unsupported dietary stipulations—their extra-Biblical "standards." "Claiming that a raw food diet is Biblical is wrong at best, tyranny at worst," the man warns.[1070]

Self-righteous raw eaters are at risk of promoting rules that have nothing to do with an authentic dedication to Christ. Like the Pharisees, who dedicated their lives to performative rituals and rules to feel superior to others, raw foodists brandish their pointless rules over others—rules that have nothing to do with godliness. Raw foodists are at risk of worshipping the false god of biological purity while committing the sin of arrogance as well. Doug Wilson, a Reformed Calvinist pastor, conservative both in politics and theology, articulates such an attitude in a reactionary book on food, spitting on concepts like food being "natural" or "organic" that underlie faith in raw foodism. "Christ and His Word are the standard, not nature," Wilson makes clear.[1071] Raw food is certainly not necessary, given that. People who fall for smug dietary fads like such a diet are either leftists, stupid, or both.

Wilson would believe that he has backing for such pronouncements, from the apostle Paul, who allowed that if food is "received with thanksgiving," it is fine to consume, "for everything God created is good."[1072] Do not let anyone judge you by what you eat or drink, Paul says in Colossians 2:16-23 and Romans 14:3. Believably, Doug Wilson is just echoing Paul.

Calvinist pastor John Piper warns that because everything is permitted, there is more moral risk in judging others unnecessarily than in dishonoring God by consuming junk food.[1073] Science, after all, he

---

139.

[1069]   Matt. 23

[1070]   Matt. 2018. "Food Pharisees | Taking Back the Bible from the Raw Food Diet." Reformed Expressions. March 8, 2018. https://reformedexpressions.com/food-pharisees/

[1071]   Wilson, D. (2016). *Confessions of a food Catholic*. Moscow, Idaho: Canonpress, 73.

[1072]   1 Tim. 4:4–5

[1073]   Desiring God. "Does Junk Food Dishonor God?" *YouTube*, 25 Apr. 2019, www.youtube.com/watch?v=MRA0nl4yWSA. Accessed 22 Apr. 2025.

claims, cannot consistently prove what is junk or not. Thus, a certain liberty of consumption is allowed for Christians when it comes to food and drink, unlike other areas of life, like sexuality.

Considering the permissive attitude toward food in the New Testament, some Christians have had fun defending dietary liberalism and have even flirted with approving junk food. In 2018, Doug Wilson was asked about health and faith, and he quipped, "Look, grease is God's gift too—fry up some bacon and quit acting like quinoa's the fifth gospel . . . Bacon is fine. [So is] bacon frying," the smell of which is like a "benediction" wafting through the air. "Refined sugar is fine," he continued.[1074] The most maligned food, the most carnivorous and high temperature-cooked taboo, in the minds of raw foodists (especially raw vegans), are considered as God's blessings by anti-hippie conservative pastors. Cook meat and prove your Christian traditionalism, manliness, and the fact that you won't fall for leftist gimmicks, the likes of Doug Wilson might say.

Numerous pastors have mocked the "idolatry" of self-conscious healthy eating and Doug Wilson's followers have mocked health-conscious Christians, framing junk food as a symbol of rejecting elitist sanctimony like that of the Pharisees. Christian blogs say things like, "God's cool with junk in moderation—don't let it own you."

Food Is Not Spiritual

"For the kingdom of God is not a matter of eating and drinking,
but of righteousness, peace, and joy in the Holy Spirit."
—Rom. 14:17

A common idea, as we've seen, among New Age raw foodists, is that food spiritually affects us. It can raise our spiritual awareness, instill a sense of harmony, improve our moods, even help form our moral values and affect how we treat other people, animals, the earth's ecology, and our own bodies.

Many Christians reject these supposed connections between the body, our diet, and spirituality. Food has no bearing on the spirit, they argue, and pastor Doug Wilson claims that God actually "cares very much that we *don't* care" about the type of food we're eating, its quality, whether something is organic, or the morality of what we eat. If Christians care too much, they might be guilty of "dislocated moralism"—

[1074] Canon Press. "Food Does Not Make You Holy | Doug Wilson." *YouTube*, 2 July 2010, www.youtube.com/watch?v=YoRSn1ec_nI. Accessed 22 Apr. 2025.

making unnecessary moral judgments about things that don't matter and falling into a mindset of false righteousness like the Pharisees of old.[1075]

Wilson argues that caring too much about the quality of your food or the strict adherence to dietary regimens subverts the importance of friendly fellowship with other Christians. If you bring your own food dishes to someone's house and refuse to eat their food, it's an insult that risks creating emotional distance between Christians.[1076] And the food you're bringing is probably just "fruity" hippie crap from some "weird diet," as Wilson might say.[1077]

Too much focus on food distracts from spiritual health and risks worshipping the body—worshipping the "created instead of the Creator" (as the phrase goes). Worshipping anything worldly is still not well regarded in certain Christian circles, similarily as in the time of the Desert Fathers.

It's clear that many Christians dismiss the claims of Christian raw foodists and have nothing in common with New Age beliefs on the connection between diet and spirituality.

According to Christian critics of raw food and dietary strictness, the Bible makes clear that food does not make or break your spiritual life. It does not imperil your salvation. You can eat anything and it should not affect your afterlife and it doesn't even affect your spirit in the here and now. Wanton gluttony, or eating excessively to the extreme, is perhaps the only dietary habit that could be considered a sin.

In summary, some people interpret the New Testament as holding that the type of food we eat is spiritually irrelevant. New Age raw foodists, of course, heartily disagree. All of their talk of food affecting quality of consciousness, energetic vibrational frequency, the chakras, karma, or our ability to harmonize with God and the universe, along with other spiritual attributes, make that clear. For New Age followers, and a few raw foodist Christians, spiritual power is accessed through nature and biology, through the energetic power of uncooked plants. But for most Christians, only the grace of Christ can empower us spiritually.

[1075] Cannon Press. "Organic or Non-Organic? Does God Care? | Doug Wilson." *YouTube*, 13 Mar. 2012, www.youtube.com/watch?v=ikNNOB-3IIo. Accessed 22 Apr. 2025.

[1076] Ibid.

[1077] Wilson, D. (2016). *Confessions of a food Catholic*. Moscow, Idaho: Canonpress, 166.

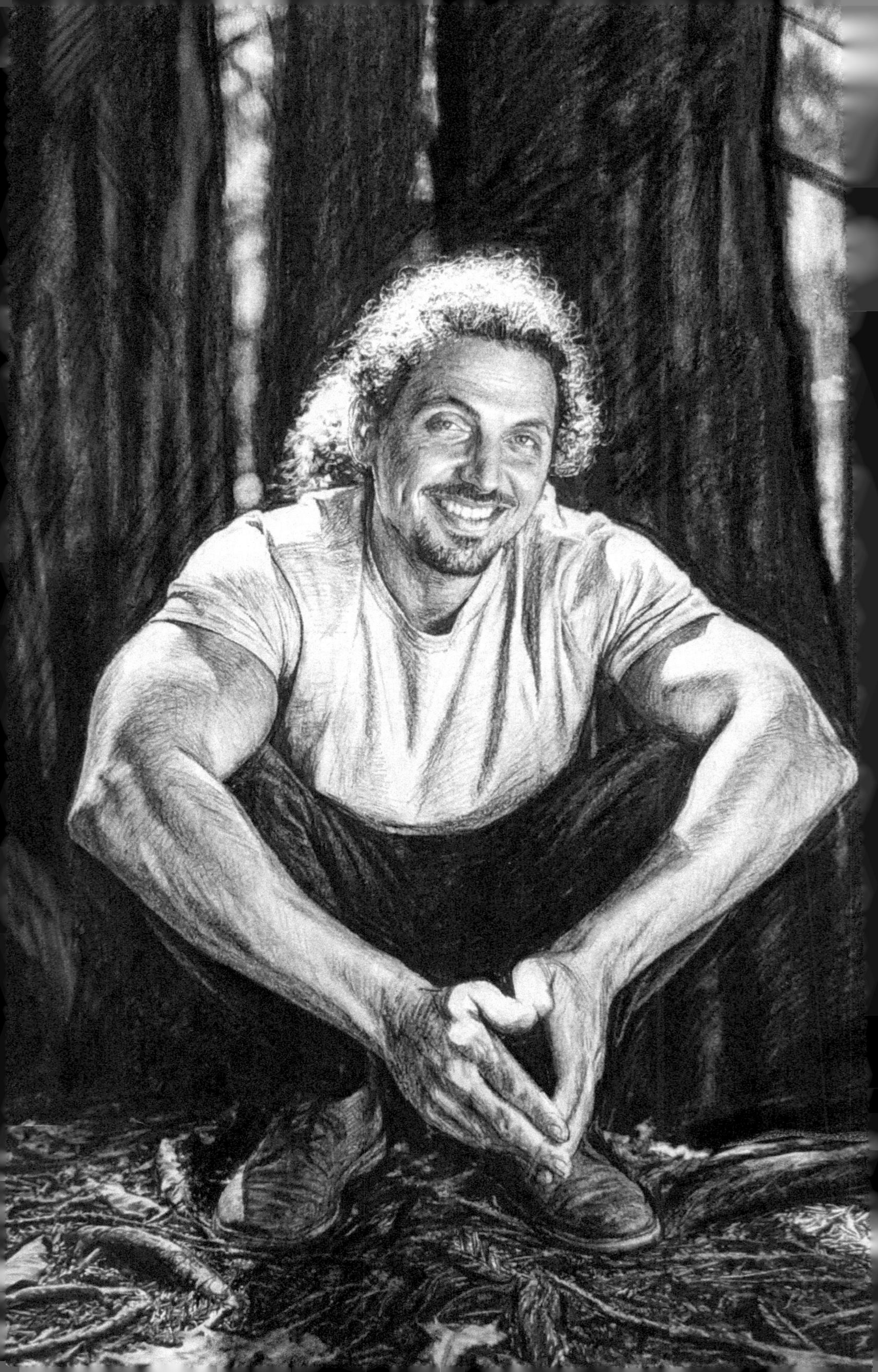

23.
Jesse J. Jacoby: Raw Food, Ecology, and Spirituality

"Mountain peaks . . . being blown to smithereens by dynamite sticks that were planted to feed more of this disease that is greed . . . calcium carbonate tears plaster the boulders that survive beneath, as birds mutter the saddest songs . . . over coal mines that pollute the air and water."
—Jesse J. Jacoby

Jesse Jacoby has a very grounded presence in YouTube interviews. His calm cadence, deep voice, long curly dark brown hair, and a beaded necklace portray an Earth-loving man in touch with traditional indigenous wisdom and New Age belief systems. Considering his tranquil demeanor and hippie vibe in interviews, it might be surprising to learn that he uses fervent war-like poetics to articulate his mission to ecologically defend the Earth and spiritually elevate humanity.

Jacoby, a raw food activist of partial Choctaw heritage, conceives of the Earth as a living being, an entity worthy of reverence and protection. Around this conception of the planet, Jacoby builds his dietary and spiritual beliefs.

The Earth earns a theology of its own, and for him, it is deemed to be "the only noble entity" that deserves our complete "allegiance," echoing Joe Alexander's beliefs on the subject.

Each human's mission, Jacoby argues, is to be a soldier defending the planet that gave humanity its life and nourishment. Tragically, he believes, "humanity has become parasitic to Earth."[1078] By being so ecologically destructive, humans have sucked the life out of the planet and many of its creatures. Western civilization has especially acted as a destructive parasite because it's treated the planet so awfully, Jacoby

---

[1078]   Jacoby, Jesse. *Gaia Speaks*. Soulspire Publishing, 5 Aug. 2019, 19.

argues. Western civilization's toxic anti-Earth mindset needs to transform before it destroys us and our terrestrial Mother.

And crucially, a raw vegan diet plays a central role in saving the planet.

EARTH SPIRIT

Caring for the environment is the highest spiritual calling, according to Jacoby. Ecology, God, and the human spirit are inextricably linked. "There is a hole in God's heart the size of Earth Mama's scars . . . the hurt will always last," he laments of environmental destruction.[1079] His dedication to environmentalism is potently emotional in his writings. The ruination of the Earth is not just a scientific question of CO_2 levels, it's a heart-wrenching tragedy that causes the suffering of billions of sentient animals and even (sentient) trees. When forests are torn down, there are "moral tears" spilled by "bobcats, mountain lions, ravens, and owls" who resided there.[1080] And trees don't just saturate the air with oxygen. "Trees are living creatures with soul. Their sap is blood."[1081] Any cruel human who clear-cuts is engaging in a massacre. At times, his appeals to remedy this unjust ecocide reaches a fever pitch and toys with property destruction: "This is the time to disfigure gas-fueled vehicles. There is no space left for hatred and the evil committed to secure crude oil."[1082] The urgency and stinging tone in Jacoby's screed follows from the importance he assigns to the sacred flora and fauna of the planet.

To heed the urgent call of the suffering of the Earth and put an end to it, we need to address how we eat and think about the world. Jacoby has written numerous books detailing the health benefits of raw foods, but what is most poetic about his work is its environmentalism and spirituality.

[1079]   Ibid., 125.
[1080]   Ibid., 126.
[1081]   Ibid., 191.
[1082]   Ibid., 128.

Raw Food as a Given

Raw vegan food, Jacoby feels, is the starting point for a meaningful life. It's the basis for being physically the way "nature intended" us to be.[1083] Many of the standard arguments for raw food's efficacy are explained in his book *The Raw Cure: Healing Beyond Medicine*. Raw food contains more enzymes and doesn't have harmful cooked compounds like heterocyclic amines, compounds that can damage DNA and are linked to cancer.[1084] Cooked food causes the pancreas to work extra hard to produce enzymes to digest it, and our bodies produce white blood cells and inflammation in response to most cooked foods, he claims.[1085]

But the spiritual effect of raw food is often the focus of his writing. On raw plant foods, we will have more energy, more positive emotions, and our "creative side will have a presence again."[1086] We will have more passion for our interests, a higher IQ, less frustration and hatred, and more of an ability to "express our true selves" than we would on toxic and cooked diets.[1087] The "dead energy" from other food makes you a slave to TV and the "mainstream media"—a passive observer rather than a participant in life.[1088] "Living foods are for living people," Jacoby summarizes. Raw plants are fuel for a vibrant life and a conscious and motivated mind that can initiate positive change in the world.[1089]

Our dietary habits, he argues, form our values and will make or break the planet's culture and ecology. Societal dysfunction, suffering, spiritual disorders, and the resulting environmental destruction occur when we make bad food choices.

[1083]   Ibid., 40.

[1084]   Jacoby, Jesse. *The Raw Cure: Healing beyond Medicine*. Soulspire Publishing, 2012, 38.

[1085]   Ibid., 39.

[1086]   Ibid., 40.

[1087]   Ibid., 25.

[1088]   Jacoby, Jesse. *Gaia Speaks*. Soulspire Publishing, 5 Aug. 2019, 103.

[1089]   Ibid., 104

INDIGENOUS VS. WESTERN PARADIGM

*"I am suffering from a disease called civilization. I keep choking on
plastic that saturates the oceans . . . I was afflicted with a mental illness
called deforestation. I am constipated with indigenous genocide."*
—Jesse J. Jacoby

*"We break free from this American dream that was
the monster hiding under our beds all along."*
—Jesse J. Jacoby

Jacoby is a prime exponent of the New Age movement's rejection of
Western values and embrace of the values of other cultures. One of the
main themes of his raw foodist spirituality is the elevation of "indigenous" values in contrast to pernicious Western principles.

Indigenous values are Earth-centric, Earth-loving, and acknowledge the planet as a sentient spirit and being. Western values, on the
other hand, are primarily anthropocentric, seeing humans as the master of the Earth, the only truly important creature who has an allowance to freely use and abuse the resources of the planet. The Earth,
according to these values, is expendable. Western values promote the
vampiric extraction of economic value from the Earth, without respecting its dignity and health.

Jacoby grew up in a cultural context that was polluted with these
unfortunate values. His childhood in late-twentieth-century Chicago
was "engulfed in a web of lies," he says. " A "police state" coexisted with
the toxic education system that "estranged" him from his Choctaw
ancestral roots. The main philosophy behind what he was taught was
simply a shallow "need to earn money."[1090] His urban neighborhood
was disconnected from nature, which caused all sorts of psychological
problems and prompted people to attempt to "fill this void" with "alcoholism, consumerism, degeneration, fast food, and sports."[1091] It was a
shallow, ignorant, toxic, and gritty mess. It was an unnatural, concrete
America, sick from cooked food.

His early life left him with a bitter taste. Western civilization, he
writes, is synonymous with "anger, arrogance, confusion, depression,
greed, [and] poor health."[1092] The West's English language, widely accepted on a global scale, "drives the agenda which is destroying man-

---

[1090]   Ibid., 9.
[1091]   Ibid., 10.
[1092]   Ibid., 17.

kind and this beautiful planet." English is the language of the world's superpower and the oppressive systems of greed and extraction that flow out of it. The values of English-speaking countries fan the flames of "human greed—a demon who haunts us all," Jacoby says as if he was not immune from this sin.[1093] These values should be consciously rejected: "If we put the dollar aside" and the avarice it represents, he says, and not hold it as the ultimate aim of our existence, we can prioritize the health and happiness of the planet.[1094]

Western society is plagued by "a disease called insatiety"—a virus of the mind and a "destructive spirit driven by excess, greed" that the American Indian Ojibwe tribe called *windigo*.[1095] This insatiety steamrolls the environment and places profit above human health. We must focus on cleaning up the "polluted mess that is known as Western culture," Jacoby says straightforwardly—a pollution that is both ecological and spiritual. We must change priorities and "banish all harmful chemicals" and other forms of environmental destruction like deforestation and fracking that are downstream consequences of the voracious culture.[1096]

In his youth, Jacoby saw many young people under a spiritual and dietary veil of ignorance, being "immersed in gang life" with "their only sources of nourishment . . . from convenience" or liquor stores "on every corner."[1097] It was a culture of "hostility" and intoxication from foods and drugs. The degrading foods and other poisons consumed reinforced degenerate attitudes, including a general anger that pervaded everything. There is a "cultivation of assholism through mechanisms . . . [like] egoic entitlement, nutricide, pharmaceuticals."[1098] Spiritual darkness was chemically-fed.

The epitome of this toxic culture was tragically seen in the life of Jacoby's brother, who, during his teens, underwent "systemic poisoning" and was experimented on by psychiatrists and doctors who force-fed him psychotropic pharmaceuticals. After a long period of mental health decline, his sibling became "a fraction of the beautiful human he was before" and eventually committed suicide by walking in front of a train.[1099]

[1093]   Ibid.,. 17.
[1094]   Ibid., 19.
[1095]   Ibid., 18.
[1096]   Ibid., 19.
[1097]   Ibid., 11.
[1098]   Ibid., 211.
[1099]   Ibid., 12.

Defeating a system that enabled such horrific destruction of human life, that could "castigate the purity and innocence of the human mind" became Jacoby's goal.[1100] The "Western regions," he felt, needed to be cleansed spiritually, physically, and ecologically.

Witnessing such a hellscape prompted Jacoby to seek a better way of life and a natural cure for the civilizational depression that his brother experienced. His insights into a better way of life began in California, during a literal tree-hugging experience. Wrapping his arms partway around enormous Redwood trees and "praying" with them, he discovered "peace within" and a broadening of the imagination. He thought of how such an experience would've uplifted his brother and other victims of Western society. It became clear how vital the role that nature plays in our peace of mind was.[1101]

Jacoby became aware that inundation in natural environments coupled with eating a colorful plant-based diet spiritually "elevated" him. He felt better than ever. He had "extracted a spiritual energy" from the Redwoods and had reconnected to his Choctaw heritage. He had to cleanse out toxic values and reclaim a "culture uninfluenced by Western society."[1102] In this new paradigm he had discovered, he would source his wisdom from "surrendering" his consciousness to nature and absorb the "ethos of the ocean, rivers, trees, and wind."[1103] By surrendering to nature, "we vacate our desire for power . . . we discard struggle, and inherit affluence."[1104] We leave the insidious culture of greed behind. Gratitude soothes us. Harmony and empathy toward all life forms take the place of egoic power struggle, the demand for control, and the lust for power.[1105]

"Native American cultures" had a strong connection with the "Spirit" of the Earth in Jacoby's mind. By reconnecting with his Choctaw heritage, he had found the antidote to the Chicago-style unhealthy American malaise. The spirit of the Earth, which was venerated in Native cultures, was the source of wisdom, of useful "downloads" to the soul.[1106] Saturated with that spirit, Jacoby believed himself to be a "soldier of consciousness" whose mission was to destroy greed and save the planet from future destruction.[1107]

[1100]   Ibid., 27.
[1101]   Ibid., 12.
[1102]   Ibid., 13.
[1103]   Ibid., 19.
[1104]   Ibid., 114.
[1105]   Ibid., 200.
[1106]   Ibid., 18.
[1107]   Ibid., 13.

On this soldierly journey, "spiritual entities" aid his purpose. In Jacoby's description of the supposed supernatural aides that guide raw foodist eco-warriors, we see some similarity with David Wolfe's beliefs. "Ancestral guides, angelic beings," Jacoby claims, "archangels . . . and tribal chiefs"—the allies of nature, provide the conscious warrior with wisdom. Mind-altering plant medicines from Mother Earth are another source of wisdom. All these forces urge Jacoby and others, he says, to "dismantle the powers that suppress us" and help regenerate the planet.[1108]

Plants and Indigenous wisdom are the fuel for the fight. Jacoby admires the sayings of Chief Seattle, an Earth-revering Native American leader who had to deal with the "savageness" of European-American invaders. A famous letter attributed (possibly falsely) to the chief details this ethos. "We are part of the Earth as Earth is part of us," Chief Seattle says.[1109] He pleads with the insatiable Westerners who are usurping Native American land to maintain its ecological "sacredness" and acknowledge humanity's connectivity with the land. Seattle says, "What befalls the earth befalls all the sons of the earth."[1110] Man does not own the Earth, he warns, the Earth owns man—a nearly impossible concept for anthropocentric European settlers to accept. The famous letter says of the white man: "The love of possessions is a disease they are sickened with . . . They claim this mother of ours, Earth, as their own."[1111] Seattle's letter serves as a mythological emblem for Jacoby's aversion to negative Western values.

The Earth-centric perspective is fully embraced by Jacoby. Man was created, he argues, "to coexist," with nature, "find equanimity . . . and improve the planet." Not to "butcher forests . . . [or] poison each other" or cause disease and suffering.[1112] Man is intertwined with the planet and made for harmony with it. As Chief Seattle said, "Whatever [a man]] does to the web [the web of life], he does to himself" and to harm the Earth is to "heap contempt" on the God who created it.

Lakota natives view nature with respect, Jacoby notes, and actually view it as having personhood—they recognize rivers as having the rights of a legal person. Western culture, however, abuses those rights and the land while poisoning our bodies with agro-chemicals. "Great Spirit tells me," Jacoby warns, "the pain will not subside unless we

---

[1108] Ibid., 20.
[1109] Ibid., 31.
[1110] Ibid., 32.
[1111] Ibid., 110.
[1112] Ibid.,. 25.

stop . . . glyphosate ["Roundup"] and pesticides."[1113] Jacoby emphasized the link between Indigenous American values, ecology, and diet.

The Spiritual Values of Raw Foodism

"Your best action is to reclaim your mind . . . out of the
hands of the cultural engineers who want to turn you
into a half-baked moron consuming all this trash being
manufactured out of the bones of a dying world."
—Terrence McKenna, as quoted by Jacoby

In an effort to discard the Western anthropocentric worldview and reclaim an Earth-centric ethos, nutrition cannot be ignored. "We can expand our spirit," Jacoby says, "through our lifestyle, through our diet, through how pure our vessel is." Conversely, our spirit can "shrink and atrophy" from consuming processed and cooked foods. Biology is again at the center of a spiritual power struggle for a raw foodist.

Those who eat in accordance with nature and treat the Earth with respect have overcome the mental conditioning of the profit-seeking engineers of toxic civilization. Spiritual and nutritional liberation go hand in hand. Raw foodists and ecologically aware people have accomplished "free-thinking" as well as the "refusal to be governed . . . to obey orders or commands from tyrants," who are thoroughly corrupted people who are practically beyond remedy, who have "been stripped of all goodness." Spiritually elevated people, especially raw vegans, have escaped the programming from education systems and media that was designed by ecocidal profiteers. They have committed themselves to "love culture"—an ethos that "contributes in no way to the suffering of other forms," other beings.[1114] There is no reason to kill other creatures for food; the spiritual seer is vegan.

Among the corruption and "delusions" of the myopically profit-seeking world, "There are good folks interspersed . . . who know no crime, experience no disease, and are thriving from plant-based purity," Jacoby explains.[1115] In Jacoby's description of those that have spiritually awakened, physical purity and dietary practices meld with mental enlightenment. Most people who are aware of the tainted ecology of the world and the toxic culture that has been devised by "profiteers"

[1113]   Ibid., 142.
[1114]   Ibid., 37.
[1115]   Ibid.

have cleaned up their bodily ecology with the right diet and are thus attuned to the Earth's "frequency" and "spirit."[1116]

Dietary purity is key. To download the right spiritual values from Earth, "no harmful chemicals can be in our sphere." We have to eat organic food with no synthetic agricultural chemicals on it—nor can we partake of "the most erroneous action" of eating the "poison" that is animal flesh.[1117] Equally as clearly, we must eat raw "living foods" to hear the Earth's moral messages because these foods have the "highest radiant frequency" or the highest energetic vibrations.[1118] To have one mind and one set of values in common with the living Earth, we must take in its unadulterated energy in the form of raw organic vegan foods.

When we eat the chemical and cooked crap that the dark forces engineer for us, we embrace unnatural and destructive forms of behavior so prevalent in disordered cultures like that of Jacoby's Chicago upbringing.[1119] We also become "visibly depressed" on "harmful diets" devoid of "raw, organic fruits [and] vegetables."[1120] But after we embrace the "rhythms of Mother Earth" by eating raw and being in nature, we can "revive morality" and generate the constructive values we need to save the planet and be well ourselves.[1121] A nutritional-spiritual whole-being cleansing takes place. Raw food becomes belief and moral habit. "We flush our system from the lies of civilization," and "stop competing for a chance to boost ego" and instead find the authentic self "trapped beneath layers of fears," Jacoby says. Our true soul and our personal talents are "buried" if we eat chemicalized and processed foods—"what corporations manufactured from evil."[1122]

Jacoby says, "When I emancipated myself from the corporate food chain, I was immediately rewarded with a stronger spiritual connection to . . . my higher power."[1123] "Plant medicines," like raw foods as well as plant hallucinogens, "generate love from our souls." With healing plants spiritually building us up, we can banish the "common diseases" of "anger and greed." and find a more perfect harmony.[1124]

[1116] Ibid., 39.

[1117] Ibid., 39.

[1118] Ibid., 40.

[1119] Ibid., 40.

[1120] Ibid., 41.

[1121] Ibid., 44.

[1122] Ibid., 197.

[1123] Ibid., 42.

[1124] Ibid., 74.

In his psychic diet plan, Jacoby doesn't go to the utmost extremes of raw foodist advocacy though. He allows steamed vegetables to be incorporated.[1125] At the least, organic plant foods, free of synthetic chemicals, help to steer the soul in the right direction.

But raw foods are where the true power is, so they should form the base of one's diet. Similar to the theories of Bircher-Benner, Jacoby acknowledges the sun "biophotons" in plant foods. When we eat colorful plants, we absorb the sun's life-giving energy. Jacoby describes the spiritual-nutritional power of the sun in a way that blurs the lines between the corporeal and incorporeal. We can find healing, he claims, by "exposing our flaws and wounds to direct sunlight in moderation." Both by exposing our skin to sunlight and receiving 'sun energy in the organic fruits and vegetables we ingest" we absorb the power to be most fully ourselves. When we take in raw food, it's an act of getting back in touch with this god-like life-giving entity. Most religions, Jacoby notes, have worshipped the sun. It's too bad that humans have become estranged from both the Earth and sun, and we lather our bodies with chemical sunscreen to protect ourselves from this "very essence of life" and treat it as an enemy.[1126] We have severed ourselves from the benevolent forces of the universe, stuffing ourselves with lifeless cooked food and shielding ourselves from the sun and its power in the form of raw plant food. These are signs of being spiritually adrift.

PREDATORY DIETS VS. GAIAN DIETS

> *"Men who cannot abdicate . . . profits, at the expense of the greater good of the planet, are criminals. Their crime is treason to Gaia—the only noble entity we are ever to pledge our allegiance to."*
> **—Jesse J. Jacoby**

> *"We will evolve into organic farms. Our immortal sorrows will feed happiness to the children of tomorrow."*
> **—Jesse J. Jacoby**

The opposite of a conscious plant-based and raw diet is the standard Western diet of the twentieth century—a diet high in refined grains, meat, and processed chemicalized food. This diet feeds the economic, spiritual, and ecological harm of the planet, Jacoby believes.

[1125]   Ibid., 41.
[1126]   Ibid., 72.

He was exposed to this tired old dietary paradigm in his upbringing. "I remember being manipulated," Jacoby recalls, "into believing that I needed to drink cow's milk to strengthen my bones, and that eggs and meat were needed" for protein. Physically, he was being poisoned by a system devoid of "the most vital nutrients—being raw fruits and vegetables."[1127]

Intertwined with the spiritual ravages of Western civilization are its dietary crimes. To expel the "violent force" of insatiable greed, "we are required" to adopt, says Jacoby, a "healthier lifestyle."[1128] If there was widespread adoption of veganism, "the end of violence and wars would soon be inevitable" as people would grow respect for the welfare of other creatures. And human health would be better: "Without meat, dairy, and eggs we would erase all disease," Jacoby claims.[1129]

A mostly raw vegan diet, of course, promotes constructive spiritual values, the apex of which involves protecting the health of the planet, Gaia, which is nearly indistinguishable from God. But to Jacoby, God is a pantheistic presence throughout nature, as opposed to the anthropocentric "Western" Biblical belief that "one man embodied God." Jacoby connects Christianity with misleading Western paradigms and dismisses "the myth of human supremacy" that God would have lived through one human, Jesus.[1130]

To care for the truest godlike entity, Mother Earth, "We begin by cleaning up our diet." By doing so, we "resurrect beauty" in Earth's ecology and in our own physiology instead of "decimation" (disease, corruption). "Gaia is waiting for you," Jacoby rallies readers, for "your health and well-being are interrelated with hers."[1131] Cellular ecology, affected by the food we eat, correlates with planetary ecology. Our individual purchasing and consumption choices help make or break the planet. We either encourage regenerative ecofriendly farming or the destruction of the environment by buying agrochemical foods.

Diseased ecology is the "root of the problem," both physically and spiritually for humans. When we realize that "our soil is sick" and that our "water is poisoned," we should choose dietary habits that not only do not contribute to this disgraceful poisoning of the outer world, but also keep the inner world of the body unpolluted.[1132] Cleaning up our planet is the only way that we can truly eliminate physical disease,

---

[1127] Ibid., 9.

[1128] Ibid., 18.

[1129] Ibid., 17.

[1130] Ibid., 124.

[1131] Ibid., 33.

[1132] Ibid., 35.

Jacoby believes, and the outer environment is analogous to our inner health. "When rivers are damned" for electricity production and thus can't cleanse the pollutants saturating them, "the planet cannot heal," just as "when humans stagnate their lymphatic system with alcohol, animal-based foods, dairy . . . [and] processed foods."[1133]

Pristine ecology and food quality, which are deeply interrelated, spiritually regenerate the world. "The real battle I aim to conquer begins within my own temple," Jacoby says in one of his poems.[1134] "I live as a purist—someone who refuses to allow impurities to enter my terrain."[1135] No synthetic chemicals and hardly any cooked crap is going to sully Jacoby's inner realm. No depressing, heavy energies, or demoralizing pesticides to drag down the mind.

Foods grown by ruthless and expedient corporations for quick profit, at the expense of healthy ecology, create a hellscape. In one of his poems, Jacoby sings a lament about such an abused world: "Orangutan numbers decline . . . We can feel the souls of these animal brothers screaming into our bones, begging us to . . . give up our addiction to flesh foods so we can eradicate factory farms, and stop trading rainforests for cattle ranches and GMO soy, corn, and wheat plantations that feed the livestock."[1136] The big corporate cooked food products we are eating are causing torment in the lives of animals and are hacking down forests.

He poetically pleads for solutions. "We pray [for humans] . . . to stop treating trees as commodities" to be torn down to make room for big agribusiness's chemicalized fields.[1137] "We pray," Jacoby continues, "to universally switch to nut-based milks" to lessen the "trillions of gallons of water annually" used to "sustain the dairy and meat industries."[1138] We can end the suffering of the planet by dumping foods created in predatory contexts like dairy, with cows, in such contexts, being considered imprisoned. Raw nut milk should replace cow's milk in the refrigerator.

Spiritual and mental health are at stake in such choices. Food affects our gut bacteria and whether benevolent or devious strains that affect our mind, thrive in our intestines. Jacoby acknowledges the common scientific parlance of gut bacteria affecting neurotransmitter levels and inflammation in the body but he goes a step further with

---

[1133]   Ibid., 35, 143.
[1134]   Ibid., 14.
[1135]   Ibid., 13.
[1136]   Ibid., 117.
[1137]   Ibid., 118.
[1138]   Ibid., 119.

his claims. "These microbes are conscious beings," he claims. They are "capable of communicating with our brains" and pathogenic bacteria fed by bad foods are "master manipulators" who "drive us to eat food laced with drugs" like non-organic food, meat, cooked junk food. These bacteria are truly malicious and seem to be self-aware in their complicity in evil. They are on a "mission to take over and destroy" our hosting bodies and "also want to destruct this planet."[1139] These hostile entities are ethical extensions of the cruel humans that concoct the toxic food that these bacteria thrive off of; they are symbiotic with the ecocidal profiteers and blind the spiritual senses of the eaters that they infect.

Deranged Food, Deranged Souls

The pernicious practices of greedy agrobusiness destroy people spiritually and serve as metaphors for our disordered inner states. The heavily pesticide and herbicide-doused genetically modified foods are "designed to withstand" a chemical assault but still "yield"—analogous to what big agriculture companies demand weak and demoralized consumers to do.[1140]

Toxified people are the collateral damage of the ruthless profit-seeking system and its noxious crops. Similar to the West's factory-farmed livestock, Westerners are "cultivated to conform to preconditioned" eating habits and follow "artificial life patterns" so as to profit the immoral food businesses.[1141] To them, the synthetic chemicals on our food are "viewed as opportunities for stock values to rise" and they don't care if they destroy people physically and spiritually.[1142]

These chemicals, as well as low quality food, are not just health concerns, They carry spiritual meanings. Glyphosate, known commonly as "Roundup," is the embodiment of "hate for all life" and "gradually poison[s] all life on the planet" by saturating the soil, the foundation of the food chain.[1143]

And our "submission to inherited dietary patterns" is responsible for reduced intelligence and moral values, Jacoby believes.[1144] Bad diet contributes to Westerners being aloof to how much harm their societies are causing to the planet.

[1139] Ibid., 18.

[1140] Ibid., 21.

[1141] Ibid., 22

[1142] Ibid., 24.

[1143] Ibid., 163.

[1144] Ibid., 21.

To fix the causes that underlie our spiritual decay—our ignorance, reduced consciousness, amorality, and depression— we need to eat raw plant foods which can "provide lasting relief from what causes sadness," Jacoby says.[1145] Only "edible plant matter in fresh, raw form" can lift us to our highest "happiness, and intelligence."[1146] From the materialist point of view, Jacoby notes, antioxidants in plants inhibit the breakdown of neurotransmitters in our brain, giving us more feel-good chemicals, and can fight inflammation that can interfere with mood.[1147] And we also need to feed beneficial bacteria in our guts, not the malicious types.

Diet has such a powerful effect on the spirit that it's even possible to heal evil humans (purveyors of environmental destruction). "Their awakening requires several ayahuasca sessions and a transition to a plant-based lifestyle," Jacoby prescribes.[1148]

To be spiritually-aware people, we must be physically pure. "No angelic beings desire attachment to those who ingest evil," Jacoby claims. Spiritual guides flee anyone who consumes meat or toxic foods. "The presence of your higher power in your life broadens and is enriched when you provide a healthy terrain . . .as we continue to ingest impurities, we are driven further from reaching our pure potential as sovereign beings," he continues.[1149] Dietary pollution obscures our spiritual vision and prevents self-empowerment.

The "spirit" of crops grown by big agriculture (soy, corn, glyphosate-soaked wheat, etc.) is "depleted of vitality." These foods pass on their impoverished state to consumers. These are spiritually unsound foods. Enclosed within raw plant food, on the other hand, are spiritual riches. Jacoby continues his descriptions of spiritual growth that are intertwined with descriptions of physical nutrition: "Be a source of light," he urges readers, "Feed the starving souls who seek true knowledge with the most nourishing fruit, plants, seeds and wisdom."[1150]

Because of the synergistic misery engendered by the feedback loop of ecological-dietary-spiritual depravity, the national emergency facing America is not a lack of healthcare (for this is yet another system that poisons people for profit) but a lack of clean food, water, and air.[1151] By cleaning up our surroundings, our diet, and embracing plants as sus-

---

[1145]   Ibid., 103.

[1146]   Ibid., 103, 114.

[1147]   Ibid., 104

[1148]   Ibid., 151

[1149]   Ibid., 125

[1150]   Ibid., 34

[1151]   Ibid., 28

tenance and medicine, we will heal our minds and bodies. Plants like cannabis are better medicines, Jacoby notes, than the high-profit synthetic drugs that keep people sick that the West calls "healthcare."[1152]

The only solution for the modern West's woes and the planet's woes is the natural medicine of mostly-raw veganism. An uncooked plant based diet is the one source of power that will heal our soil, oceans, air, bodies, and souls.

[1152] Ibid., 31

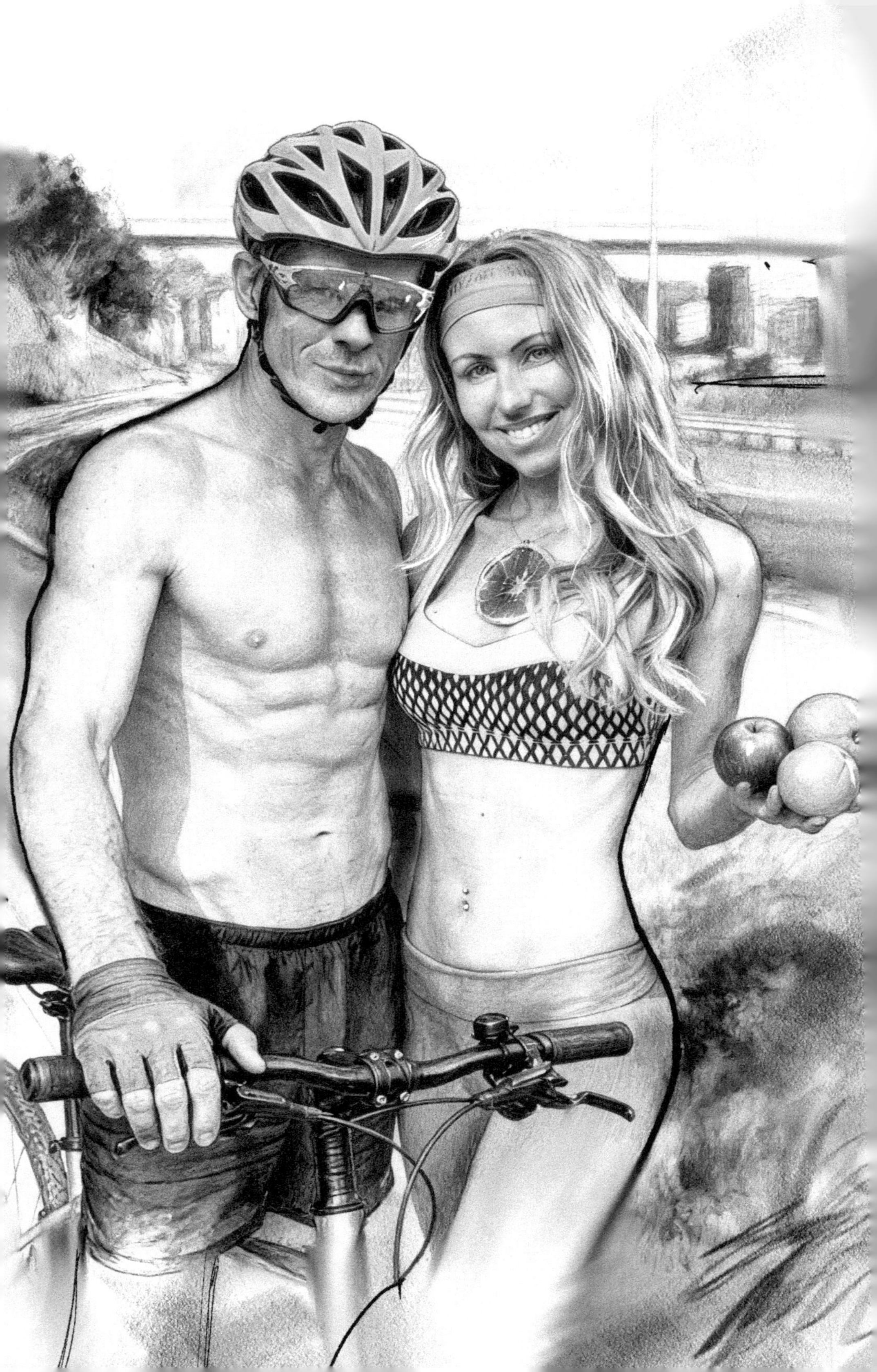

24.
Masculinizing and Feminizing Raw Food

Raw food, somehow, is incorporated into nearly every human concern. Raw foodists have even used their diet to bolster their own gender identity. A few notable twenty-first-century raw vegans have claimed that their uncooked plant based diet has reinforced their perceived feminine or masculine traits.

Some men on this diet have felt the need to defend the compatibility of raw vegan food with modern conceptions of masculinity, since both cooking (like barbecuing) and meat consumption, in America especially, has been culturally associated with masculinity. Occasionally, male raw advocates redefine masculinity, countersignaling conditioned conceptions of manhood, but more often, they argue that raw veganism enhances traditionally-defined male traits of muscular strength, sexual virility, self-sufficiency, and other characteristics. Raw vegan women similarly discuss how a raw diet enhances their femininity, physically and mentally.

Tonya Zavasta's blog post from 2004, on her "Beautiful on Raw" website is a small illustration of the interplay of gender and raw food. She argues that raw veganism reinforces ideal masculine traits in men and feminine traits in women as they age. Usually, as people grow old, she notes, they slide, in appearance, toward the center of the physical spectrum, they become androgynous or even resemble the opposite sex in an unattractive way. There are "women whose broadening bodies and faces take on a vaguely masculine look, and men whose appearance loses its masculine edge, including facial and muscle definition, softening to a kind of vague femininity." Men become softer and women harder. But raw food, she promises, is a good solution because it helps balance hormones at any age. Uncooked food preserves "those distinguishing feminine and masculine features so prevalent during younger years when hormones are at their peak."[1153] For both men and women, in other words, their unique and ideal features are maintained..

Raw food, advocates claim, makes us more manly and more womanly. Or in rare cases, it can help us to transcend the limited confines of shortsighted conceptions of what a man or women should be.

RAW FOOD AND MASCULINITY

One evening in Chicago, raw foodist Jesse J. Jacoby sat in a dingy tavern, watching his friend order "a plate of fried chemicals in the form of some sort of cheese stick, to go along with an alcoholic cocktail." Jacoby had reluctantly joined his friend that evening, despite his aversion to alcohol and highly processed food.[1154] However, he felt fairly comfortable, having been satiated by his raw food dinner he had eaten earlier in the evening. But all of a sudden, he was confronted by a patron.

"Sitting next to me was a sorry mistake for a man," Jacoby later wrote. Taking a break from guzzling down mixed drinks and shouting approval for a performing musician, the raucous older man approached the out-of-place raw foodist. "What's wrong with you? Where is your drink? Where is your food?" the man cross-examined Jacoby. After Jacoby's brief explanation, the seemingly incensed man, stumbling "while his eyes rolled back in his head," chastised Jacoby's supposed lack of manhood. "Be a man! You are a pussy! Be a man. You need to wake the fuck up and be a man," he taunted.[1155]

This incident highlighted a conflict between raw veganism and American cultural constructions of masculinity. In the minds of many men, their consumption of alcohol, meat, and high-temperature cooked food like fried foods is important to their sense of manhood. "Many guys believe poor lifestyle choices are somehow masculine," Jacoby explains. "I cannot count how many times I have listened to fat guys and degenerates," he complains with bite, "insist that they eat meat [because] as they say: 'I am a man.'"[1156] What a deranged and senseless excuse for manhood, a raw vegan might think.

Because of these ingrained notions of masculinity in Western culture, raw vegans in modern America have had an uphill battle in gaining cultural acceptance among men. As a result of this cultural

---

[1153] "How Raw Foods Make You Different | Beautiful on Raw." *Beautifulonraw.com*, Feb. 2004, www.beautifulonraw.com/the-ten-biomarkers-of-a-long-term-raw-foodist.html. Accessed 9 Apr. 2025.

[1154] Jacoby, Jesse. *The Raw Cure: Healing beyond Medicine*. Soulspire Publishing, 2012, 168

[1155] Ibid., 169

[1156] Ibid., 169

resistance, numerous raw vegans have felt the need, in order to convince others and perhaps themselves of the compatibility of their diet with masculinity, to use traditional manly virtues to argue that carnivorous barbecues, booze, and French fries should be ditched in favor of eating only uncooked plants.

But Jacoby has lambasted what he considers to be stupid notions of masculinity and has argued for a reframing of what a self-actualized man should be.

CHALLENGING COMMON DEFINITIONS OF MASCULINITY

One way of defending the plausible masculinity of raw veganism is to point out the functional failings or perceived anti-masculine qualities of cooked or junk food diets. Jacoby asks, is being flaccid both in the tone of your body and in your erectile function really masculine? Are clogged arteries, higher body fat and thus higher estrogen levels (since fat cells can produce estrogen), really masculine?

"The whole cultural aspect of being a man," which Jacoby critiques, has promoted immorality and severely damaged men's characters, he feels. Men think it's manly to belittle others in order to pump up their own egos, their shallow sense of self. Men think it's manly to "control" or "abuse" women. Men think it's masculine to get into fist fights. But all of these distorted notions of manhood, Jacoby argues, showcase a man's "insecurities and desperation for approval" along with their mistaken value judgments.[1157]

"It is not manly to hide behind a phony caricature," Jacoby declares. It is not masculine to kill animals; it is not even "feminine," because that would be an insult to the female gender, he says. "It is not manly to eat steak dinners . . . to be 'the fat guy' who wakes up one day and cannot even see his sex organ, because he let his stomach get so big from allowing the food industry to rid him of his manhood." No way is it masculine to have been duped by advertisements for toxic food, to have lost one's mental sovereignty. Nor is it manly to have squandered your strength and virility, to have "deteriorated organs, weak bones, and disease" or to be unable to have an erection.[1158]

Consuming cooked and toxic foods, men actually become "lost, shadows of men," They become disempowered: spiritually blind to

---

[1157]   Ibid., 170
[1158]   Ibid.,. 171

their true purpose and physically decrepit. They become, overall, "flaccid" because of "the poisons of meat, dairy, eggs, sugars, fats, flours."[1159]

In Jacoby's scheme, true masculinity is being a warrior-guardian of Mother Earth. True manhood involves mindful dietary and lifestyle choices that regenerate the injured planet and do no harm to other creatures. A real man is a nurturer and protector. He is physically vibrant, alive with purpose, having the courage to fight the powerful destructive forces that are assailing Mother Earth. A real man is acutely alive and unusually conscious. And he is constantly fueled with the raw energetic force of the Earth's plants.

Other raw foodists articulate more conventional compatibilities between their diets and masculinity. They highlight physical endurance, strength, high libido, or other perceived masculinizing effects of their diet.

Extolling Traditional Masculine Virtues

A viral early YouTube video by Markus Rothkranz entitled "Go Raw Now Trailer," dated 2008, opens with a deeply tanned Rothkranz, wearing a torso-exposing unbuttoned white dress shirt and sporting long bleached-blond hair, posing and confidently twirling onstage as hair-metal music plays and pyrotechnic special effects explode in front of a green screen background. Female backup singers sing something along the lines of "living like a star." Rothkranz, seeking to portray raw food as fun, exciting, sexy, and youthful, holds a microphone up to his mouth and explains to the green-screened audience how "primitive" peoples with neither stove nor electricity have much more vitality than technologically advanced Americans: "They're a hundred years old and still having sex. You tell me who's better off!" he challenges.[1160] Men from traditional civilizations who eat more naturally, are brimming with virility and still horny in their last years of life.

Later, there's a shot of a shirtless Rothkranz in the gym, showing off his defined muscles and brushing off the need for animal products. "The biggest, most powerful animals on the planet don't eat meat!" Rothkranz emphasizes.[1161] Elephants, rhinoceros, and gorillas get huge on raw plants. Clips of his friends boasting about their deadlift and

---

[1159]   Ibid., 170.
[1160]   Dharmaboost. "Go Raw Now Trailer." *Youtube.com*, 2008, youtu.be/z3xOU2tLl-7g?si=57YwsaPwZE0x4Tbt. Accessed 10 Apr. 2025.
[1161]   Ibid.

bench press weights drill in the supposed energizing, muscle boosting, and masculinizing effects that raw food has on men.

Through YouTube videos like these, which frequently feature muscle building, testosterone boosting, and libido enhancing tips, Rothkranz has striven to prove the compatibility between traditionally masculine characteristics and raw veganism. Often wearing tank tops that reveal his bulky arms, he attempts to show how raw eaters can not only preserve their manly characteristics but can actually easily surpass the manliness of cooked food eaters.

In a 2010 YouTube video, Rothkranz showcased how a 53 year old cab driver in Las Vegas and how the man accomplishes a body-building physique on a completely uncooked diet composed mostly of greens, fruit, raw potatoes and sprouted nuts. It's easy to build muscle on raw food, Rothkranz claims. The cab driver points out that typically ignored muscle-building foods like avocado have more "usable" protein, than you'd think.[1162] Raw food, it's claimed, even gives each weight-lifting session more potent muscle-building effects than it would on a cooked food diet. Rothkranz does note, however, that if you only eat primarily low-protein fruit, you're going to be scrawny. You need veggies, nuts, and seeds to build manly bulk.

Similarly, a 2015 video shows Rothkranz vigorously lifting weights as an electric guitar riffs in the background, interspersed with clips of him drinking green vegetable juice.[1163] He's no scrawny, weak hippie. Raw amino acids that make up protein are more absorbable than cooked protein, because of intact co-factors, like enzymes, vitamins, and minerals, and other compounds that make protein more usable, he argues. Rothkranz points out that raw algae, fava beans, natto, seeds, and nuts are packed with protein.

Rothkranz continues his argument for the muscle-enhancing effects of raw food in another video about raw vegan bodybuilders. "These guys don't cook their food," he touts. Rothkranz explains, as clips of middle-aged raw body builders appear on the screen, "Eating food in its natural uncooked state gives us one hundred times the [lifting] power."[1164] The body builders, who undoubtedly have huge muscles, also claim that less protein is needed to build muscle on a

[1162] The Healthy Life. "RAW FOOD VEGAN BODYBUILDER Cab Driver Eats No Meat." *YouTube*, 16 Sept. 2010, www.youtube.com/watch?v=SbEUHCU_GtM. Accessed 10 Apr. 2025.

[1163] The Healthy Life. "Bodybuilding Set with Plant-Based Protein." *YouTube*, 21 Feb. 2021, www.youtube.com/watch?v=vmHyq-a02F8. Accessed 10 Apr. 2025.

[1164] The Healthy Life. "Raw Vegan Muscle Bodybuilding DVD Set Now Available !" *Youtube*, 2010, youtu.be/_IlgWnwgEak?si=7i7-nzUGsX-yqUTX. Accessed 10 Apr. 2025.

raw diet because your body utilizes the nutrients more efficiently than cooked food.

Rothkranz and the bodybuilders tout the efficiency of the diet, telling men they can build more muscle on less food and will require less sleep. Viewers can optimize their efficiency in their masculine quest to build muscle and brim with energy.

Higher libido, Rothkranz tells men, is another supposed benefit of a raw food diet. A YouTube clip entitled, "How to Raise Testosterone Naturally" shows him winking and holding an upraised cucumber. "Food controls your hormones," he emphasizes.[1165] If you eat too much, especially cooked refined carbs, you produce a lot of insulin, which diminishes your human growth hormone levels. These could typically help build muscles. More fiber from raw plant foods also "equals less estrogen" because fiber moves it out of your body. Testosterone is preserved and counterproductive extra estrogen is washed away.

Rothkranz details the raw dried herbs he sells and how they can increase testosterone. Celery, he notes, helps the production of androgens and reduces estrogen production—eat two raw celery stalks daily, he urges.[1166] If you want higher estrogen levels, he warns, and want to be a chubby, less virile male, then eat dairy products.[1167]

Cooked animal fats are no good but raw plant fats, like olive oil, coconut, nuts, and seeds have the highest quality fats, and the best building blocks for steroid hormones like testosterone, he says.[1168] Olive oil, he claims, may be responsible for the stereotypical extreme virility of Mediterranean men, who are rumored to father children at advanced ages.

A diverse, nutrient-dense raw food diet makes you ooze youthful sexual energy, according to Rothkranz and other raw foodists—a far cry from the self-chastising, severely limited, and self-weakening diets of the raw foodist Desert Fathers.

[1165]   The Healthy Life. "How to Raise Testosterone Naturally." *YouTube*, 26 May 2024, www.youtube.com/watch?v=ZNCQJ8pR39w. Accessed 10 Apr. 2025.

[1166]   Ibid.

[1167]   The Healthy Life. "The Importance of Using the Right Protein." *YouTube*, 6 July 2022, www.youtube.com/watch?v=Ht6nXkMLCmo. Accessed 10 Apr. 2025.

[1168]   The Healthy Life. "How to Raise Testosterone Naturally." *YouTube*, 26 May 2024, www.youtube.com/watch?v=ZNCQJ8pR39w. Accessed 10 Apr. 2025.

ON FEMININITY

Rothkranz doesn't shy away from his opinion on how diet affects women's gender expression and sexual experience.

In his book on female sexual health, Rothkranz lays out what he sees as a typical problematic timeline for a woman. As they enter their thirties, they start to worry more about their life situation, their future, and losing their beauty in middle age—all of which causes them to increase their intake of junk food and cooked food, which clogs their liver and diminishes their energy and sex drive along with sullying their beauty.[1169] The liver, Rothkranz points out, is a major producer of hormones. When it's not healthy from cooked and junk food consumption, the feminine sexual experience collapses, a woman feels less motivation in general, and potential partners aren't as interested in her increasingly unhealthy physique. Food is connected to the other areas of her life. Without a focus on raw food, a woman loses her feminine edge and the power to seduce people.

Before adopting a raw food diet, Rothkranz instructs, women should fast to "revitalize" their "sex and endocrine glands" in order to boost their hormones. After that, they are to make use of raw vegetable juices like what he calls "sex juice"—celery mixed with a little bit of ginger and honey. Celery contains the hormone androsterone, he says, which makes women more "playful." "Just smelling" raw ginger "is enough" to get the "female parts stimulated!" Raw seaweed, the densest source of nutrients around, boosts the sex drive like crazy.

Cooked junk food clogs not only the liver but even the breast tissue. The animal products women eat can accumulate fat-soluble toxins like pesticides, steroids, hormones, in breasts, and hips. These disrupt natural sex hormone production and increase breast cancer risk, it's claimed.[1170]

According to Rothkranz, women "especially" look their best while eating raw. Raw food clears the skin, brightens your eyes, and makes women look alive again. Women notice they don't need makeup anymore because their complexion is flawless and texture defects fade. In another book, co-written with his raw food chef girlfriend, he says that women tell him they feel lighter, more confident, and beautiful.[1171]

[1169] Rothkranz, Markus. *SEX—WOMENS' EDITION (78 Page E-Booklet)*. markusebooks. com. Accessed 2025.

[1170] Ibid.

[1171] Rothkranz, Markus, and Cara Brotman. *Love on a Plate*. Rothkranz Publishing, 1 Jan. 2015.

Female raw foodists also have things to say about how uncooked food has affected their life and self-image.

Kristina Carrillo-Bucaram is known online as FullyRaw Kristina, and she has over three million followers across platforms. As a very popular raw food influencer, she speaks largely to a female audience, giving tips to optimize their physical and mental health. In the mid 2000s, when she was eighteen years old, she had a chance encounter with a "raw food coach" in a Whole Foods store. He convinced her to try out a raw vegan diet to see if that would help her hypoglycemia, migraines, and other health issues.[1172] From then on, she became an advocate for the diet that allegedly cured her ills.

Since that fateful day, she has become a relatively viral YouTube personality, with over 100 million views across her 800+ video catalog. She started numerous successful raw food–inspired businesses.

She is known for her smiley demeanor but also her emotional vulnerability, her focus on "mind, body, and spirit," and her embrace of such concepts like self-love, in addition to her extremely colorful featured fruit dishes.

Her work touches on how raw food plays into womanhood. In a 2013 video, "Empowering Women with Raw Food," Kristina Carrillo-Bucaram explains how raw veganism empowers women in their femininity. This is "one of the most important topics," she says, related to diet and how it affects women. "Women in particular have a very unique relationship with food," she says.[1173] In a sense, it can make or break a woman's relationship with herself.

As the camera pans to images of flowers in a field, Kristina explains that food "cannot only bring us confidence but it can bring us power and happiness." The key to gaining this power is to "feel confident" in one's body. Raw food can help a woman "feel confident in her skin and shine bright like a diamond," she preaches. There is an obvious implication that physical beauty especially matters for women, as opposed to men, and that confidence and self-love are tied into a woman's relationship with her raw food-built body. You can make "rooms light up" if you have a "glow" and "aura," she argues.[1174] Colorful raw plant foods can help women attract attention.

[1172]   Huynh, Dai. "Uncooked Food Leads to Better Health, Devotees Say." *Chron*, 5 Jan. 2009, www.chron.com/life/food/article/Uncooked-food-leads-to-better-health-devotees-say-1732174.php. Accessed 24 Apr. 2025.
[1173]   FullyRaw Kristina. "Empowering Women with Raw Food." *YouTube*, 17 Apr. 2013, www.youtube.com/watch?v=TMqdQbTELpI. Accessed 24 Apr. 2025.
[1174]   Ibid.

A woman's confidence increases when she knows she's doing the right thing for her body by eating raw. And she also feels "beautiful" and like she can accomplish anything, Kristina argues. Food builds a positive self-image and how one feels about life. In her own life, she says that she began to "feel alive" when she started eating raw, including embodying her own sense of femininity more comfortably.[1175] Kristina connects eating raw food to being inspired to find "success," and she aims to inspire other women to feel the same. She certainly found success in the raw food niche and credits her new self-confidence to eating that way.

MASCULINE DURIANRIDER AND FEMININE FREELEE

A telling illustration of how gender is seen within a raw foodist context is the advocacy of two prominent high-carb low-fat mostly raw vegans and former lovers—Harley Johnstone (known online as Durianrider) and Leanne Ratcliffe (known online as Freelee the Banana Girl). They rose to fame within the nutrition world in the late 2000s and early 2010s. They've long been vocal, confrontational, and controversial commentators on diet and gender issues. They've utilized a mixture of comedy and aggressive critiques of other raw foodists or dieters who don't follow their mostly fruit diet.

Freelee and Durianrider have largely promoted a "Raw 'Till 4 Diet." Energizing raw fruit is recommended until four p.m. or later in the day, at which point, cooked vegan food is allowed. Raw food is emphasized but doesn't comprise all of their diet. Durianrider states that, fruit is essential to feel one's best but a 100% raw food diet isn't.[1176]

Australian ultra-cyclist, vegan advocate, and YouTube content creator Harley Johnstone, born in 1977, adopted Durianrider as his online persona, in honor of both his love of cycling and his favorite fruit, the Southeast Asian durian, often described as foul-smelling.

This feisty high-sugar semi-raw food advocate has garnered controversy as well kudos for his bad boy reputation and disputed nutritional tips. Occasionally, he has unapologetically poured refined sugar on his cereal when he can't access quality fruit. Durianrider practically

---

[1175]   Ibid.

[1176]   Johnstone, H. (2022, August 22). Rawfood diet vs Durianrider protocol for health and performance? [Audio podcast episode]. In *Durianrider Raw Truth*. iVoox. https://www.ivoox.com/en/rawfood-diet-vs-durianrider-protocol-for-health-audios-mp3_rf_74397220_1.html

worships sugar but he does prefer to ingest it in the form of raw fruit. He claims that sugar is key to having more energy and even an enhanced sense of masculinity.

Durianrider is known for his macho persona, blunt tips on relationships and sexual performance, advice for men in dealing with women, and the routine featuring of pictures of his scantily-clad girlfriends in his video thumbnails.

He has often framed veganism and his high-raw-food-diet as being hypermasculine. He urges followers to adopt a high-carbohydrate and low-fat mostly fruit diet for improved physical performance and libido and attempts to define the spiritual values that helped generate his own fulfilled masculinity.

Physical Masculinity

"You want to be like carbed-up, virile, energetic,
high blood flow—if you know what I mean."
—Durianrider

Durianrider discusses multiple aspects of physical masculinity in his YouTube videos. In one titled "Why Masculine Presence is a DRUG women live for," he details postures that women will perceive as confident, focused, relaxed, masculine—and conversely, physical postures that women will perceive as weak, distracted, and lacking in masculinity. Masculine "presence," featuring "open" and unafraid body language is recommended.[1177]

Athleticism, though, and sexual vigor are the main focuses of Durianrider's conception of physical masculinity. In one video, he posits that sugar, especially from raw fruit, is a better "performance enhancer" in extreme cycling than supplemented testosterone.[1178] Fruit sugar, hydration, and sleep are the most critical things, he argues, for efficient recovery from hard workouts.

Protein holds athletes back, Durianrider claims. He believes that he has superior biking endurance because he's fueled by raw fruit. In his book *Carb the Fcuk Up Lifestyle and Dietary Guide*, he explains that protein is overrated and, when it comes to biking, he's "outclimbed" meat-eaters on bananas alone. Carbs fuel his impressive performances, he believes. More sugar equals more stamina. Nevertheless, there have

---

[1177]   Durianrider. "Why Masculine Presence Is a DRUG Women Live For." *YouTube*, 4 May 2021, www.youtube.com/watch?v=Z4t5Rs8WpPc. Accessed 20 Apr. 2025.

[1178]   Durianrider. "Is Sugar REALLY More Powerful than Testosterone for Recovery and Performance??" *YouTube*, 31 Jan. 2025, www.youtube.com/watch?v=29oHpLMuhys

been rumors of Durianrider using performance-enhancing drugs to improve his athletic performance.

But those drugs, he'd argue, can't compete with raw sugar in the long term. This ultimate fuel for a highly performing athlete quickly builds a cyclist's glycogen stores, so that they can use this complex carbohydrate that's released from their muscles and liver during intense activity. No other food fills our bodies' sugar stores like raw fruit, he argues. That's why he can bike for hours and overcome fatigue.[1179] He's beaten thousands of meat eating cyclists and runners in competitions, since becoming vegan, he notes. And some of them were decades younger than him.[1180]

Durianrider also believes that the invigorating effects of a fruit diet are responsible for his insatiable libido and allegedly exceptional sexual performance. He certainly has never been interested in starving out the passions from the body, as the Desert Fathers or Johnny Lovewisdom were.

In a 2012 video on the ideal diet for sexual performance, he cheekily turns the camera to his girlfriend and asks her for some thoughts on his sexual skills. She responds, "My pelvis is a little sore, maybe later."[1181]

Eating mostly fruit keeps his libido through the roof and gives him plenty of blood flow down below. Fruit is the natural Viagra—raw veggies are less important and plant fats are hardly on his menu. Eating low-fat vegan is how he's still pulling models at forty plus, he explains.

Eating fruit is crucial for a man to have the increased "sexual stamina" needed to thoroughly satisfy a woman. In her own videos, Freelee acknowledges, to men, that "You're going to get more oxygen and blood flow to your penis" when you eat mostly fruit.[1182]

More carbs equal more energy in the sack. His girlfriends never complain. There's nothing complex to figure out; it's just fruit, he claims.

[1179] Johnstone, H. (2013, April 17). Interview with vegan Harley Johnstone aka Durianrider. Rawsomehealthy.com. https://www.rawsomehealthy.com/interview-vegan-harley-johnstone-aka-durianrider/

[1180] Johnstone, H. (n.d.). Durianrider podcast [Audio podcast episode]. In *Durianrider Raw Truth*. Spotify for Creators. https://podcasters.spotify.com/pod/show/durianrider

[1181] Durianrider "TANTRIC SEXUALITY + Best Diet for Sexual Performance?" *YouTube*, 4 Feb. 2012, www.youtube.com/watch?v=7EopRCp-wTA. Accessed 20 Apr. 2025.

[1182] Freelee and Durianrider. "10 Sexual Benefits of a High Fruit Diet." *YouTube*, 11 Dec. 2013, www.youtube.com/watch?v=kVHABB4pq5A. Accessed 20 Apr. 2025.

"When your carbs are strong, so is your dong," Durianrider summarizes.[1183] It's no surprise that in India, the mango is seen as an aphrodisiac, he says. Meat on the other hand, is a sex-killer. "It's hard to attract a faerie when you're dining on roadkill."[1184.] Meat, it's implied, makes you uglier, smell bad, and potentially impotent. Sugar from fruit keep the testosterone pumping. Women, he claims, can tell he's got that "edge."[1185]

Spiritual Masculinity

Raw sugar-rich fruit is the physical foundation for spiritual masculine values, Durianrider believes, in addition to manly physical traits. Fruit uplifts one's mood and gives men energy to realize a masculine sense of "freedom" and agency in their lives. In one video, Durianrider portrays himself as a happy and fit cyclist, brimming with energy and enjoying a "hot" girlfriend. He contrasts himself with angry anti-cyclist car drivers he comes into contact with on the road. Those car drivers are sedentary cooked food miserable folks, whose life "sucks" because they probably "just got a fat chick pregnant."[1186]

These people don't have the frequent inspired attitudes or emotional strength to live out their best lives and assert themselves. They aren't strong enough to live their dreams. They're unlike the energized and oxygenated raw vegan, always on the go around town, speedily cycling by society's lethargic masses.

Durianrider also cherishes his unapologetic boldness, assertiveness, and willingness to offend as emblematic masculine characteristics. Nice guys definitely finish last, according to him. Feminine women want an aggressive, confident man, he often says in his videos. Beta guys who lack assertiveness aren't pulling the chicks. "I refuse to sit back and be a spineless, gutless wimp," he says in reference to his willingness to fight for his dietary beliefs and his brave ambassadorship for the life-changing power of fruit.[1187] He has been emboldened by

[1183]   Durianrider "TANTRIC SEXUALITY + Best Diet for Sexual Performance?" *YouTube,* 14 Feb. 2012, www.youtube.com/watch?v=7EopRCp-wTA. Accessed 20 Apr. 2025.

[1184]   Durianrider "TANTRIC SEXUALITY + Best Diet for Sexual Performance?" *YouTube,* 14 Feb. 2012, www.youtube.com/watch?v=7EopRCp-wTA. Accessed 20 Apr. 2025.

[1185]   Johnstone, H. (2020, March 2). Harley Johnstone (Durianrider) talks testosterone, fruit, and cycling (A. Dixon, Host). *The Love Fruit Podcast.* Simplecast. https://love-fruit-podcast. simplecast.com/episodes/harley-johnstone-durianrider-talks-testosterone-fruit-and-cycling

[1186]   Durianrider. "Testosterone & What EVERY Man Needs to Know!" *YouTube,* 20 June 2024, www.youtube.com/watch?v=Bz8k_1riWcY. Accessed 20 Apr. 2025.

[1187]   Durianrider. "Why is Durianrider so Aggressive? (Warning: Content May Offend the

fruit, he believes. Eating copious amounts of energizing fruit sugar, he thinks, gives guys the edge they need to have the motivation to maintain their confidence and assertiveness.

Individualism and authenticity are also central to Durianrider's masculine self-image. He thinks of himself as a "health vigilante" who isn't afraid to speak taboo truths about diet and societal norms. One podcast host describes him as being a "lightning rod for controversy," which is "a role he relishes."[1188] He isn't afraid to take on the advocates of "fad diets" like the paleo, keto, or carnivore diets, nor is he afraid to criticize the mediocrity of omnivorism or even attack the way that other raw foodists are living (like low-energy raw foodists who prefer greens over fruit). Raw fruit gave Durianrider the spirit to be his true self.

FREELEE

As the yin to Durianrider's yang, but never lacking in boldness, Freelee has argued that raw foodism liberated her to fulfill her ideal femininity.

A fruit-based diet, she argues, helped her develop a healthier and more authentic femininity by opening her eyes to discard oppressive feminine norms like makeup and restrictive dieting. Fruit helped to clear her skin of acne and other troubles, which rendered cosmetics unnecessary.[1189]

She also believes that a high-carb raw fruit diet helped her realize a new sense of "strong" physical femininity unlike the weakening effects of other restrictive weight-loss diets. In her view, an ideal feminine body is very thin with a vigorous cardiovascular fitness potential, not a more sedentary or overly curvy body type. She lost forty pounds eating unlimited fruit and she had dumped what she deemed a typical frail or fake female body.

Glucose Deficient)." *YouTube*, 9 May 2013, www.youtube.com/watch?v=3goYA0TOnPI. Accessed 20 Apr. 2025.

[1188] "How to Thrive & Perform Athletically on a High-Carb, Low-Fat Vegan Diet." *Rich Roll*, 30 Sept. 2013, www.richroll.com/podcast/rrp-53-durianrider-how-to-thrive-perform-athletically-on-a-high-carb-low-fat-vegan-diet/. Accessed 20 Apr. 2025.

[1189] Ratcliffe, Leanne. *Go Fruit Yourself.* 2nd ed., Leanne Ratcliffe, 2020. ISBN: 1092785531.

Feminine Aesthetics, Physiology,
and Sexual Performance

Freelee feels that raw fruit changed her aesthetics, her feminine self-image, and her relationship to the opposite sex. After her dietary change, she noticed no more pimples or "pregnant" bloated belly. Men found her more attractive. "When I was forty pounds heavier, guys were not finding me physically attractive. It just wasn't the same," Freelee says.[1190] She didn't have "that fruity physique," the alleged ideal body that women get when they eat primarily fruit. In addition to better skin, she started to grow silky hair and develop improved proportions and more balanced hormones, she claims.

Before she was on a mostly raw diet, a former boyfriend once asked her why her eyes were so yellow. It horrified her that her eyes were indeed that color because, in her mind, she had been eating too much cooked food and animal protein.[1191]

Freelee also believes that raw food has improved her menstrual health. In a 2019 book, she wrote that her periods went from painful and heavy to light and easy on raw vegan diet. Before, her periods were a nightmare. Cramps, bloating, etc. After switching to mostly fruit, it was a breeze and she barely needed a pad.[1192]

She contrasted animal proteins with raw veganism. "Dairy wrecked my cycle—acne, mood swings, clots. Raw vegan fixed it in months. My period's a non-event now, and that's freedom every woman deserves," says Freelee.[1193] Meat-eaters would tell her that their periods were torture, while she hardly suffered. Raw carbs cured the pain and things flowed smoothly, she claims. Freelee also says that the water content in fruit helps "moisturize" female genitalia for enhanced sexual pleasure and less irritation.[1194]

Fruit also raises women's self-esteem and their relationship to their own bodies, she argues. Fructose is conducive to greater sexual openness because it increases serotonin, which makes women feel bet-

---

[1190]   Freelee and Durianrider. "Raw Food Vegan SEX." *YouTube*, 12 Dec. 2013, www.youtube.com/watch?v=RCna06lImno. Accessed 20 Apr. 2025.

[1191]   Durianrider. "SEXY HOT Body for Life Diet Tips with Fruitarian Vegan Freelee." *YouTube*, 16 Nov. 2012, www.youtube.com/watch?v=zTqEXoGq2nQ. Accessed 20 Apr. 2025.

[1192]   Ratcliffe, Leanne. *Go Fruit Yourself*. 2nd ed., Leanne Ratcliffe, 2020. ISBN: 1092785531.

[1193]   Freelee the Banana Girl. "Why Dairy Destroys Your Hormones." TheBananaGirl.com, undated but active as of 2025, thebananagirl.com/why-dairy-destroys-your-hormones.

[1194]   Freelee and Durianrider. "10 Sexual Benefits of a High Fruit Diet." *YouTube*, 11 Dec. 2013, www.youtube.com/watch?v=kVHABB4pq5A. Accessed 20 Apr. 2025.

ter about themselves "in the bedroom."[1195] Women have more self-esteem and feel more comfortable in their own skin. On a fruity diet, her "brain function" has been better—she's happier and more confident and those traits are more "sexually attractive" to potential partners.[1196]

Freelee, like Durianrider, doesn't shy away from glorying in her fruit-fueled sexual aptitude. In *The Raw Till 4 Diet*, she writes: "Eating this way has my energy through the roof—my sex drive's never been higher. No more sluggish nights; I'm ready to go anytime."[1197]

Genders Severed: The Breakup of Durianrider and Freelee

Despite all its benefits on body, spirit, and their gendered selves, the high-raw diet of Durianrider and Freelee could not save their relationship. The fruit-fueled love affair eventually ended, leaving an acrimonious gap between them.

On a July 2022 YouTube video, Freelee announced that she was "making a public record that my ex-boyfriend Harley is stalking me." Video footage showed Durianrider (Harley) entering Freelee's isolated jungle property in Queensland, Australia.[1198] Wearing his trademark bright biking gear, Durianrider stood firm as Freelee's boyfriend attempted to push Durianrider's bicycle away from their property. Freelee said that Durianrider cried for a long while shortly after, but she did not release the footage, considering he was mentally unwell. Durianrider claimed that he had announced to Freelee he was visiting multiple times and did not try to "sneak" onto property.[1199]

This video was preceded by years of mutual accusations of emotional and physical abuse between the former lovers. Durianrider had made dozens of videos about Freelee since their breakup in the mid 2010s. He calls her his "biggest enemy" on the internet and complains that she was making "millions" off of his diet and training protocol.[1200]

[1195]   Ibid.

[1196]   Freelee and Durianrider. "Raw Food Vegan SEX." *YouTube*, 12 Dec. 2013, www.youtube.com/watch?v=RCna06lImno. Accessed 20 Apr. 2025.

[1197]   Ratcliffe, L. (n.d.). *What is the Raw Till 4 Diet?* The Banana Girl. https://thebananagirl.com/pages/what-is-the-raw-till-4-diet[](https://thebananagirl.com/pages/the-raw-till-4-diet)

[1198]   The Frugivore Diet. "Durianrider Is Stalking Me (Trespassing, Slander, Harassment)." *YouTube*, 2 July 2022, www.youtube.com/watch?v=qfQ1WaQ9qgE. Accessed 20 Apr. 2025.

[1199]   Ask Durianrider. "Freelee the Banana Girl Won't Tell You the Truth so I Will." *YouTube*, 5 July 2022, www.youtube.com/watch?v=G-6gjbF2kcg. Accessed 20 Apr. 2025.

[1200]   Ask Durianrider. "Freelee the Banana Girl Is She OK?" *YouTube*, 6 July 2024, www.youtube.com/watch?v=clsweVDSSTE. Accessed 20 Apr. 2025; Ask Durianrider. "Freelee the

Durianrider has claimed that Freelee physically abused him in the past and pulled a kitchen knife on him. "I tried to move on," says Durianrider of the relationship, but he claims that Freelee was constantly spreading false accusations against him."[1201]

Freelee's Rejection of Constructed Femininity

After her very public and acrimonious breakup, Freelee's tone changed about femininity and she became a vocal critic of traditional Western gender norms. In her videos, she made a point of posing with visible armpit hair and proclaimed her desire to be free of razors and the need for external validation of her beauty.

In her post-relationship blog posts and ebooks, she cried out against the psychological and physical constrictions of supposedly arbitrary concepts of femininity. She declared in one blog post, in which she introduced her popular ebook, *My Naked Lunchbox*, that women "not only crave tasty, nutritious food but also have a ravenous appetite to be their true self, which involves not conforming to useless norms."[1202] This ebook, she said, is for "the rebellious ones" who want to break the shackles of harmful gender norms.

Raw food, Freelee now emphasizes, can help women break out of patriarchal oppression. Women are brought up to believe that they are "born ugly" and must rely on artificial beauty treatments like makeup, painful fashion like high heels, and even cosmetic surgeries.[1203] All of this artificial attention to beauty, she claims, keeps women preoccupied with their efforts and submissive to male demands about their appearances and life in general. For example, she criticizes high heels for making women "physically vulnerable" and reliant on men's "steady flat-footed support."[1204] Eating a mostly raw fruit diet helps women look their natural best, erasing the need for the time, effort, and discomfort of practicing beauty treatments that men demand of them.

This breaking free from patriarchal oppression also involves a redefining of femininity or even a rejection of the concept. "You are not a gender to be manipulated for \$\$\$ and power. I am neither mascu-

Banana Girl Won't Tell You the Truth so I Will." *YouTube*, 5 July 2022, www.youtube.com/watch?v=G-6gjbF2kcg.

[1201]   Ask Durianrider. "Freelee the Banana Girl Won't Tell You the Truth so I Will." *YouTube*, 5 July 2022, www.youtube.com/watch?v=G-6gjbF2kcg. Accessed 20 Apr. 2025.

[1202]   Freelee. "What Is My Naked Lunchbox?" *Freelee the Banana Girl* , 2025, thebananagirl.com/pages/my-naked-lunchbox?srsltid=AfmBOorU_gMIrm9T3ZJRp4lbQZoz-f6nmJZqxN-SQDG74nM8-ytv7EVEZ. Accessed 20 Apr. 2025.

[1203]   Freelee, Ms. Banana Girl. *My Naked Lunchbox: The Most Controversial Cookbook Ever Written*. E-book ed., Independently published, 2019.

[1204]   Ibid.

line nor feminine, I am just me. Fuck femininity," she writes in a blog post.[1205]

Freelee had changed her perception of femininity over time. In her earlier years, raw food was the gateway to enhancing femininity, in later years, raw food, she claimed, helped her transcend femininity as defined by others. Durianrider's perception of masculinity, however, appears not to have altered. Though both of them have used the power of raw food to form their gendered sense of self.

[1205]   Freelee the Banana Girl. "The Femininity Lie." *Freelee the Banana Girl Blog*, thebananagirl.com, 1 Apr. 2019, https://thebananagirl.com/blogs/freelees-blog/the-femininity-lie.

Conclusion:
The Longing for Paradise

Raw foodism has been an expression of human longing. By eating uncooked food, people have sought to radically enhance their health, spiritual power, political aims, aesthetics, and sexual prowess, as well as the ecological health of the planet.

All of the advocates of raw foodism discussed in this book have seen biology and diet as a conduit through which they would find empowerment in this life—empowerment that was often of a spiritual nature, which they believed only possible by feeding the physical body in the optimal way. In this way, the story of raw foodism is a story of materialism. Spirituality and practically the entire experience of life was thought to depend on biology—on one's physical and nutritional state.

There is a certain melancholy embedded in raw foodism's quest for power, as some raw foodists have seen their far-flung hopes—hopes for an Edenic paradise, for environmental rejuvenation, for exceptional personal longevity—dashed when facing life's hard realities.

Some who have dared to dream, some who have publicly expressed a childlike faith in a revitalized world, fed on the nearly magical properties of raw plants, some who have hoped to reclaim God's original desire for this planet to be a paradise or to protect Mother Earth from the poisonous ecological destruction by sick cooked-food humanity, have ended up knocked dead on a sidewalk or trapped in a burning building, without seeing any widespread change that they had fought for. Many have failed in their valiant pursuit, having left this life without making a substantial mark in the way society views food or without many people adopting their worldview. Many failed in extending their own lifespan. Some raw advocates are still with us, though, and their story has yet to fully play out.

In the quest for self-optimization and power over health, raw foodism is still adhered to by niche groups but its influence is overshadowed by rapid technological advances of the twenty-first century.

As our understanding of the human body accelerates, AI-driven diagnostics and treatment, nanotechnology, evidence-based nutraceuticals, regenerative and gene-editing therapies, and other developments may supplant the importance of the health world's previous focus on dietary naturalism.

Considering this, raw food can be seen as a precursor to the present and coming revolutionary age in human physiology. Perhaps it will be seen in the future as an archaic preamble to vast gains in knowledge and power over our bodies. Perhaps health-focused raw foodism will be seen as a rudimentary indication of the human desire for more control over the fate of our bodies.

And indeed, in much of the modern history of raw foodism, advocates have been, scientifically speaking, grasping in semi-darkness. Their dietary beliefs have been led largely by intuition and personal observation. Nevertheless, they could've had vague insights into nutritional and spiritual truths that science has not caught up to yet.

Earlier modern raw foodists of the nineteenth and twentieth centuries like Bircher-Benner, Christian, Ehret, and Wigmore had a fraction of the scientific information that is available to us in the internet age. But to their credit, they knew that something was off with the way people around them were eating. Their raw foodism was, at the least, an intuitive realization that eating processed foods was doing tremendous damage to health. They at least brought to the attention of those who would listen that eating whole (unprocessed) colorful plant foods was the basic starting point of caring for the body.

But perhaps more weighty than raw food's effects on the body were its spiritual effects. Raw foodism revived a faith in the Earth as the source of all metaphysical good. It is our spirits that the Earth heals above all, New Agers claimed. Our terrestrial Mother gives us wisdom and instructions that we can only absorb if we consume her raw, in the form of a fruit or leafy green. You weren't just taking in medicine for your body, you were taking in the deepest intelligence of the universe into your soul. Raw food gave you instructions on how to live. Raw food was a communion rite.

The devotion to our planet intensified to a point where some New Age raw foodists would assert that humans live only to serve our great Mother. We are like the worms of the dirt, who, when fulfilling their proper role, serve the ecosystem through which they wriggle. But if a human pollutes too much, eats cooked food, and lives for herself, she is blind to the most sacred purpose of her existence: serving Gaia. For, after all, raw food gives us the instructions on how to care for Her.

In the case of Hitler's raw foodist reveries, the Earth took on a crueler hue. It was not an all-loving sentient nurturer but the cold overseer of a giant contest of strength. Whichever creature followed its laws best would overcome (or slaughter) other creatures. If a person ate right, he would be strong and would have a better chance of defeating any threat, whether viral or human. Raw food was, in Hitler's mind, fuel for the warrior in proving that might was right.

The fact that someone as malevolent as Hitler could have a soft spot for raw eating demonstrates the amorality of the diet. Like so many things, raw foodism could service good or ill. The diet's proponents thought they were imbibing power but what if that power, if real, was used for evil? Perhaps some raw foodists would claim that it's impossible to be immoral on the diet.

Of course, it wasn't only those in modern times who felt that ingesting raw food had spiritual meaning. The ancient Hindu and Christian ascetics found purifying value in uncooked food. Their sense of its power didn't take on as magical a flavor as the New Agers, but raw food to them had the power to strip away the carnal ties that bind us to sin and ignorance. The ancient seekers felt they were imbibing humility and shedding the corruption of civilization.

For most raw advocates, raw food was the starting point to solving everything. Through it, corruption could be cleansed from the world, be it spiritual, physical, sociological, aesthetic, or ecological. Time and time again, in the writings of raw foodists, cooked food was blamed for causing all of this corruption in the first place. The adoption of cooked food mirrored the story of Eden. Once a forbidden type of food was consumed, all of our problems began.

Cooked food was responsible for suffering and raw food would be responsible for salvation. Changing our biology through diet was the gateway to solving all of our own personal problems as well as all of the larger problems that plagued the world.

The yearning for paradise, the mythology of Eden, the reclaiming of careless sunny days of some primordial tropic were themes etched into the hearts of raw foodists. There would be no more suffering if the only food we consumed was that from some utopian garden. Our bodies, our environment, and our minds would be saved from harm. Leaves, fruit, nuts, and seeds in their natural state had the power, more than anything else, to heal the wounds of our flesh, our societies, and our souls. Many of the raw foodists may not have succeeded in their hopes but their fervency was a testimony to that intense human drive to make things right, to heal our brokenness.

Bibliography

"Ann Wigmore." *Vegetarian Times*, Apr. 1994, p. 18.

—. "Verse 2.23.18 Shri Chaitanya Bhagavata." Wisdomlib.org, 28 Mar. 2022, www.wisdomlib.org/hinduism/book/chaitanya-bhagavata/d/doc1107781.html. Accessed 9 Feb. 2025.

Aboul-Enein, B. H. (2013). Preventive Nutrition in Nazi Germany: A Public Health Commentary. Journal of Health Ethics, 9(1).

Albala, Ken. (2015). The SAGE Encyclopedia of Food Issues, Volume 1. Sage Publications. p. 1176.

Albanese, Catherine, ed. (2016). The Spiritual Journals of Warren Felt Evans from Methodism to Mind Cure. Indiana University Press.

Alexander, Joe. Blatant Raw Foodist Propaganda!, Or, Sell Your Stove to the Junkman and Feel Great!, Or, Consider Your True Nature. Blue Dolphin Publishing, 1990. Pg. 6

Alvaro, Carlo. Raw Veganism : The Philosophy of the Human Diet. Abingdon, Oxon, Routledge, 2020.

Amsden, Matt, and Janabai Amsden. The RAWvolution Continues: The Living Foods Movement in 150 Natural and Delicious Recipes. New York, Atria Books, 2013.

Anonymous. (1923). Journal of the American Medical Association 81: 768.

Ask Durianrider. "Freelee the Banana Girl Is She OK?" YouTube, 6 July 2024, www.youtube.com/watch?v=clsweVDSSTE. Accessed 20 Apr. 2025.

Ask Durianrider. "Freelee the Banana Girl Wont Tell You the Truth so I Will." YouTube, 5 July 2022, www.youtube.com/watch?v=G-6gjb-F2kcg.

Aurelius, Marcus. Meditations. 180 AD. Penguin, 2019.

Beskow, Per. (1983). Strange Tales about Jesus: A Survey of Unfamiliar Gospels. Fortress Press. pp. 84-89.

Bircher-Benner, Max. The Physician of the Future. Germany, Bircher-Benner, 2015.

Bob McCauley ND. God's Path to Disease-Free Living. WestBow Press, 7 Apr. 2017.

Bronkhorst, Johannes. "Historical Context of Early Asceticism." The Oxford History of Hinduism (2020): n. pag. Print.

Burton, Tony. "The Visionary Guru Edmond Szekely Lived and Wrote at Lake Chapala in the 1970s – Lake Chapala Artists and Authors." Lakechapalaartists.com, 2017, lakechapalaartists.com/?p=8837. Accessed 25 Apr. 2025.

Byrom, Thomas. The Heart of Awareness: A Translation of the Ashtavakra Gita. Shambhala Publications, 1 Dec. 1990.

Cannon Press. "Organic or Non-Organic? Does God Care? | Doug Wilson." YouTube, 13 Mar. 2012, www.youtube.com/watch?v=i-kNNOB-3IIo. Accessed 22 Apr. 2025.

Canon Press. "Food Does Not Make You Holy | Doug Wilson." YouTube, 2 July 2010, www.youtube.com/watch?v=YoRSn1ec_nI. Accessed 22 Apr. 2025.

Christian, E., & Christian, M. G. (1904). Uncooked foods and how to use them: A treatise on how to get the highest form of animal energy from food, with recipes for preparation, healthful combinations and menus. The Health-Culture Co. Pg. 8

Clement, Brian R, and Theresa Foy DiGeronimo. Living Foods for Optimum Health. Prima Lifestyles, 1996.

Clement, Brian. Hippocrates LifeForce: Superior Health and Longevity. Book Publishing Company, 2007, p. 83.

Cornélio, Alianda M., et al. "Human Brain Expansion during Evolution Is Independent of Fire Control and Cooking." Frontiers in Neuroscience, vol. 10, 25 Apr. 2016, https://doi.org/10.3389/fnins.2016.00167. Accessed 19 Feb. 2020.

Cousens, Gabriel. Spiritual Nutrition : Six Foundations for Spiritual Life and the Awakening of Kundalini. Berkeley, Calif., North Atlantic Books, 2005.

Cramp, Arthur J. (1936). . Press of American Medical Association. pp. 57-59

Desiring God. "Does Junk Food Dishonor God?" YouTube, 25 Apr. 2019, www.youtube.com/watch?v=MRA0nl4yWSA. Accessed 22 Apr. 2025.

Dharmaboost. "Go Raw Now Trailer." Youtube.com, 2008, youtu.be/z3xOU2tLl7g?si=57YwsaPwZE0x4Tbt. Accessed 10 Apr. 2025.

Diogenes Laertius and Charles Duke Yonge. The Lives and Opinions of Eminent Philosophers. United States?, Andesite Press, 2015. p. 47

Doniger, Wendy. "Food and Asceticism in Ancient India," Journal of the American Oriental Society, vol. 100, no. 3, 1980, pp. 233–240, doi:10.2307/601803.

Ehret, Arnold. Arnold Ehret Works (3 Books in 1): Mucusless Diet Healing System & Rational Fasting & 49 Day Fasting Experiment . Independently Published, Oct. 2023.

Emerson, Ralph Waldo. "Self-Reliance." Essays: First Series, Project Gutenberg, 8 Feb. 2006,. Accessed 27 Apr. 2025.

Emerson, Ralph Waldo. Nature: Original. Independently Published, 2023.

Emerson. Nature

Eva Loves Raw. "Matt Monarch Heartfelt Candid Interview." YouTube, 10 Apr. 2022, www.youtube.com/watch?v=ePy5k3rHyII. Accessed 16 Apr. 2025.

Flavius Josephus. The Antiquities of the Jews. BoD – Books on Demand, 23 May 2018, p. Book 18, chapter 1.

Freelee and Durianrider. "10 Sexual Benefits of a High Fruit Diet." YouTube, 11 Dec. 2013, www.youtube.com/watch?v=kVHABB-4pq5A. Accessed 20 Apr. 2025.

Freelee and Durianrider. "Raw Food Vegan SEX." YouTube, 12 Dec. 2013, www.youtube.com/watch?v=RCna06lImno. Accessed 20 Apr. 2025.

Freelee the Banana Girl. "The Femininity Lie." Freelee the Banana Girl Blog, thebananagirl.com, 1 Apr. 2019,.

Freelee the Banana Girl. "Why Dairy Destroys Your Hormones." The-BananaGirl.com, undated but active as of 2025, thebananagirl.com/why-dairy-destroys-your-hormones.

Freelee the Banana Girl. "Why Vegan Women Have Better Periods." YouTube, uploaded circa 2017, youtube.com/freeleethebananagirl (exact date fuzzy; searchable by title).

Freelee, Ms. Banana Girl. My Naked Lunchbox: The Most Controversial Cookbook Ever Written. E-book ed., Independently published, 2019.

Freelee. "What Is My Naked Lunchbox?" Freelee the Banana Girl, 2025, thebananagirl.com/pages/my-naked-lunchbox-?srsltid=AfmBOorU_gMIrm9T3ZJRp4lbQZoz-f6nmJZqxN-SQDG74nM8-ytv7EVEZ. Accessed 20 Apr. 2025.

FullyRaw Kristina. "Empowering Women with Raw Food." YouTube, 17 Apr. 2013, www.youtube.com/watch?v=TMqdQbTELpI. Accessed 24 Apr. 2025.

Gaius Julius Solinus, and Theodor Mommsen. Collectanea Rerum Memorabilium. Berolini, Weidmann, 1958.

Gambhirananda, Swami, translator. Eight Upanishads. Vol. 2, Advaita Ashrama, 2006.

Gandhi, Mahatma. A Guide to Health. Translated by A. Rama Iyer, S. Ganesan, 1921.

Gandhi, Mahatma. Collected Works of Mahatma Gandhi. LXXXV, July 16, 1946-October 20, 1946. New Delhi, The Publications Division, Ministry Of Information And Broadcasting, Govt. Of India, 1982.

Gandhi, Mahatma. Hind Swaraj. Delhi, Rajpal & Sons, 1909.

Ganguli, Kisari Mohan, translator. The Mahabharata of Krishna-Dwaipayana Vyasa, vol. 3, Vanaparva, sections 25–26. Munshiram Manoharlal Publishers, 2001.

Genuis, Stephen J., and Kasie L. Kelln. "Toxicant Exposure and Bioaccumulation: A Common and Potentially Reversible Cause of Cognitive Dysfunction and Dementia." Behavioural Neurology, vol. 2015, 2015, pp. 1–10, https://doi.org/10.1155/2015/620143. Accessed 20 Apr. 2022.

Gerald James Larson, and Īśvarakr̥ṣṇa. Classical Sāṃkhya : An Interpretation of Its History and Meaning. Delhi, Motilal Banarsidass Publishers, 2014, pp. 10–18, 49, 163.

Ginsburg, Christian D. The Essenes. Lettel Books, 20 Feb. 2024. p.2

Goddard, Neville, and Mitch Horowitz. Feeling Is the Secret. Gildan Media LLC aka G&D Media, 17 Dec. 2020.

Goddard, Neville. Feeling Is the Secret. Martino Fine Books, 2010.

Graham, Douglas. "Interview on Raw Food and Lifestyle." Get Fresh!, 2006,

Griffith, Ralph T.H., translator. The Rámáyan of Válmíki, book 3, Aranyakanda, cantos 11.23–24. Trübner & Co., 1872.

Hamilton, Edith. The Greek Way. New York ; London, W.W. Norton & Company, 2017.

Harrison, Paul. Elements of Pantheism : A Spirituality of Nature and the Universe. Colorado (Colo.), Paul Harrison, 2013.

Hau, Michael. "Constitutional Therapy and Clinical Racial Hygiene in Weimar and Nazi Germany." Journal of the History of Medicine and Allied Sciences, vol. 71, no. 2, 4 Sept. 2015, pp. 115–143, https://doi.org/10.1093/jhmas/jrv034. Accessed 16 Apr. 2021.

Hicks, Angela. The Huangdi Neijing: The Yellow Emperor's Classic of Medicine. Singing Dragon, 2013.

Hicks, Stephen R. C. Nietzsche and the Nazis: A Personal View. Ockham's Razor Publishing, 2010.

Hippocrates Health Institute Magazine, Spring 2011 issue, p. 12.

Hitler, Adolf, et al. Hitler's Table Talk, 1941-1944 : His Private Conversations. New York, Enigma Books, 2008.

Hitler. Mein Kampf. Translated by James Murphy, London, Pimlico, 18 July 1925.

Huynh, Dai. "Uncooked Food Leads to Better Health, Devotees Say." Chron, 5 Jan. 2009, www.chron.com/life/food/article/Uncooked-food-leads-to-better-health-devotees-say-1732174.php. Accessed 24 Apr. 2025.

Jacoby, Jesse. Gaia Speaks. Soulspire Publishing, 5 Aug. 2019. Pg. 19

Jacoby, Jesse. The Raw Cure: Healing beyond Medicine. Soulspire Publishing, 2012. Pg. 168

Johann Chapoutot. "The Nazis and Nature: Protectors or Predators?" Vingtième Siècle. Revue D'histoire, vol. 113, no. 1, 2024, pp. 29–39, shs.cairn.info/journal-vingtieme-siecle-revue-d-histoire-2012-1-page-29?lang=en.

Johnstone, H. (2013). Carb the fcuk up lifestyle and dietary guide. Harley Johnstone.

Johnstone, H. (2013, April 17). Interview with vegan Harley Johnstone aka Durianrider. Rawsomehealthy.com.

Johnstone, H. (2016). Durianrider's lean body bible. Harley Johnstone.

Johnstone, H. (2020, March 2). Harley Johnstone (Durianrider) talks testosterone, fruit, and cycling (A. Dixon, Host). The Love Fruit Podcast. Simplecast.

Johnstone, H. (2022, August 22). Rawfood diet vs Durianrider protocol for health and performance? [Audio podcast episode]. In Durianrider Raw Truth. iVoox.

Johnstone, H. (n.d.). Durianrider podcast [Audio podcast episode]. In Durianrider Raw Truth. Spotify for Creators.

Kulvinskas, Viktoras H. Survival in the 21st Century. Book Publishing Company (TN), 1 Jan. 2010.

Li, Gao, and Bob Flaws. Li Dong-Yuan's Treatise on the Spleen & Stomach : A Translation of the Pi Wei Lun. Boulder, Co, Blue Poppy Press, 2004.

Linge, Heinz. With Hitler to the End. Simon and Schuster, 1 Sept. 2009.

Lovewisdom, Johnny. Spiritualizing Dietetics ""Vitarianism."" Createspace Independent Pub, 5 June 2014.

Lovewisdom, Johnny. The Ascensional Science of Spiritualizing Fruitarian Dietetics. CreateSpace, 20 Mar. 2014.

Lukacs, John. The Hitler of History. New York, Vintage Books, 1998.

Mahatma 1869-1948 Gandhi. Key to Health. Hassell Street Press, 9 Sept. 2021.

Mahatma Gandhi. Story of My Experiments with Truth. Popular Prakashan Ltd, In, 2013.

Malkmus, George H. Why Christians Get Sick. 1995. Treasure House Edition ed., Shippensburg, PA, Treasure House, 1997. Pg 120

Malkmus, George. Back to the Garden, vol. 11, no. 1, Spring 2001, Hallelujah Acres.

Matt Monarch. "23 Year Ex-Raw Vegan Comes out about Raw Vegan Diet." YouTube, 26 Sept. 2023, www.youtube.com/watch?v=_H2Ppcv1HUU. Accessed 15 Apr. 2025.

Matt Monarch. "I Had Surgery for Irreversible Ulcerative Colitis." YouTube, 5 May 2021, www.youtube.com/watch?v=ECgenBMir10. Accessed 16 Apr. 2025.

Matt. "Food Pharisees | Taking Back the Bible from the Raw Food Diet." Reformed Expressions, 8 Mar. 2018, reformedexpressions.com/food-pharisees/. Accessed 25 Mar. 2025.

McCauley, Bob. Honoring the Temple of God - a Christian Health Perspective. SE, Inc, 5 June 2008. Pg. 4

McLachlan, Michael S., et al. "Bioaccumulation of Organic Contaminants in Humans: A Multimedia Perspective and the Importance of Biotransformation." Environmental Science & Technology, vol. 45, no. 1, 11 Aug. 2010, pp. 197–202, https://doi.org/10.1021/es101000w. Accessed 14 Feb. 2025.

Meyer-Renschhausen, Elisabeth, and Albert Wirz. "Dietetics, Health Reform and Social Order: Vegetarianism as a Moral Physiology. The Example of Maximilian Bircher-Benner (1867–1939)." Medical History, vol. 43, no. 3, July 1999, pp. 323–341, doi:10.1017/S0025727300065388.

Miller, Rob . "Raw Vegan vs Cooked Vegan." All-Creatures.org, 2006, www.all-creatures.org/articles/rawvegan.html. Accessed 7 Mar. 2025.

Monarch, M. (2005). Raw spirit: What the raw food advocates don't preach.

Monier Williams (1872). . Clarendon Press, Oxford. p. 363.

Ms.FitVegan. "MY Interview with 23 Year EX-RAW VEGAN Matt Monarch! | a MUST WATCH 😳." YouTube, 28 Sept. 2023, www.youtube.com/watch?v=dS6t8x1NAHQ. Accessed 16 Apr. 2025.

Müller, F. Max, translator. The Upanishads. Part II, Oxford University Press, 1884.

Nevill Drury. The New Age: A History of the Movement. New York, Thames & Hudson, Inc., C, 2004.

Nietzsche , Friedrich . Thus Spoke Zarathustra. Evergreen Books, 2017.

Nietzsche, Friedrich. Daybreak: Thoughts on the Prejudices of Morality. Translated by R. J. Hollingdale, Cambridge UP, 1997, p. 153.

Nietzsche, Friedrich. Thus Spoke Zarathustra. Translated by Walter Kaufmann, Penguin Books, 1978.

Nikhilananda, Swami, translator. The Upanishads: A New Translation. Vol. 1, Ramakrishna-Vivekananda Center, 2003.

Ohler, Norman, and Shaun Whiteside. Blitzed : Drugs in the Third Reich. Boston, Houghton Mifflin Harcourt, 2017.

Olivelle, Patrick, and Richard W Lariviere. Dharmasūtra Parallels : Containing the Dharmasūtras of Āpastamba, Gautama, Baudhāyana, and Vasiṣṭha. Delhi, Motilal Banarsidass Publishers, 2005.

Olivelle, Patrick. The Ascetics of Ancient India. Oxford University Press, 1998, 126.

Overcoming AIDS and Other "Incurable Diseases" the Attunitive Way Through Nature

Palladius, Bishop Of Aspuna, and John Wortley. Palladius of Aspuna : The Lausiac History. Athens, Ohio, Cistercian Publications ; Collegeville, Minnesota, 2015. p. 46

Prabhupada, A.C. Bhaktivedanta Swami, translator. Srimad-Bhagavatam, book 11, chapter 6, verse 16. Bhaktivedanta Book Trust, 1982.

Proverbs 13:25

Quill, Ed. "STATE SUES to STOP WOMAN OFFERING REM-
    EDIES for AIDS." Archive.org, The Boston Globe (Boston, MA),
    2015,   web.archive.org/web/20150924200656/www.highbeam.
    com/doc/1P2-8045670.html. Accessed 4 Mar. 2025.

Ralph Waldo Emerson. Nature. 1841. Woodland Hills, Cailf., Regatta
    Press, 2010.

Ratcliffe, L. (n.d.). What is the Raw Till 4 Diet? The Banana Girl.

Ratcliffe, Leanne. Go Fruit Yourself. 2nd ed., Leanne Ratcliffe, 2020.
    ISBN: 1092785531.

Ratcliffe, Leanne. My Naked Lunchbox. Leanne Ratcliffe, 2019.
    ISBN: 1092770453.

Ratcliffe, Leanne. The Raw Till 4 Diet. Leanne Ratcliffe, 2017. ISBN:
    1976960312.

Rehmannia Dean Thomas, and Janabai Owens Amsden. Raw Chi :
    Balancing the Raw Food Diet with Chinese Herbs. Berkeley, Cal-
    ifornia, Evolver Editions, 2014.

Richards, John, translator. Ashtavakra Gita. John Richards, 1994,.

Rothkranz, Markus, and Cara Brotman. Love on a Plate. Rothkranz
    Publishing, 1 Jan. 2015.

Rothkranz, Markus. Heal Yourself 101 : Get Younger & Never Get
    Sick Again. Rothkranz Pub, 2009.

Rothkranz, Markus. SEX - WOMENS' EDITION (78 Page E-Book-
    let). markusebooks.com. Accessed 2025.

Satchidananda, Swami, translator. The Yoga Sutras of Patanjali. Inte-
    gral Yoga Publications, 2012.

Slate, Nico. Gandhi's Search for the Perfect Diet. University of Wash-
    ington Press, 28 Feb. 2019.

Smetana, Sergiy, et al. "Meat Substitutes: Resource Demands and
    Environmental Footprints." Resources, Conservation and Re-
    cycling, vol. 190, no. 106831, Mar. 2023, p. 106831, https://doi.
    org/10.1016/j.resconrec.2022.106831.

Smith, George Davey. "Lifestyle, Health, and Health Promotion in
    Nazi Germany." BMJ, vol. 329, no. 7480, 16 Dec. 2004, pp. 1424–

1425, https://doi.org/10.1136/bmj.329.7480.1424. Accessed 4 Apr. 2020.

Solomon, Robert C, and Kathleen M Higgins. What Nietzsche Really Said. New York, Schocken Books, 2001.

Solomon, Robert C., and Kathleen M. Higgins. What Nietzsche Really Said. Schocken Books, 2000.

Sooke, Alastair. "The Discobolus: Greeks, Nazis and the Body Beautiful." Www.bbc.com, 24 Mar. 2015, www.bbc.com/culture/article/20150324-hitlers-idea-of-the-perfect-body.

Szekely, Edmond, and Barry Peterson. The Essene Gospel of Peace: The Complete 4 Books in One Volume. Audio Enlightenment , 26 May 2018.

The Boston Globe. "JUDGE SAYS WOMAN CAN CLAIM AIDS CURE." Archive.org, 2025, web.archive.org/web/20150810033341/www.highbeam.com/doc/1P2-8050504.html. Accessed 4 Mar. 2025.

The Frugivore Diet. "Durianrider Is Stalking Me (Trespassing, Slander, Harassment)." YouTube, 2 July 2022, www.youtube.com/watch?v=qfQ1WaQ9qgE. Accessed 20 Apr. 2025.

The Healthy Life. "How to Raise Testosterone Naturally." YouTube, 26 May 2024, www.youtube.com/watch?v=ZNCQJ8pR39w. Accessed 10 Apr. 2025.

The Healthy Life. "Bodybuilding Set with Plant-Based Protein." YouTube, 21 Feb. 2021, www.youtube.com/watch?v=vmHyq-a02F8. Accessed 10 Apr. 2025.

The Healthy Life. "Do I Have Plastic Surgery." Youtube, 24 Feb. 2021, www.youtube.com/watch?v=lZj2xR2dCGU. Accessed 2025.

The Healthy Life. "RAW FOOD VEGAN BODYBUILDER Cab Driver Eats No Meat." YouTube, 16 Sept. 2010, www.youtube.com/watch?v=SbEUHCU_GtM. Accessed 10 Apr. 2025.

The Healthy Life. "Raw Vegan Muscle Bodybuilding DVD Set Now Available !" Youtu.be, 2010, youtu.be/_IlgWnw-gEak?si=7i7-nzUGsX-yqUTX. Accessed 10 Apr. 2025.

The Healthy Life. "The Importance of Using the Right Protein." YouTube, 6 July 2022, www.youtube.com/watch?v=Ht6nXkMLCmo. Accessed 10 Apr. 2025.

The Healthy Life. "The Outer Is Not Superficial- the Key to Staying Young." YouTube, 8 June 2018, www.youtube.com/watch?v=qdrs-loMyb9s. Accessed 17 Mar. 2025.

Timothy Holt. "Hallelujah Diet with Reverend George Malkmus." YouTube, 16 Feb. 2013, www.youtube.com/watch?v=GrNW1l-S96pQ. Accessed 7 Apr. 2025.

Vishvanáth Náráyan Mandlik, et al. Mānava-Dharma-Śāstra [Vol. 3] with the Commentary of Govindarāja : Being a Supplement to Mānava-Dharma Śāstra with the Commentaries of Medhātihi, Sarvajñanārāyaṇa, Kullūka, Rāghavānanda, Nandana, and Rāmachandra in 2 Volumes. New Delhi Munshiram Manoharlal Publishers, 1992.

Wigmore, Ann . Overcoming AIDS and Other "Incurable Diseases" the Attunitive Way through Nature. A. Wigmore, 1 Jan. 1987.

Wigmore, Ann. Why Suffer? Book Publishing Company, 18 Jan. 2013.

Wigmore, Ann. Why Suffer? Book Publishing Company, 18 Jan. 2013. Pg. 149

Wigmore, Ann. Why Suffer? How I Overcame Illness & Pain Naturally. Avery Publishing Group, 1985.

Wilson, Douglas. Confessions of a Food Catholic. Moscow, Idaho, Canonpress, 2016.Pg. 139

Wolfe, David, and Charles Nicholas Good. Amazing Grace : The Nine Principles of Living in Natural Magic. San Diego, Calif., Sunfood Pub.; Berkeley, Calif, 2008.

Wolfe, David, and Nick Good. Amazing Grace. North Atlantic Books, 18 May 2010.

Wolfe, David. Eating for Beauty : For Women & Men. Berkeley, Calif., North Atlantic Books, 2009.

Wortley, John. An Introduction to the Desert Fathers. Cambridge, United Kingdom; New York, Ny, Cambridge University Press, 2019.

Yang, Jizhou, and Sabine Wilms. The Great Compendium of Acupuncture and Moxibustion : Zhēn Jiǔ Dà Chéng. Volume 1. Portland, Oregon, Chinese Medicine Database, 2010.

Young, Richard A. (1999). Is God a Vegetarian?: Christianity, Vegetarianism, and Animal Rights. Open Court. p. 5.

Zavasta, Tonya. Your Right to Be Beautiful : How to Halt the Train of Aging & Meet the Most Beautiful You. Memphis, Tenn., Br Pub, 2003.

Zavasta, Tonya. Your Right to Be Beautiful : How to Halt the Train of Aging & Meet the Most Beautiful You. Memphis, Tenn., Br Pub, 2003. P. 37

durianrider "TANTRIC SEXUALITY + Best Diet for Sexual Performance?" YouTube, 14 Feb. 2012, www.youtube.com/watch?v=7EopRCp-wTA. Accessed 20 Apr. 2025.

durianrider. "Is Sugar REALLY More Powerful than Testosterone for Recovery and Performance??" YouTube, 31 Jan. 2025, www.youtube.com/watch?v=29oHpLMuhys. Accessed 20 Apr. 2025.

durianrider. "SEXY HOT Body for Life Diet Tips with Fruitarian Vegan Freelee." YouTube, 16 Nov. 2012, www.youtube.com/watch?v=zTqEXoGq2nQ. Accessed 20 Apr. 2025.

durianrider. "Testosterone & What EVERY Man Needs to Know!" YouTube, 20 June 2024, www.youtube.com/watch?v=Bz8k_1riWcY. Accessed 20 Apr. 2025.

durianrider. "Why Is Durianrider so Aggressive? (Warning: Content May Offend the Glucose Deficient)." YouTube, 9 May 2013, www.youtube.com/watch?v=3goYA0TOnPI. Accessed 20 Apr. 2025.

durianrider. "Why Masculine Presence Is a DRUG Women Live For." YouTube, 4 May 2021, www.youtube.com/watch?v=Z4t5Rs8WpPc. Accessed 20 Apr. 2025.

www.wisdomlib.org. "Bhaktavijaya: Stories of Indian Saints." Wisdomlib.org, 26 May 2024, www.wisdomlib.org/history/book/bhaktavijaya-stories-of-indian-saints. Accessed 9 Feb. 2025.

www.wisdomlib.org. "Verse 2.23.17 Shri Chaitanya Bhagavata." Wisdomlib.org, 28 Mar. 2022, www.wisdomlib.org/hinduism/book/chaitanya-bhagavata/d/doc1107780.html. Accessed 9 Feb. 2025.

Ms.FitVegan. "MY Interview with 23 Year EX-RAW VEGAN Matt Monarch! | a MUST WATCH 🤢." YouTube, 28 Sept. 2023, www.youtube.com/watch?v=dS6t8x1NAHQ. Accessed 16 Apr. 2025.

"Arnold_Ehret." Bionity.com, 2025, www.bionity.com/en/encyclopedia/Arnold_Ehret.html. Accessed 19 Mar. 2025.

"Hallelujah Acres History — 1997-2001." Hallelujah Diet , 31 Jan. 2012, myhdiet.com/blogs/healthnews/hallelujah-acres-history-1997-2001. Accessed 7 Apr. 2025.

"Health Minister Training Online - Now Available!" Hallelujah Diet , 28 Apr. 2012, myhdiet.com/blogs/healthnews/health-minister-training-online-now-available. Accessed 7 Apr. 2025.

"How Raw Foods Make You Different | Beautiful on Raw." Beautifulonraw.com, Feb. 2004, www.beautifulonraw.com/the-ten-biomarkers-of-a-long-term-raw-foodist.html. Accessed 9 Apr. 2025.

"How to Thrive & Perform Athletically on a High-Carb, Low-Fat Vegan Diet." Rich Roll, 30 Sept. 2013, www.richroll.com/podcast/rrp-53-durianrider-how-to-thrive-perform-athletically-on-a-high-carb-low-fat-vegan-diet/. Accessed 20 Apr. 2025.

"Johnny Lovewisdom." Wikibin.org, 2025, wikibin.org/articles/johnny-lovewisdom-3.html. Accessed 23 Apr. 2025.

"Palladius, the Lausiac History (1918) Pp. 35-180. English Translation." Tertullian.org, 2025, www.tertullian.org/fathers/palladius_lausiac_02_text.htm. Accessed 14 Feb. 2025.

"Remembering Rev. George Malkmus." Hallelujah Diet , 2024, myhdiet.com/pages/remembering-rev-george-malkmus. Accessed 7 Apr. 2025.

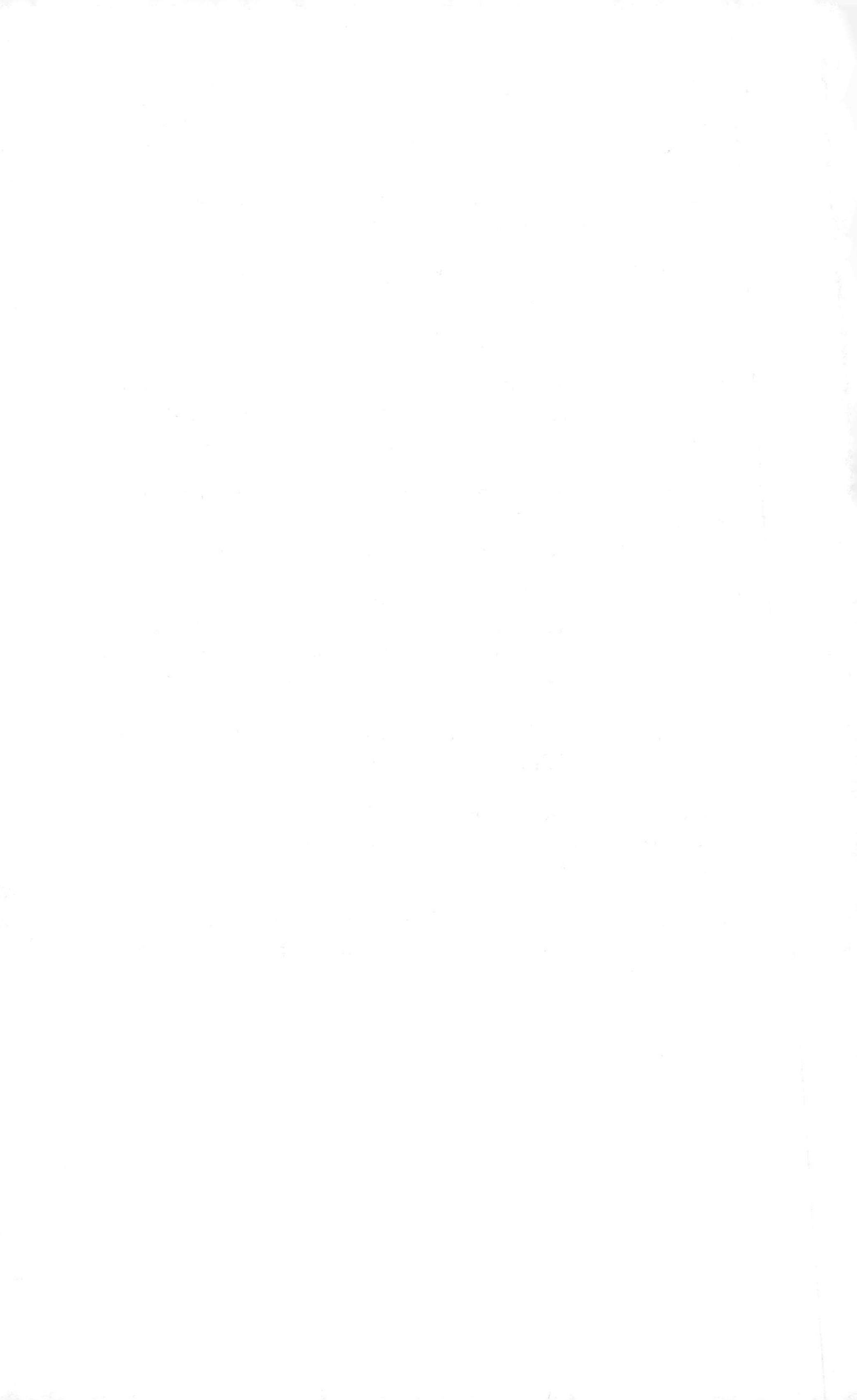

About the Author

E van has a lifelong interest in history and a master's degree in holistic nutrition, though this book is not intended to share any of his personal beliefs about nutrition.

www.ingramcontent.com/pod-product-compliance
Lightning Source LLC
Chambersburg PA
CBHW051754050726
47598CB00006B/2276